Blueprints

CLINICAL CASES
OBSTETRICS &
GYNECOLOGY

Blackwell's *Blueprints* series offers medical students the complete study package.

Blueprints **Clinical Cases** feature symptom-based clinical cases that lead the student through steps to a diagnosis. Each book is written by residents and complements the *Blueprints* core books and *Blueprints* Q&A series.

> Blueprints Clinical Cases in Medicine
> Blueprints Clinical Cases in Pediatrics
> Blueprints Clinical Cases in Psychiatry
> Blueprints Clinical Cases in Obstetrics & Gynecology
> Blueprints Clinical Cases in Surgery
> Blueprints Clinical Cases in Neurology
> Blueprints Clinical Cases in Emergency Medicine
> Blueprints Clinical Cases in Family Medicine

The original Blueprints and *Blueprints* **Specialty** books provide the essentials you need during rotations and as a review before Steps 2 and 3 of the United States Medical Licensing Examination (USMLE):

Blueprints in Medicine   Blueprints in Family Medicine
Blueprints in Pediatrics   Blueprints in Emergency Medicine
Blueprints in Psychiatry   Blueprints in Neurology (specialty)
Blueprints in Obstetrics   Blueprints in Cardiology (specialty)
  & Gynecology
Blueprints in Surgery   Blueprints in Radiology (specialty)

Blueprints **Q&A Step 2** provides review questions and complete answer options for content *most likely covered on the USMLE Step 2:*

> Blueprints Q&A Step 2: Medicine
> Blueprints Q&A Step 2: Pediatrics
> Blueprints Q&A Step 2: Psychiatry
> Blueprints Q&A Step 2: Obstetrics & Gynecology
> Blueprints Q&A Step 2: Surgery

Blueprints **Q&A Step 3** offers the current board format practice questions with complete answer options for review before USMLE Step 3:

> Blueprints Q&A Step 3: Medicine
> Blueprints Q&A Step 3: Pediatrics
> Blueprints Q&A Step 3: Psychiatry
> Blueprints Q&A Step 3: Obstetrics & Gynecology
> Blueprints Q&A Step 3: Surgery

Blueprints

CLINICAL CASES

SECOND EDITION

OBSTETRICS & GYNECOLOGY

Aaron B. Caughey, MD, MPP, MPH (Series Editor)
Assistant Professor in Residence
Department of Obstetrics and Gynecology
University of California, San Francisco
San Francisco, California

Arzou Ahsan, MA, MD
Department of Obstetrics and Gynecology
Alta Bates Hospital
Berkeley, California

Linda Margaret Hopkins, MD
Fellow, Maternal-Fetal Medicine
Department of Obstetrics, Gynecology and Reproductive Sciences
University of California, San Francisco
San Francisco, California

Juan E. Vargas, MD
Chief of Obstetrics, San Francisco General Hospital
Department of Obstetrics and Gynecology
University of California, San Francisco
San Francisco, California

O.W. Stephanie Yap, MD
Assistant Professor, Gynecologic Oncology
Department of Obstetrics and Gynecology
Morehouse School of Medicine
Atlanta, Georgia

Susan H. Tran, MD (Contributing Editor)
Fellow in Genetics and Maternal-Fetal Medicine
Departments of Pediatrics and Obstetrics and Gynecology
University of California, San Francisco
San Francisco, California

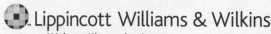
Lippincott Williams & Wilkins
a Wolters Kluwer business
Philadelphia · Baltimore · New York · London
Buenos Aires · Hong Kong · Sydney · Tokyo

Acquisitions Editor: Nancy Anastasi Duffy
Managing Editor: Selene Steneck
Marketing Manager: Jennifer Kuklinski
Associate Production Manager: Kevin P. Johnson
Design Coordinator: Stephen Druding
Compositor: International Typesetting and Composition
Printer: R.R. Donnelley & Son's - Crawfordsville

Printed in the United States of America

First Edition, 2002
Second Edition, 2007

Library of Congress Cataloging-in-Publication Data

Obstetrics & gynecology. — 2nd ed./Arzou Ahsan ... [et al.]
    p.; cm. — (Blueprints. Clinical cases)
  Rev. ed. of: Blueprints clinical cases in obstetrics & gynecology /
Arzou Ahsan ... [et al.]. c2002.
   Includes index.
   ISBN 1-4051-0490-2
   1. Obstetrics—Case studies. 2. Obstetrics—Examinations, questions, etc.
   3. Gynecology—Case studies. 4. Gynecology—Examinations, questions, etc.
   5. Physicians—Licenses—Examinations—Study guides.
  I. Ahsan, Arzou. II. Title: Obstetrics and gynecology. III. Series.
   [DNLM: 1. Obstetrics—Case Reports. 2. Obstetrics—Examination Questions.
   3. Genital Diseases, Female—Case Reports. 4. Genital Diseases, Female—
   Examination Questions. 5. Pregnancy Complications—Case Reports. 6. Pregnancy
   Complications—Examination Questions. WQ 18.2 O142 2006]
  RG106.B585 2006
  618.076—dc22 2006000718

To purchase additional copies of this book, call our customer service department at **(800) 638-3030** or fax orders to **(301) 223-2320.** International customers should call **(301) 223-2300.**

Visit Lippincott Williams & Wilkins on the Internet: http://www.LWW.com. Lippincott Williams & Wilkins customer service representatives are available from 8:30 am to 6:00 pm, EST.

06 07 08 09 10
1 2 3 4 5 6 7 8 9 10

Dedication

We would all like to thank the staff at both Blackwell and LWW, particularly Selene Steneck, for their untiring work on this project. We also would like to thank our family, friends, and colleagues, including the residents and faculty in the Department of Obstetrics and Gynecology at UCSF, particularly Drs. A. Eugene Washington, Mary E. Norton, Miriam Kuppermann, and Peter Callen. Thanks also to my family, Aidan, Ashby, and, of course, Susan, whose patience and support during all of my projects keep me on task and productive.
    Aaron

For Strayer, Oriane, and Judas
    Arzou

For Alex, Eli, and Sam . . .
    Love, Linda

For Holly, for everything and beyond
    Juan

Thank you, Robert and Alex, for everything!
    Stephanie

Preface

The *Blueprints* Clinical Cases series has been developed to complement clinical rotations during the third and fourth years of medical school and for use as a review when preparing for in-service and Board exams. The cases describe common and important presentations of patients seen in the outpatient and inpatient settings. The design of the cases is meant to parallel the clinical thought process. Because the diagnosis is not revealed immediately, students must think through the presentations as they unfold. Once the diagnosis is made, a discussion of treatment and other management issues follows.

Blueprints Clinical Cases in Obstetrics & Gynecology has been designed to take you, the student clinician, through a variety of settings in the clinic, triage, labor and delivery, emergency department, and operating room. The book has two sections. The first half consists of obstetric cases, and the second half consists of gynecologic cases. The presentations are mostly common complaints seen in our patients and cover the gamut of most obstetric issues, gynecologic cancers, and general gynecology. There are a few other variations between this book and the rest in the series, as well as additional considerations you need to make while reading these cases.

These cases have been designed to take you through the thought process of assessing and diagnosing a patient presenting with the given chief complaint. The emphasis is on common patient complaints and prevalent or important disease processes. Case-based learning is an effective and enjoyable educational tool, but it requires an approach different from conventional learning methods. Following is a description of the overall format of the cases and suggestions on how to get the most out of this book.

ID/CC: The case titles and chief complaints (CC) are based on common presenting symptoms, signs, and lab or diagnostic test findings. In general, they represent the common reasons physicians are consulted to see patients and suggest a broad differential diagnosis to begin the case.

HPI (HPP): The history of present illness (HPI) contains additional descriptive history regarding the patient's chief complaint. In addition, it usually includes a brief review of pertinent systems. At the end of the HPI, you should consider the differential diagnosis, what to look for on the physical exam, and which diagnostic tests should be ordered. Some of these items have been formalized in the thought questions.

The HPI in obstetrics is also known as the HPP (history of present pregnancy). Obstetric patients are always presented with their gravidity and parity, as well as their gestational age and pregnancy dating criteria. *Gravidity* refers to the number of pregnancies a patient has had and *parity* to the number of births. Parity is further broken down into term, preterm, aborted, and living children, resulting in a four-digit description. Multiple gestations count as only a single pregnancy and birth but obviously result in more living children. Aborted pregnancies include spontaneous and elective abortions as well as ectopic pregnancies. When the difference among these three is significant, additional descriptors are supplied. Dating of the pregnancy is done using the patient's last menstrual period and confirmed with physical exam and ultrasound. Ultrasound dating can vary by 8% to 12%; thus, the variation from the actual dating increases as the pregnancy progresses.

Past Hx: The past medical, surgical, and social histories along with medications and allergies further supplement the HPI. In some cases, this section contains crucial information regarding the patient's baseline medical status or social situation. Consider how these issues in conjunction with current medications impact the differential diagnosis and eventual treatment plans. In addition to the past medical and surgical histories, obstetrician-gynecologists include sections of past obstetric history (PObHx) and past gynecologic history (PGynHx). PObHx includes the number of pregnancies and births, gestational age at delivery, birthweight, mode of delivery, and any complications. PGynHx includes frequency and regularity of menses, menarche, age at onset of menopause, pelvic infections, and history of any gynecologic surgeries.

VS/PE: Vital signs (VS) and physical exam (PE) provide further clarifying information regarding the patient's illness. In these cases, only the pertinent positive and negative findings are mentioned. If a system or finding is not described, it can be assumed to be normal and does not contribute to the final diagnosis. Information gained from the physical exam should further narrow the differential diagnosis and list of desired diagnostic tests. In many of our patients who are young and healthy, the PE noted in these cases focuses on the abdominal and pelvic exams. Please note that your notes in an actual clinical setting should reflect a full physical exam; only the pertinent positives and negatives are presented here to save space.

Labs/X-ray: Again, we include only the pertinent positive and negative findings. Common abbreviations are used as well as the standard format for the complete blood count (CBC) and electrolyte panels. We include photos and radiographic images in many of the cases to further enhance the skill of incorporating these visual tools into diagnosis. Certainly the most common imaging modality used in obstetrics/gynecology is ultrasound. Real-time ultrasound allows clinicians to visualize the uterus and ovaries in their patients and, of course, the fetus and placenta in obstetric patients. The images included with cases are representative of common images seen, and you should familiarize yourself with these images as well as the strengths and limitations of the different imaging modalities.

Thought Questions and Answers: These open-ended questions are meant to stimulate ideas regarding diagnosis, pathophysiology, and treatment and to help plan further workup. In order to get the most out of these questions, spend some time reflecting on possible answers. We suggest writing the answers down or, if working in a group, discussing the possibilities with other students. The answers to the thought questions follow immediately, so try not to read ahead. The thought questions often follow the HPI or the PE, but occasionally they are used throughout the cases to help stimulate thought regarding how to proceed in the workup.

Case Continued: These sections may give further bits of diagnostic information in the middle of a case or give the final diagnosis, and often treatment or follow-up, at the end of the case.

Multiple Choice Questions: There are four multiple choice questions at the end of every case. These questions are meant to be in-service or Board-style questions, and they should be done at the end of each case. These questions and answers provide additional information about the case diagnosis and often address other important conditions in the differential diagnosis.

Obstetrics: Gynecology is truly a surgical subspecialty, and these patients can be considered in a similar way to those in medicine and surgery, but obstetric patients are unique within medicine. Several key differences need to be considered when caring for obstetric patients. First, the baseline physiology is different from that of all other patients, and it may change throughout pregnancy. Second, two patients must be considered: the mother and the fetus. Thus, both the diagnosis and treatment may differ from those of nonpregnant patients. Finally, pregnancy itself is not an illness. In general, these patients are well and, therefore, need to be treated and considered in that light. For educational purposes, many of the patients in our cases undergo complications of pregnancy, but for the majority of patients, pregnancy is an uncomplicated process.

We hope you enjoy and benefit from the cases we have created. We believe that these cases and the questions and answers will be useful to the novice student, the more experienced subintern, and even junior physicians in training.

Aaron B. Caughey, MD, MPP, MPH
Arzou Ahsan, MA, MD
Linda Margaret Hopkins, MD
Juan E. Vargas, MD
O.W. Stephanie Yap, MD

Reviewers

LoRissa R. Autery
4th year student
Howard University College of Medicine
Washington DC

Sarah Katel
4th year student
Drexel University College of Medicine
Philadelphia, Pennsylvania

Christie Messenger
4th year student
University of Missouri–Columbia–College of Medicine
Columbia, Missouri

Jennifer Zil
4th year student
Medical University of South Carolina
Charleston, South Carolina

Contents

Abbreviations/Acronyms

A	aborta (abortions)
ABG	arterial blood gas
ACE	angiotensin-converting enzyme
ACS	antenatal corticosteroids
ACTH	adrenocorticotropic hormone
ADA	American Diabetes Association
ADH	antidiuretic hormone
AF	anteflexed
AFI	amniotic fluid index
AFLP	acute fatty liver of pregnancy
AFP	α-fetoprotein
AGUS	atypical glandular cells of undetermined significance
AIDS	acquired immunodeficiency syndrome
All	allergies
ALT	alanine transaminase
approx	approximately
ARC	AIDS-related conditions
AROM	artificial rupture of the membranes
ASCUS	atypical squamous cells of unknown significance
AST	aspartate transaminase
AV	anteverted
BC	birth control
β-hCG	beta human chorionic gonadotropin
BID	*bis in die* (two times a day)
BME	bimanual exam
BP	blood pressure
bpm	beats per minute
BPP	biophysical profile
BSO	bilateral salpingo-oophorectomy
BUN	blood urea nitrogen
BV	bacterial vaginosis
BX	biopsy
Ca	calcium
CAH	congenital adrenal hyperplasia
cAMP	cyclic adenosine monophosphate
CBC	complete blood count
cc	cubic centimeter
CC	chief complaint
CCE	no clubbing, cyanosis, and edema

CF	cystic fibrosis
CMT	cervical motion tenderness
CMV	cytomegalovirus
CNS	central nervous system
Cor	coronary
CPP	chronic pelvic pain
Cr	creatine
C/S	cesarean section
CST	contraction stress test
CT	computed tomography
CTAB	clear to auscultation bilaterally
Ctxns	contractions
CVAT	costovertebral angle tenderness
CVS	chorionic villus sampling
D&C	dilation and curettage
D&E	dilation and evacuation
DES	diethylstilbestrol
DEXA	dual x-ray absorptiometry
DHEAS	dihydroepiandrosterone sulfate
DHT	dihydrotestosterone
DMPA	medroxyprogesterone acetate
DUB	dysfunctional uterine bleeding
dx	diagnosis
EBL	estimated blood loss
EFW	estimated fetal weight
EGA	estimated gestational age
EGBUS	external genitalia, Bartholin's, urethra, and Skene's
ESR	erythrocyte sedimentation rate
EtOH/ETOH	ethanol use
FDA	Food and Drug Administration
FHR	fetal heart rate
FHT	fetal heart tracing
FHx	family history
FIGO	International Federation of Gynecology and Obstetrics
FSBG	finger stick blood glucose
FSH	follicle-stimulating hormone
FTP	failure to progress
G	gravida (pregnancies)
GA	gestational age
GBS	Group B *Streptococcus*
GDM	gestational diabetes mellitus
Gen	general
GERD	gastroesophageal reflux disease
GI	gastrointestinal
GLT	glucose loading test
GnRH	gonadotropin-releasing hormone
GTD	gestational trophoblastic disease
GTT	glucose tolerance test

Abbreviations/Acronyms xix

GU	genitourinary
HA	headache
Hb	hemoglobin
hCG	human chorionic gonadotropin
Hct	hematocrit
HEENT	head, ears, eyes, nose, throat
HELLP	hemolysis, elevated liver enzymes, low platelets syndrome
HGSIL	high-grade squamous intraepithelial lesion
HIV	human immunodeficiency virus
h/o	history of
HPI	history of present illness
hPL	human placental lactogen
HPV	human papillomavirus
HR	heart rate
HRT	hormone replacement therapy
HSG	hysterosalpingogram
HSM	hepatosplenomegaly
HSV	herpes simplex virus
Hx	history
ID	identification
Ig	immunoglobulin
IHCP	intrahepatic cholestasis of pregnancy
IM	intramuscular
IOL	induction of labor
IUD	intrauterine device
IUGR	intrauterine growth restriction
IUI	intrauterine insemination
IUP	intrauterine pregnancy
IUPC	intrauterine pressure catheter
IV	intravenous
IVDA	intravenous drug abuse
IVF	in vitro fertilization
IVH	intraventricular hemorrhage
KOH	potassium hydroxide
labs	laboratory tests
LAD	lymphadenopathy
lb	pound
LDH	lactate dehydrogenase
LEEP	loop electrosurgical excision procedure
LFT	liver function test
LGA	large for gestational age
LGSIL	low-grade squamous intraepithelial lesion
LH	leuteinizing hormone
LLQ	lower left quadrant
LMP	last menstrual period
LOT	left occiput transverse
MCV	mean corpuscular volume
Meds	medicines/drugs

MgSO$_4$	magnesium sulfate
MIF	müllerian-inhibiting factor
MIU	milli-international units
MoM	multiples of the median
MRI	magnetic resonance imaging
MRKH	Meyer-Rokitansky-Kuster-Hauser
MSAFP	maternal serum α-fetoprotein
mu	milliunits
MV	Montevideo units
NAD	no acute distress
ND	no distension
NKDA	no known drug allergies
NPO	*nil per os* (nothing by mouth)
NSAID	nonsteroidal anti-inflammatory drug
NST	nonstress test
NSVD	normal spontaneous vaginal delivery
NT	nontender, nuchal translucency
NTD	neural tube defect
N/V	nausea and vomiting
OCP	oral contraceptive pill
OCT	oxytocin challenge test
Δ OD 450	deviation of optical density at 450
OR	operating room
P	para (births of viable offspring)
Pap smear	Papanicolaou smear
PCOS	polycystic ovary syndrome
PCR	polymerase chain reaction
PE	physical examination
PGE$_{1M}$	prostaglandin E$_{1M}$ (misoprostol [Cytotec])
PGE$_2$	prostaglandin E$_2$
PGF$_{2\alpha}$	prostaglandin F$_2$-alpha
PID	pelvic inflammatory disease
PIH	pregnancy-induced hypertension
Plts	platelets
PMDD	premenstrual dysphoric disorder
PMHx	past medical history
PNV	prenatal vitamins
PO	*per os* (by mouth, orally)
POb/GynHx	past obstetric and/or gynecologic history
POC	products of conception
POP	pelvic organ prolapse
PPD	purified protein derivative
PPH	postpartum hemorrhage
PPROM	preterm premature rupture of the membranes
PRL	prolactin
PRN	*pro re nata* (as needed)
PROM	premature rupture of membranes
PSHx	past surgical history

PT	prothrombin time
PUBS	percutaneous umbilical blood sampling
PUPPP	pruritic urticarial papules and plaques of pregnancy
QID	*quater in die* (four times a day)
RBC	red blood cell
RDS	respiratory distress syndrome
RLQ	right lower quadrant
ROS	review of systems
RPR	rapid plasma reagin
RR	respiratory rate
RR&R	regular rate and rhythm
RUQ	right upper quadrant
S > D	size greater than dates
SAB	spontaneous abortion
SC	subcutaneous
SCA	sickle cell anemia
SEM	systolic ejection murmur
SGA	small for gestational age
SHx	social history
SLE	systemic lupus erythematosus
SQ	subcutaneous
SROM	spontaneous rupture of the membranes
SSE	sterile speculum exam
STD	sexually transmitted disease
STI	sexually transmitted infection
SVE	sterile vaginal examination
TAB	therapeutic abortion
Tbili	total bilirubin
TCA	trichloroacetic acid application
Temp	temperature
TOA	tubo-ovarian abscess
TOC	tubo-ovarian complex
Toco	(related to labor)
TOLAC	trial of labor after cesarean
TSH	thyroid-stimulating hormone
UA	urinalysis
UC	uterine contraction
URI	upper respiratory infection
US	ultrasound
UTI	urinary tract infection
V/Q	ventilation/perfusion ratio
VAS	vibroacoustic stimulation
VBAC	vaginal birth after cesarean
VIN	vulvar intraepithelial neoplasia
VS	vital signs
VZV	varicella-zoster virus
WBC	white blood cell
WNL	within normal limits

I

Early Pregnancy

First Prenatal Visit

ID/CC: A 29-year-old G_1P_0 woman presents for her first prenatal visit.

HPI: This is a desired pregnancy for P.C., who is 18 weeks from her last menstrual period (LMP). She had a positive urine pregnancy test 12 weeks ago. She is worried because she has not yet felt any quickening (fetal movement).

PMHx: None

Meds: Prenatal vitamins (PNV)

All: No known drug allergies (NKDA)

POb/GynHx: Irregular menses, every 45 to 60 days

SHx: Denies use of tobacco, ethanol, or recreational or intravenous drugs.

FHx: 25-year-old brother is mentally retarded with autistic behavior. P.C. and her husband are a nonconsanguineous couple of Italian descent.

VS: Afebrile, BP 110/62, HR 86

PE: *Gen:* pleasant adult female in no acute distress. *Abdomen:* soft, nontender, gravid, with uterus palpable 4 cm below the umbilicus. *Pelvic:* long and closed cervix, gravid uterus. No palpable adnexal masses. *Doppler:* positive fetal heart tones in the 150s.

Labs: Urine dipstick: no proteinuria, no glucosuria

THOUGHT QUESTIONS

- Which antenatal diagnostic evaluations are appropriate for this patient?
- Should an obstetric ultrasound be ordered? Why?
- Given the patient's family history, which inherited disorders should be considered?

All pregnant women should undergo routine prenatal testing (Box 1-1). Additional testing may be indicated based on personal and family history and/or ethnic background. Routine prenatal laboratory tests on the first visit should include complete blood count (CBC), blood group and Rh, antibody screen, rapid plasma reagin (RPR), hepatitis B surface antigen, rubella titer, Papanicolaou (Pap) smear, cervical studies for *Neisseria gonorrhoeae* and *Chlamydia trachomatis*, HIV, and urinalysis. Subsequent tests include maternal serum triple or quad screen at 15 to 20 weeks, a repeat hematocrit, and glucose screens at 24 to 28 weeks. In this case, because of the ethnic background of the patient and of the baby's father, screening for β-thalassemia is in order, which can be done simply by obtaining a CBC and hemoglobin electrophoresis. A normal MCV in at least one of the parents rules out the possibility of β-thalassemia major, the homozygous state of this recessive disorder, in the baby.

Because this patient has irregular menses, her dates are uncertain. Therefore, an ultrasound is needed to verify gestational age (GA). Obstetric ultrasound performed in the first trimester can estimate GA via a crown–rump length measurement, which has an error of less than ±7 days. In the second trimester, GA can be estimated to within 10 to 14 days based on calculations using the biparietal diameter, head circumference, abdominal circumference, and femur length measurements. Thereafter, intrinsic and extrinsic factors contribute to greater growth variations in the fetus, making estimation of GA by ultrasound less accurate.

Given this patient's family history of mental retardation, chromosomal abnormalities and fragile X as well as other inherited disorders should be considered. Ideally, further information about the patient's brother would be most helpful in establishing a diagnosis and deciding which, if any, testing is indicated for your patient.

BOX 1-1 Routine Tests in Prenatal Care

Initial Visit and First Trimester

Hematocrit

Blood type and screen

RPR

Rubella antibody screen

Hepatitis B surface antigen

Gonorrhea culture

Chlamydia culture

PPD+

Pap smear

Urinalysis and culture

Cystic fibrosis screen

VZV titer in patients with no history of exposure

HIV test offered

Second Trimester

MSAFP/triple screen

Ultrasound

Amniocentesis in AMA women

Third Trimester

Hematocrit

RPR

GLT

Chest x-ray if PPD+

Group B Streptococcus culture

CASE CONTINUED

Obstetric ultrasound reveals a single live fetus at 16 weeks GA. Routine prenatal labs are normal except for a mild microcytic, hypochromic anemia. Review of records from the patient's brother revealed normal karyotype based on testing performed when he was 5 years old. Maternal serum triple screen correlated with the ultrasound dating is normal.

QUESTIONS

1-1. The most appropriate next step in the management of this patient's mild anemia with low MCV is:
   A. Do nothing because this represents physiologic anemia of pregnancy
   B. Iron sulfate 325 mg BID, repeat CBC in 4 to 6 weeks
   C. Hemoglobin electrophoresis, iron studies
   D. Amniocentesis, DNA testing for β-thalassemia
   E. None of the above

1-2. Given this patient's family history, you recommend which of the following?
   A. Repeat chromosome analysis and DNA for fragile X testing on her brother.
   B. If her brother cannot be tested, she can undergo karyotype analysis and DNA testing for Fragile X.
   C. No further workup needed because ultrasound findings and triple screen are normal.
   D. Chromosome analysis of the mother.
   E. A and B are correct.

1-3. Which of the following statements concerning GA assessment is correct?
   A. Maternal perception of fetal movements first occurs between 14 to 16 weeks.
   B. At 20 weeks of gestation, the uterine fundus should be palpable at the level of the symphysis pubis.
   C. An intrauterine pregnancy can be seen by transvaginal ultrasound by 5 weeks GA.
   D. The uterine fundus usually can be palpated at the symphysis pubis by 8 weeks.
   E. Fetal heart tones can be heard with Doppler after 8 weeks.

1-4. Which of the following prenatal screening evaluations should be offered to the populations described?
   A. Cystic fibrosis (CF), Canavan disease, and Tay-Sachs disease in Ashkenazi Jews
   B. CF in a Hispanic couple with no family history of CF
   C. Sickle cell anemia (SCA) in African-Americans
   D. A and C are correct
   E. A, B, and C are correct

ANSWERS

1-1. C. This couple's ethnic background places them at risk for β-thalassemia. Therefore, the anemia should be evaluated in both parents. "Physiologic anemia" of pregnancy occurs because of the relatively greater expansion of plasma volume compared to the increase in total RBC mass. As a result, the hematocrit decreases and reaches a nadir at approximately 32 weeks GA. However, this anemia is not associated with hypochromia and microcytosis. Although iron deficiency anemia is the most common anemia seen in pregnancy, empiric treatment for iron deficiency anemia without simultaneous diagnostic workup is inappropriate. Because amniocentesis is an invasive procedure with associated risks, direct testing of the fetus for β-thalassemia is not indicated unless the parents are known carriers.

1-2. E. Optimal assessment of a potentially heritable disorder in a family is best achieved by evaluation of the known affected individual. In this case, because chromosomal analysis was performed 20 years earlier and the resolution of karyotypes is far greater today, it is reasonable to repeat an analysis in addition to investigating the possibility of fragile X, which should be ruled out in any male with mental retardation of unknown cause, particularly if he has traits associated with the syndrome, such as autistic behavior. In cases where evaluation of the affected family member is not possible, the patient, herself can undergo karyotype analysis and DNA screening for the Fragile X premutation or mutation. However, a normal ultrasound and a normal triple screen test, while reassuring, do not invalidate the need for the workup outlined above. Usually the results of these two tests are normal in fragile X as well as in unspecified mental retardation.

1-3. C. Transvaginal ultrasound can detect an intrauterine gestational sac as early as 4.5 weeks GA and an embryo by 6 weeks GA. Fetal movements can be felt on average at approximately 18 weeks GA and typically 1 or 2 weeks sooner in multiparous women. Between approximately 18 and 36 weeks GA, the fundal height in centimeters is roughly equal to weeks of GA. Hence, the uterine fundus should be palpable at the umbilicus by 20 weeks GA. At 12 weeks GA, the uterine fundus should be palpable transabdominally at the symphysis pubis. With the aid of Doppler, fetal heart tones can be heard as early as 11 weeks, if not a bit sooner with more modern equipment. Failure to detect fetal heart tones at 12 weeks GA or later should warrant further investigation with ultrasound.

1-4. D. CF, Canavan disease, and Tay-Sachs disease are autosomal recessive disorders that can affect individuals from any ethnic background. However, their incidence is higher among Ashkenazi Jews. In addition, genetic screening is facilitated among Ashkenazi Jews because of the "founder effect," that is, common gene mutations existing within the group. Universal screening should be offered for CF, although the detection rate of mutations is different for each ethnic group. With current mutation panels, less than 60% of CF mutations can be detected among Latinos, who have a low prevalence of CF. Among African-Americans, the carrier rate for SCA is 8%. SCA prenatal screening via hemoglobin electrophoresis is routinely offered to African-Americans.

 ## SUGGESTED ADDITIONAL READING

Chou R, Smits AK, Huffman LH, et al. US Preventive Services Task Force. Prenatal screening for HIV: a review of the evidence for the U.S. Preventive Services Task Force. *Ann Intern Med.* 2005;143:38–54.

Morgan MA, Driscoll DA, Mennuti MT, et al. Practice patterns of obstetrician-gynecologists regarding preconception and prenatal screening for cystic fibrosis. *Genet Med.* 2004;6:450–455.

ACOG committee opinion. Number 298, August 2004. Prenatal and preconceptional carrier screening for genetic diseases in individuals of Eastern European Jewish descent. *Obstet Gynecol.* 2004;104:425–428.

Screening Tests in Pregnancy

ID/CC: A 35-year-old G_1P_0 woman at 16 weeks gestational age (GA) presents for her second-trimester visit.

HPI: M.A. currently has resolution of the nausea and vomiting that were problematic through 12 weeks of gestation. She has no contractions, bleeding, or dysuria. She recently saw a genetic counselor and, despite the counselor's recommendation to obtain an amniocentesis, would prefer to avoid the risk of this procedure if possible. You validate her decision, and ask if she would like to obtain a triple-marker screening test for Down syndrome, which has 80% sensitivity in women 35 years and older. She is interested in this test because it involves only a blood draw, and she is quite happy to avoid the amniocentesis if the test is negative.

PMHx: Migraine headaches

PSHx: Tonsillectomy

Meds: PNV

All: NKDA

POb/GynHx: Unremarkable. No STIs or PID, normal Pap smears.

SHx: M.A. is an economics professor, and her partner is a psychologist. No ethanol, tobacco, or recreational drug use.

THOUGHT QUESTIONS

- What is the answer to M.A.'s question?
- What are the sensitivity and specificity of a screening test?

- What are the positive and negative predictive values?
- What are the likelihood ratios?

Often in medicine there are two possible pathways to a diagnosis. One method, illustrated by amniocentesis, involves a risky, often more expensive, diagnostic test. The second often involves using a much less risky, often less expensive, screening test to identify the high-risk patients within a population in order to determine who should undergo the more invasive test. Which pathway to use is dependent on the importance of the diagnosis, the baseline risk of the patient, the risk of the diagnostic procedure, and the test characteristics of the screening test. The two classic test characteristics reported usually are sensitivity and specificity, and these characteristics, in addition to the other attributes of the situation, are used to determine whether a patient will benefit from screening.

Sensitivity is defined as the percentage of cases identified by a screening test. If a screening test identifies 93 of 100 cases, then the test has 93% sensitivity. In a 2 × 2 table, sensitivity is the number of true positives divided by the total number of individuals with disease (Table 2-1). *Specificity* is the percentage of people without disease who are correctly identified as not having disease. For example, if in the same population 100 people were not cases and 96 of them were identified as not being cases, then the test has 96% specificity. In a 2 × 2 table, specificity is the number of true negatives divided by the total number of individuals without disease (see Table 2-1). Of importance is the relationship between sensitivity and specificity. Most screening tests return a value that is either above or below a threshold. Where the threshold is set determines the sensitivity and specificity. If the threshold of the test is set quite low, then the sensitivity will be high but the specificity low. Conversely, if the threshold is set quite high, then the sensitivity will be low but the specificity high. When sensitivity versus

TABLE 2-1 Sensitivity and Specificity in a 2 × 2 Table

| | Disease | |
Test Result	*Present*	*Absent*
Positive	a = TP True positive	b = FP False positive
Negative	c = FN False negative	d = TN True negative

Sensitivity = a/(a+c)
Specificity = d/(b+d)

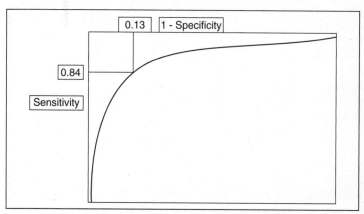

FIGURE 2-1. Receiver Operator Characteristic (ROC) curve. The ROC diagram illustrates the trade-off between sensitivity and specificity. In this ROC, the point chosen illustrates where sensitivity is 84% and specificity is 87%.

1 – specificity is plotted for a series of possible threshold values for a test, the result is called a *receiver operator characteristic* (ROC) curve. The ROC curve can be examined to locate an optimal point where the trade-off between sensitivity and specificity is reasonable (Figure 2-1).

Predictive Value of Screening Tests

The trade-off between sensitivity and specificity is an important consideration, but another is how useful the test is in differentiating individuals with a diagnosis from those without. One way to use the results of a screening test is to use its predictive value. The *positive predictive value* (PPV) is the proportion of screen-positive patients who actually have the diagnosis. These are the true-positive patients divided by all those who test positive, or $a/(a+b)$ in a 2×2 table (Table 2-2). The *negative predictive value* (NPV) is the proportion of screen-negative patients who do not have the diagnosis. These are the true negatives divided by all who test negative, or $d/(c+d)$ in a 2×2 table (see Figure 2-1). In the example of the triple-marker screen, because the test is positive for all women with a risk ≥1:190, the PPV is poor, only approximately 1%. On the other hand, NPV is quite good at 1:700 or better because the baseline risk in the population is low.

Likelihood Ratios

The PPV and NPV of tests also can be calculated by using likelihood ratios (LRs). An LR is the probability of a particular test finding in a patient with disease divided by the probability of the same test finding in a patient without the disease. Thus, LR can be calculated for

TABLE 2-2 Calculating Predictive Value

	Disease	
Test Result	*Present*	*Absent*
Positive	a = TP True positive	b = FP False positive
Negative	c = FN False negative	d = TN True negative

PPV = a/(a+b)
NPV = d/(c+d)

both positive and negative tests. A positive LR test, LR(+), is equal to the sensitivity divided by 1 − specificity. A negative LR test, LR(−), is equal to 1 − sensitivity divided by specificity. This is shown as follows:

$$LR(+) = \frac{\text{Prob (Pos test given disease)}}{\text{Prob (Pos test given no disease)}} = \frac{a/(a+c)}{b/(b+d)} = \frac{\text{Sensitivity}}{1 - \text{Specificity}}$$

$$LR(-) = \frac{\text{Prob (Neg test given disease)}}{\text{Prob (Neg test given no disease)}} = \frac{c/(a+c)}{d/(b+d)} = \frac{1 - \text{Sensitivity}}{\text{Specificity}}$$

Now that we know how to calculate LRs, we need one more concept in order to use them to calculate posttest probabilities. What we need is odds as opposed to probability. *Odds* is a ratio of probabilities, defined as the probability of an event occurring divided by the probability of the event not occurring.

$$\text{Odds} = p/(1 - p)$$
$$p = \text{Odds}/(\text{Odds} + 1)$$

LR is actually multiplied by the pretest odds to calculate the posttest odds. Thus, the pretest probability can be converted to odds using the first equation, then multiplied by LR and converted back to probability using the second equation. Of note, when the pretest probability is small (<1%), odds and probability are almost equal.

 CASE CONTINUED

You explain to M.A. that, despite a negative test result, there still is a small chance that her baby has Down syndrome, although using an LR(−) of 0.5, the probability is only half what it was prior to having the test. Because M.A. had not wanted an amniocentesis at the beginning and now her probability is lowered, she decides to do without the diagnostic test.

QUESTIONS

2-1. Assume you are given the following 2 × 2 table for Down syndrome screening (Table 2-3). What are the sensitivity, specificity, PPV, and NPV of this screening test?
  A. 0.5, 0.99, 0.1, 0.90
  B. 0.5, 0.99, 0.01, 0.90
  C. 0.5, 0.90, 0.01, 0.999
  D. 0.5, 0.90, 0.11, 0.001
  E. 0.90, 0.5, 0.999, 0.01

TABLE 2-3 Theoretical Screening Test for Down Syndrome

Test Result	Disease	
	Present	Absent
Positive	a = 10	b = 980 False positive
Negative	c = 10	d = 9,000 True negative

2-2. A screening test is performed, and there are ten positive results. Of these, six are false positives. Of note, there are exactly ten people with disease in the population screened. Which of the following is true?
  A. This test has 40% sensitivity.
  B. This test has 60% sensitivity.
  C. This test has 100% sensitivity.
  D. This test has 60% specificity.
  E. This test has 40% specificity.

2-3. A screening test for gestational diabetes is being tested. You know that 900 nondiabetics and 100 diabetics are being screened. There are 100 positive tests, and of these, 90 individuals have diabetes. Which of the following is true in this population?
  A. NPV of the test is 0.9.
  B. NPV of the test is 0.5.
  C. NPV of the test is 0.1.
  D. PPV of the test is 0.1.
  E. PPV of the test is 0.9.

2-4. In the screening test in Question 3, what is the LR(+)?
   A. 1
   B. 8
   C. 81
   D. 99
   E. 990

ANSWERS

2-1. C. In the 2 × 2 table shown, the sensitivity, specificity, PPV, NPV, LR(+), and LR(−) values can be readily calculated as shown. As with many poor screening tests, although having a positive value on this test increases an individual's risk of having the disease fivefold [LR(+) = 5], the sensitivity of the test is only 50%. Thus, only half of the cases will be identified using such a screening test. These test characteristics are commonly seen in obstetric ultrasound screening for Down syndrome, as approximately 40% of Down syndrome fetuses will have a normal ultrasound (Table 2-4).

TABLE **2-4** Theoretical Screening Test for Down Syndrome

Test Result	Disease	
	Present	*Absent*
Positive	a = 10	b = 980 False positive
Negative	c = 10	d = 9,000 True negative

Sensitivity = a/(a + c) = 10/(20) = 0.5
Specificity = d/(b + d) = 9,000/(9,980) = 0.90
PPV = a/(a + b) = 10/(990) = 0.01
NPV = d/(c + d) = 9,000/(9,010) = 0.999
LR(+) = Sensitivity/(1 − Specificity) = 0.5/(0.1) = 5
LR(−) = (1 − Sensitivity)/Specificity = 0.5/0.9 = .56

Example of Using LR(+)
In this case, the pretest probability is 20/10,000 = 0.002
Odds = 0.002/(1 − 0.002) = 0.002
Posttest Odds = 0.002 × (5) = 0.01
Posttest Prob = 0.01/(1.01) = 0.01 = PPV

2-2. A. We only know three of the four boxes in the 2 × 2 table. We know that there are six false positives; thus, the remaining four positive tests must be true positives. Because there are exactly ten people with disease, there must be six false negatives. Using this information, we can calculate the sensitivity but not the specificity. Sensitivity = a/(a + c) = 4/10 = 0.4 (or 40%).

2-3. E. In the diabetes screening test, we know only three of the four boxes in the 2 × 2 table. Ninety of the 100 positive screens have diabetes, so they must be true positives. The remaining ten must be false positives. Because there are 100 people with diabetes, there must be ten false negatives as well. Thus, we can calculate PPV but not NPV. PPV = 90/100 = 0.9.

2-4. C. Remember that:

$$LR(+) = \frac{\text{Prob (Pos test given disease)}}{\text{Prob (Pos test given no disease)}} = \frac{a/(a + c)}{b/(b + d)} = \frac{\text{Sensitivity}}{1 - \text{Specificity}}$$

To determine LR(+), one must first calculate the sensitivity and specificity. In this screening test, 90 of the 100 diabetics were identified, giving sensitivity of 0.9 (or 90%). The specificity is all of the true negatives over the nondiabetics, which is 890/900 = 0.9889 (or 98.89%). Thus, LR = 0.9/0.0111 = 81.081.

 SUGGESTED ADDITIONAL READING

Caughey AB, Lyell DJ, Filly RA, Washington AE, Norton ME. Targeted ultrasound as a screen for Down syndrome in high risk women: How many missed diagnoses? *Prenat Diagn.* 2006;26:22–27.

Caughey AB, Lyell DJ, Filly R, Washington AE, Norton ME. The impact of the use of echogenic intracardiac focus as a screen for Down syndrome in women under the age of 35. *Am J Obstet Gynecol.* 2001;85:1021–1027.

Friedland DJ, Go AS, Devoren JB, Shlipak MG, SW Bent, Subak LL, Mendelson T. *Evidence-Based Medicine: A Framework for Clinical Practice* (Paperback). McGraw-Hill Medical; 1st edition, 1998.

Vaginal Bleeding in Pregnancy I—With Associated Cramping

ID/CC: A 36-year-old G_4P_2 woman at 9 weeks GA by LMP presents with complaints of menstrual-like bleeding and cramping.

HPI: A.A. now is 9 weeks into her current pregnancy (dated by an LMP) and had a positive self-administered urine pregnancy test approximately 3 weeks ago. She notes that she had been doing well in this pregnancy and actually had felt less nausea over the past week than during the preceding few weeks. However, this evening she started having some abdominal cramping. Approximately 1 hour later she noted that she was having vaginal spotting, which increased to menstrual-like flow over the past couple of hours.

PMHx/PSHx: None

Meds: PNV

All: NKDA

POb/GynHx: Two prior term vaginal deliveries, uncomplicated, 4 and 6 years ago. One first-trimester therapeutic abortion (TAB) 13 years ago. Regular menses, every 29 to 30 days. No STIs, no pelvic surgery, no infertility.

SHx: Lives with husband and two children; no domestic violence. No tobacco, recreational drug, or social ethanol use.

VS: Temp 98.8°F, BP 118/72, HR 84, RR 16

PE: *Abdomen:* soft, nontender, no distension, no peritoneal signs. *SSE:* cervix closed, small amount of blood coming from os. *BME:* uterus anteverted (AV) and anteflexed (AF), approx

7 to 8 weeks in size and slightly tender; no cervical motion tenderness (CMT); no palpable adnexal masses.

Labs: Urine pregnancy test positive; Hct 37.4; β-hCG 24,122 mIU/mL

US: Pending

THOUGHT QUESTIONS

■ What is in this patient's differential diagnosis?

■ How does the beta human chorionic gonadotropin (β-hCG) value help in this clinical situation, other than confirming the positive urine pregnancy test?

■ How will the results of the pelvic ultrasound help in the diagnosis?

Mrs. A's differential diagnosis includes ectopic pregnancy, complete spontaneous abortion (SAB), and threatened abortion. She has no risk factors for ectopic pregnancy, but this remains the most dangerous possible diagnosis. It is estimated that approximately 15% to 20% of known pregnancies result in SAB (known to the layperson as a *miscarriage*). The percentage of all pregnancies that result in SAB probably is higher. The primary etiology for first-trimester SABs is abnormal karyotype, with the most common being 45,XO (Turner syndrome). Other known etiologies for first-trimester SABs include uterine abnormalities (e.g., bicornuate uterus, submucosal fibroids), luteal phase defect (believed to result from corpus luteum progesterone production that is inadequate to maintain pregnancy), thrombophilias (e.g., antiphospholipid antibody syndrome, systemic lupus erythematosus), infections (e.g., cytomegalovirus, varicella-zoster virus, herpes simple virus), and balanced translocation of a chromosome in one of the parents. Despite these numerous possible etiologies as well as extensive testing, most SABs are idiopathic.

The value of β-hCG helps to predict what can be seen on ultrasound. With transvaginal ultrasound, an intrauterine pregnancy can be seen with a β-hCG of 1,600 to 2,000, and fetal heart motion can be seen with a β-hCG of 5,000 to 6,000. Thus, in this patient with a β-hCG >20,000, the pregnancy should be easily seen by ultrasound, provided it is normal. An intrauterine pregnancy, if seen, rules out ectopic pregnancy, except in the extremely rare case of

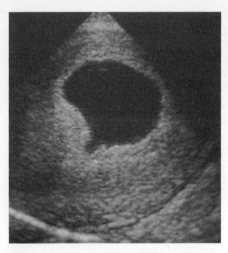

FIGURE 3-1.
An intrauterine gestational sac that, although large enough, has no evidence of fetal pole. *(Image Provided by Departments of Radiology and Obstetrics and Gynecology, University of California, San Francisco).*

heterotopic pregnancy (one pregnancy in the uterus and one ectopic). Fetal heart motion also should be seen; if it is present, the risk of miscarriage is decreased to <5%.

CASE CONTINUED

US: Intrauterine gestational sac seen (Figure 3-1); however, no fetal pole is identified. No adnexal masses and no free fluid in the cul-de-sac.

Upon returning from ultrasound exam, the patient has increased vaginal bleeding. Now when examined, the cervix is slightly dilated, and there is continued bleeding from the os. A dilation and curettage (D&C) is performed, and the bleeding stops at the end of the procedure. Tissue sent for pathologic exam reveals trophoblastic tissue but no fetal tissue.

QUESTIONS

3-1. Upon initial presentation with a closed cervix and a nonviable pregnancy, this patient's diagnosis was:
   A. Missed abortion
   B. Complete abortion
   C. Incomplete abortion
   D. Inevitable abortion
   E. Threatened abortion

3-2. When she returned from ultrasound exam with a dilated cervix, her diagnosis was:
- A. Missed abortion
- B. Complete abortion
- C. Incomplete abortion
- D. Inevitable abortion
- E. Threatened abortion

3-3. If the patient had not begun to dilate upon returning from ultrasound exam, which of the following management options would not be reasonable?
- A. Expectant management at home
- B. D&C
- C. Schedule D&C for 1 week later
- D. Misoprostol given vaginally
- E. Expectant management in the hospital

3-4. Given that this patient now has had one SAB, what is the probability of having another SAB in her next pregnancy?
- A. 15% to 20%
- B. 25%
- C. 30%
- D. 35%
- E. 40%

ANSWERS

3-1. A.; **3-2.** D. The diagnosis of SAB is made for any pregnancy that terminates itself prior to 20 weeks GA. The subcategories based on the clinical situation are as follows: (1) threatened abortion, intrauterine pregnancy with vaginal bleeding; (2) missed abortion, closed cervix, but a nonviable gestation based on absent fetal heart motion or absent fetal pole when one should be present based on GA or β-hCG; (3) inevitable abortion, intrauterine pregnancy, but dilated cervix; (4) incomplete abortion, a portion of the pregnancy has already passed, but often the trophoblastic tissue is still in situ; and (5) complete abortion, the entire pregnancy has passed through the cervix.

3-3. E. Patients who are diagnosed with a missed abortion can be managed in a variety of ways. Expectant management is commonly practiced and leads to 60% to 70% of patients passing the pregnancy on their own. However, this can be uncomfortable and can take several days to several weeks to occur. Thus, many patients prefer an intervention, which can range from an immediate D&C or a D&C scheduled the next day or several days later, to a less invasive approach of giving vaginal misoprostol to help induce uterine contractions and the expulsion of the pregnancy. If the patient opts for expectant management, the process usually is done at home. The only reason for hospital observation of a patient is if there is concern regarding an ectopic pregnancy.

3-4. A. A patient who has had one SAB does not have much of an increased risk for SAB over that of the general population. Thus, the risk remains between 15% and 20%. In patients with two consecutive SABs, 25% to 30% risk of SAB is quoted for the next pregnancy. In patients with three consecutive SABs, 35% to 45% risk of SAB has been quoted, though it depends enormously on the cause of the SABs and the patient's age.

 SUGGESTED ADDITIONAL READING

Barnhart KT, Simhan H, Kamell SA. Diagnostic accuracy of ultrasound above and below the beta-hCG discriminatory zone. *Obstet Gynecol.* 1999;94:583–587.

US Department of Health and Human Services. *Reproductive impairment among married couples.* US Vital and Health Statistics Series 23, vol. 11. Hyattsville, Md: National Center of Health Statistics; 1982:5.

Nausea and Vomiting of Pregnancy

ID/CC: A 21-year-old G_2P_1 woman at approximately 11 weeks GA by sure LMP complains of irregular vaginal bleeding, nausea, and vomiting.

HPI: M.P. is excited and happy about this pregnancy but notes worsening nausea and vomiting over the last 2 weeks, which is unlike her prior pregnancy. She feels nauseated most of the day and is unable to keep anything down other than the occasional water and saltine crackers. She also reports the onset of vaginal spotting and bleeding over the last few days. She denies any abdominal or back cramps.

PMHx: Hypothyroidism

PSHx: None

Meds: L-thyroxine, PNV

All: NKDA

POb/GynHx: One normal vaginal delivery 2 years ago. Regular menses every 28 days. No STIs or prior pelvic or abdominal surgery.

SHx: She is married and lives with her husband and son. No use of ethanol, tobacco, or recreational drugs.

VS: Temp 97.8°F, BP 120/65, HR 90, RR 20

PE: *Neck:* supple, mobile, no masses. *Abdomen:* soft, non-tender, no distension. *Pelvic:* no cervical polyp or lesion; 15-week size uterus, nontender, no adnexal masses. *Doppler:* no fetal heart sounds by Doppler tones.

Labs: hCG 170,000 mIU/mL

US: Pending

THOUGHT QUESTIONS

- What does the differential diagnosis include for this patient?
- Which diagnostic tests would be most useful?
- Does the hCG value help?

The differential diagnosis of larger than expected uterine size and bleeding includes multiple gestations, inaccurate dating, uterine leiomyomas (fibroids) or adenomyosis, and gestational trophoblastic disease (GTD). If the uterus is enlarged because of fibroids or baseline adenomyosis, the differential diagnosis includes threatened miscarriage, ectopic pregnancy, and normal intrauterine pregnancy. The hCG level and a transvaginal ultrasound would help evaluate the state of the pregnancy. An abnormally high hCG level and a "snowstorm" pattern on ultrasound are diagnostic of GTD. Thyroid function tests would rule out hyperthyroidism as a cause of the excessive nausea and vomiting.

CASE CONTINUED

The radiologist calls you with the findings of no evidence of a fetus but a "snowstorm" pattern of swollen chorionic villi within the uterine cavity (Figure 4-1). You tell the patient that she has a molar pregnancy and explain some of the differences between a complete and an incomplete molar pregnancy (Table 4-1). Her thyroid function tests are normal, and a chest x-ray film is negative for metastases. You arrange for a suction curettage to be performed.

Note: Gestational trophoblastic disease is most often a sporadic disease; however, rare cases of what appears to be an inherited susceptibility within the egg genome to having repeat complete molar pregnancies have been reported. In these rare multiple molar pregnancy cases, biparental chromosomal constitutions have been demonstrated. It is postulated that in these cases, abnormal maternal imprinting results in complete moles of biparental origin. However, almost all cases of incomplete molar pregnancies are diandric, with the additional chromosomal set paternally derived.

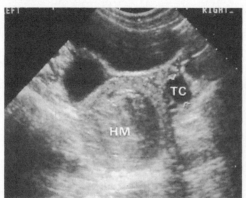

FIGURE 4-1.
Complete molar pregnancy on ultrasound. Note the hydropic villi (*Black Lucent Areas*) and the general snowstorm appearance. (*From Hamilton-Fairley D. Lecture Notes: Obstetrics and Gynaecology, 2nd ed. Oxford: Blackwell Publishing, 2004.*)

TABLE 4-1 Differences Between Complete and Incomplete Molar Pregnancies

Factor	Complete	Incomplete
Proportion	90%	10%
Karyotype	Paternal; 46,XX (mainly); 46,XY	Diandric; triploid or trisomic (mainly); diploid
Products of conception	Absent fetus, diffuse hydropic trophoblast	Abnormal fetus/embryo, focal hydropic trophoblast
Malignancy	15%–20% trophoblastic sequelae	4%–11% trophoblastic sequelae
Medical complications	Yes	Rare

QUESTIONS

4-1. What is the most common presenting symptom of a complete molar pregnancy?
A. Hyperemesis
B. Bilateral enlarged theca lutein cysts
C. Vaginal bleeding
D. Uterine enlargement greater than expected for GA
E. Pregnancy-induced hypertension

4-2. The diagnosis of a complete hydatidiform mole has been confirmed following the suction curettage. What is the most appropriate management for this patient now?
  A. Weekly and then monthly hCG testing
  B. Hysterectomy
  C. Transvaginal ultrasonographic examination
  D. Repeat suction curettage
  E. Prompt chemotherapy

4-3. At 5 and 6 weeks after evacuation of the molar pregnancy, her hCG levels are 10,900 and 12,100 mIU/mL, respectively. You now are worried about malignant GTD. Which of the following treatment would you initiate?
  A. Begin a course of single-agent chemotherapy
  B. Begin a course of combination chemotherapy
  C. Continued observation with repeat hCG testing in 1 week
  D. Hysterectomy and then methotrexate
  E. CT of the brain, chest, abdomen, and pelvis

4-4. What hormone is proposed as the cause of hyperemesis associated with a molar pregnancy?
  A. Estrogen
  B. hCG
  C. Progesterone
  D. Total thyroxine (T_4)
  E. Luteinizing hormone (LH)

 ANSWERS

4-1. C. The clinical presentation of a complete molar pregnancy has changed dramatically over the years. The diagnosis now is usually made in the first trimester, with vaginal bleeding occurring in >84% of cases. Hyperemesis is a less frequent complaint, occurring in 8% of patients. Excessive uterine size for a given GA occurs in 30% to 50% of patients with a complete mole because of retained blood and excessive trophoblastic proliferation. Bilateral theca lutein cyst enlargement occurs in approximately 15% of cases secondary to ovarian hyperstimulation by high levels of hCG. Infrequently, patients present with pregnancy-induced hypertension (1%). Of note, patients with partial moles usually do not exhibit the classic clinical features of complete moles, although vaginal bleeding remains the primary presenting symptom.

4-2. A. Following suction evacuation of a molar pregnancy, serial hCG titers must be monitored weekly until normal (<5 mIU/mL) for 3 weeks and then monthly until normal for 6 months to 1 year. Trophoblastic sequelae (invasive mole or choriocarcinoma) occur in 15% to 20% of patients with complete hydatidiform mole. The patient must receive concurrent reliable contraception to prevent pregnancy during this time period so that hCG titers can be followed. Persistently elevated hCG titers suggest persistent trophoblastic disease, at which time chemotherapy is indicated. Hysterectomy is not indicated in this disease entity, which is exquisitely sensitive to chemotherapy. Repeat suction evacuation or transvaginal ultrasonography is of little use or benefit in the treatment of a molar pregnancy in the immediate period after an evacuation.

4-3. A. The risk of subsequent GTD associated with a complete mole is 15% to 20%, whereas the risk of subsequent GTD following a partial mole ranges from 4% to 11%. Malignant GTD can be classified as nonmetastatic or metastatic for the purposes of treatment planning and prognosis. A metastatic workup includes evaluation for liver, brain, or lung metastases. Because this patient had no evidence of metastatic disease 6 weeks ago, it is reasonable to begin single-agent chemotherapy at this time. Nevertheless, some practitioners will do a complete workup to rule out metastatic disease prior to initiating chemotherapy. Surgery does not have a role in the management of her disease at this point, particularly because GTD is extremely chemosensitive. Single-agent chemotherapy with methotrexate or dactinomycin is the treatment of choice. Approximately 85% to 90% of patients are cured by the initial chemotherapy regimen. Multiagent chemotherapy is rarely needed.

4-4. A. Approximately 8% of patients with complete moles present with hyperemesis requiring antiemetic therapy. It usually is associated with markedly elevated hCG values from trophoblastic proliferation and growth and an excessively enlarged uterus. Nevertheless, it is the high circulating levels of estrogen that are thought to be the cause of hyperemesis. Data on whether hCG is a thyroid stimulator in these patients are conflicting, but today it is relatively uncommon for women with molar pregnancies to have clinical evidence of hyperthyroidism.

SUGGESTED ADDITIONAL READING

Berkowitz RS, Goldstein DP. Chorionic tumors. *N Engl J Med.* 1996;335:1740–1748.

Berkowitz RS, Goldstein DP. Gestational trophoblastic diseases. In: Hoskins WJ, Perez CA, Young RC, eds. *Principles and practice of gynecologic oncology.* 4th ed. Philadelphia, Pa: Lippincott Williams & Wilkins; 2005:1055–1076.

McNeish IA, Strickland S, Holden L, et al. Low-risk persistent gestational trophoblastic disease: outcome after initial treatment with low-dose methotrexate and folinic acid from 1992 to 2000. *J Clin Oncol.* 2002;20:1838–1844.

CASE 5

Pregnant at the Age of 40

 ID/CC: A 40-year-old G_2P_0 woman at 7 weeks GA by LMP at her first prenatal visit.

HPI: A.M. conceived spontaneously after trying for 2 years. She is excited about the pregnancy but at the same time is concerned about potential age-related risks to herself as well as to the baby. Her husband is 52 years old and healthy, and he fathered two children from a prior marriage. The week prior to the visit, she experienced spotting that lasted 3 days and then resolved. Currently she has no complaints.

PMHx/PSHx: None

POb/GynHx: Regular menses, every 30 days

Meds: PNV and folic acid

SHx: Lawyer and active tennis player, lives with husband and two cats. Denies tobacco or alcohol use.

FHx: Noncontributory

Labs: Normal prenatal labs

THOUGHT QUESTIONS

- What adverse perinatal outcomes are associated with advanced maternal age?
- What adverse perinatal outcomes are associated with advanced paternal age?
- Is advanced maternal age associated with increased maternal morbidity?
- What would be the appropriate test for fetal evaluation for this patient?

The risk of aneuploidy increases with age, rising exponentially after age 37 years. As a result, there is an increased risk for spontaneous abortion, fetal demise and stillbirth, and a liveborn child with a chromosomal abnormality (aneuploidy). Advanced paternal age (>40 or 45 years of age) is associated with an increased risk for autosomal dominant conditions due to spontaneous mutations. Because chronic illnesses such as hypertension, obesity, and diabetes mellitus type 2 are age related, there is increased maternal morbidity associated with advanced maternal age (>35 years). In addition, advanced maternal age has been associated with increased risk for preeclampsia, gestational diabetes, and cesarean delivery.

Diagnostic prenatal diagnosis for fetal aneuploidy, via chorionic villus sampling (CVS) between 10 and 13 weeks GA or amniocentesis from 16 to 20 weeks GA, is routinely offered to women who will be 35 years or older at the time of delivery. The *a priori* risk of a 35-year-old woman having a fetus with aneuploidy at the time of amniocentesis is approximately 1:200. The risk of pregnancy loss secondary to amniocentesis is estimated at 1:200. CVS has the advantage of providing a diagnosis earlier than amniocentesis, potentially providing psychological advantages for the woman. In addition, termination procedures are technically simpler and associated with less morbidity at earlier GAs. However, CVS has a slightly higher procedure-related pregnancy loss rate (1:150) than a 16-week amniocentesis.

CASE CONTINUED

The patient was offered an amniocentesis at 16 weeks GA, but she declined because of the concern for miscarriage. Instead, she chose to have a level II ultrasound (detailed ultrasound survey of fetal anatomy) and maternal serum screening.

Her estriol, hCG, and α-fetoprotein (AFP) levels were low. At 18 weeks from her LMP, ultrasound showed a fetus consistent with 16-week size, increased amniotic fluid, clubfeet, omphalocele, choroid plexus cyst, and possible heart defect (Figure 5-1).

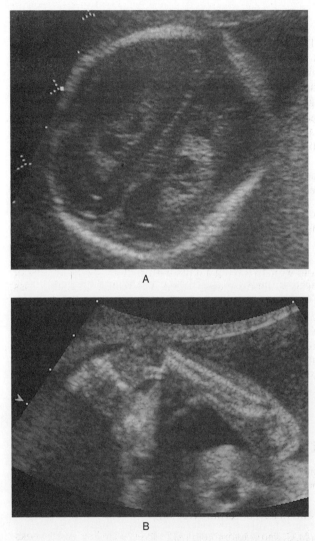

FIGURE 5-1. A: Choroid Plexus Cyst—Note the bilateral choroid plexus cysts in the lateral ventricles of the brain. **B:** Club Foot—Note that you can see the leg straight on with both the tibia and fibula, but the foot is off at an angle from these long bones. *(Image Provided by Departments of Radiology and Obstetrics and Gynecology, University of California, San Francisco).*

QUESTIONS

5-1. Based on the patient's history and data provided, what is the most likely diagnosis?
- A. Trisomy 21
- B. Trisomy 13
- C. Trisomy 18
- D. X-linked ichthyosis
- E. Beckwith-Wiedemann syndrome

5-2. The risks of amniocentesis include which of the following?
- A. Alloimmunization of an Rh-negative woman carrying an Rh-positive fetus
- B. Small risk of fetal injury with the needle
- C. Premature rupture of membranes
- D. All of the above
- E. None of the above

5-3. Of the following statements regarding ultrasound in the detection of chromosomal abnormalities, select the best answer.
- A. Ultrasound has a sensitivity of 90% for detection of Down syndrome when performed between 16 and 23 weeks.
- B. Nuchal translucency has a sensitivity >70% for detection of trisomy 21 when used between 11 to 14 weeks.
- C. A normal, detailed fetal ultrasound excludes the possibility of trisomy 21.
- D. Increased nuchal thickness, short femur, pyelectasis, and echogenic cardiac foci are excellent sonographic predictors of Down syndrome.

5-4. Which of the following conditions is associated with advanced paternal age?
- A. 47,XXX
- B. Neurofibromatosis I (NF-I)
- C. Trisomy 21
- D. Cystic fibrosis
- E. Patau syndrome

ANSWERS

5-1. C. Trisomy 21 as well as trisomy 13 can be associated with growth retardation and omphalocele but not as commonly as seen in trisomy 18. In fetuses with Down syndrome, maternal serum

AFP and estriol levels are low, but the hCG level usually is elevated. Trisomy 13 is generally not detected by maternal serum screening. The pattern of the maternal serum screen with all three values decreased is typical for trisomy 18, which can detect up to 50% of affected fetuses. The malformations listed are typical of trisomy 18. X-linked ichthyosis is caused by a deletion of the steroid sulfatase (STS) gene, leading to almost undetectable estriol levels and dry, scaly skin. However, maternal serum hCG and AFP levels usually are normal, and this condition usually is not associated with malformations. Beckwith-Wiedemann syndrome is characterized by macrosomia, omphalocele, and macroglossia.

5-2. D. An Rh-negative woman can become sensitized at the time of amniocentesis. Therefore, Rh_0 (D) immune globulin (RhoGAM) is indicated at the time of the procedure in these patients. Pregnancy loss, premature rupture of membranes, prematurity, and fetal injury are the more common risks associated with amniocentesis. The risk of pregnancy loss secondary to genetic amniocentesis in the midtrimester is 1:200 (0.5%).

5-3. B. During midtrimester ultrasound, 50% of scans of Down syndrome fetuses are read as "normal"; the other half have major malformations and/or ultrasound markers that are associated with, but not diagnostic of, Down syndrome. A nuchal translucency scan between 11 and 14 weeks has a sensitivity comparable or superior to that of second-trimester maternal serum screen for detection of Down syndrome ($\geq$70% vs. 65%). A number of morphologic variants or "ultrasound markers" have been proposed for the detection of Down syndrome, including those mentioned; however, the validity of screening low-risk populations with midtrimester ultrasound has been questioned because of poor sensitivity and specificity.

5-4. B. Trisomy 21, trisomy 13 (Patau syndrome), and trisomy X are all correlated with advanced maternal age rather than paternal age. NF-I, like other autosomal dominant disorders, rises exponentially with increasing paternal age. Cystic fibrosis is an autosomal recessive condition and is not associated with increasing paternal age.

SUGGESTED ADDITIONAL READING

Jacobsson B, Ladfors L, Milsom I. Advanced maternal age and
   adverse perinatal outcome. *Obstet Gynecol.* 2004;104:727–733.
ACOG Practice Bulletin. Clinical management guidelines for
   obstetrician-gynecologists. Prenatal diagnosis of fetal
   chromosomal abnormalities. *Obstet Gynecol.* 2001;97(5 pt 1):
   suppl 1–12.
Brambati B, Tului L. Chorionic villus sampling and amniocentesis.
   Curr Opin Obstet Gynecol. 2005;17:197–201.
Caughey AB, Lyell DJ, Washington AE, et al. Targeted ultrasound
   as a screen for Down syndrome in high risk women: How many
   missed diagnoses? *Prenat Diagn.* 2006;26:22–27.

Vaginal Bleeding in Pregnancy II—With Left Lower Quadrant Pain

ID/CC: 21-year-old G_1P_0 woman presents with complaints of vaginal bleeding and left lower abdominal pain for 1 day.

HPI: D.P. was in her usual state of health until approximately 18 hours prior to presenting to the emergency department. At that time, she noted that she had started vaginal spotting and had some crampy, nonradiating, left lower quadrant abdominal pain. Because she was several weeks late for her period, she assumed that it was beginning. However, over the ensuing 12 to 18 hours, the pain became worse than her normal menses, while the bleeding remained spotting. She notes some mild nausea, but no vomiting, anorexia, fever or chills, bowel symptoms, or dysuria.

PMHx/PSHx: None

Meds: None

All: NKDA

POb/GynHx: Menarche age 12, regular menses every 28 days until this cycle. Currently sexually active in a monogamous relationship; condoms for birth control (BC); normal Pap smear 7 months ago.

SHx: Junior at local university, lives in college dormitory; half-pack per day cigarette smoker; recreational ethanol use; no other recreational drugs.

VS: Temp 98.2°F, BP 110/58, HR 76, RR 16

PE: *Abdomen:* soft with mild tenderness in lower left quadrant, no peritoneal signs, no distension. *SSE:* cervix closed, small amount of old blood in vault. *BME:* uterus AV/AF, slightly enlarged and slightly tender. No CMT. No palpable adnexal masses, but some mild left adnexal tenderness.

Labs: Urine pregnancy test positive

Blood: Pending

US: Pending

THOUGHT QUESTIONS

- What is included in the differential diagnosis at this point?
- What is the most dangerous possible diagnosis in this patient?
- What lab tests are the most important for this patient?
- What findings on the ultrasound will help sort out the diagnosis?
- What further history might be helpful?

This young woman's differential diagnosis includes ectopic pregnancy, spontaneous abortion, threatened abortion, and ruptured corpus luteum. The most dangerous diagnosis she could have is ectopic pregnancy. The quantitative β-hCG level is an important measurement to obtain because it will help determine what should be seen on pelvic ultrasound. A CBC is important to ensure that she is not anemic from internal bleeding.

Patients who are pregnant and bleeding with abdominal pain should be treated as if they might have an ectopic pregnancy until it is ruled out by an intrauterine pregnancy (IUP) seen on ultrasound. A viable IUP will confirm pregnancy and make the diagnosis of threatened abortion. An IUP that is not viable or has partially passed confirms the diagnosis of missed abortion or incomplete abortion, respectively. An IUP plus moderate free fluid in the cul-de-sac is consistent with a hemorrhagic cyst, usually the corpus luteum.

In patients who are ruled out as ectopic pregnancy candidates, it is essential to obtain a history of possible ectopic risk factors and to carefully tease out the gestational age using LMP dating. Ectopic pregnancy occurs in approximately 1% to 2% of all pregnancies, and its incidence has increased over the past few decades. Ectopic risk factors include prior ectopic pregnancy, pelvic inflammatory disease (PID), prior tubal or pelvic surgery, infertility, assisted reproduction, age ≤25, cigarette smoking, and current intrauterine device (IUD) use.

CASE CONTINUED

Labs: β-hCG 824, WBC 9.7, Hct 35.4

US: No IUP seen, no adnexal masses seen, small amount of free fluid in cul-de-sac

Upon further questioning, the patient reports PID at age 17. Her LMP was 7 weeks ago. Because the diagnosis of ectopic pregnancy cannot be ruled out for this patient and she is hemodynamically stable and unsure whether this pregnancy is desired, it is appropriate to discharge the patient with instructions to return in 2 days for another quantitative β-hCG test or to return sooner if the pain increases.

She returns in 2 days and her β-hCG level is now 1,462. Her vitals signs are normal. Repeat ultrasound is identical to the first one, and she continues to have mild lower left quadrant pain. With the normal rise in her β-hCG level (it should approximately double every 48 hours), the patient is instructed to return again in 48 hours for repeat testing.

QUESTIONS

For questions 6-1 and 6-2, select from the following diagnoses and corresponding management:
- A. Rule out ectopic, uterine aspiration
- B. Rule out ectopic, treat with methotrexate
- C. Normal pregnancy, follow up in 48 hours
- D. Spontaneous abortion, dilation and evacuation (D&E)
- E. Spontaneous abortion, expectant management

6-1. If her second β-hCG level had increased to 1,026, what would be the diagnosis and plan?

6-2. If her second β-hCG level had fallen to 422, what would be the diagnosis and plan?

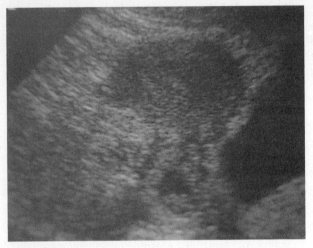

FIGURE 6-1.

6-3. If a patient presents similarly to patient D.P. with the exception of having the pelvic ultrasound shown in Figure 6-1 in addition to cervical motion tenderness, which of the following is the most appropriate management if the pregnancy is desired?
A. Exploratory laparotomy
B. Exploratory laparoscopy
C. Treat with methotrexate
D. Expectant management
E. Dilation and curettage (D&C)

6-4. A patient presents with β-hCG 1,160, Hct 36, and moderate lower left quadrant pain, but no peritoneal signs. An ultrasound shows no IUP but a small 1-cm adnexal mass distinct from the ovary. D&C is performed and reveals no villi. The next step in her management is:
A. Exploratory laparotomy
B. Exploratory laparoscopy
C. Treat with methotrexate
D. Treat with methotrexate and misoprostol
E. Treat with misoprostol

 ANSWERS

6-1. A; **6-2.** E. The β-hCG value should increase by at least 65% every 48 hours in a normal gestation. This has led to the "rule of doubling." Thus, hemodynamically stable patients with a diagnosis of "rule out ectopic pregnancy" are followed with laboratory tests and clinical exams every 48 hours, and the β-hCG level is expected to approximately double. In case of lab error and a time lapse of less than 48 hours in a desired pregnancy of a stable patient, if the increase in β-hCG is 30% to 60%, the β-hCG level is followed for an additional 48 hours to see if the rise normalizes. However, with an increase of only 25% in this patient with left lower quadrant pain, an abnormal pregnancy is presumed and the uterus should be evacuated either with a manual vacuum aspirator or via D&E to determine whether this is an IUP. If the pathology report is negative for IUP, then she would be diagnosed with ectopic pregnancy. If she remained stable and without evidence of fetal cardiac activity, she would be a candidate for pregnancy termination with IM methotrexate. If the patient was unstable, had a large adnexal mass, or had a large volume of blood in the pelvis, she would be considered a poor candidate for medical management and would undergo laparoscopic surgery for the presumed ectopic pregnancy.

If the β-hCG level was actually falling, then the diagnosis of spontaneous abortion is more likely. However, because an ectopic pregnancy still is possible, the β-hCG levels should be followed serially until they are negative. If the patient is diagnosed with spontaneous abortion and is bleeding or has an intrauterine sac on ultrasound, she often is offered expectant management instead of D&C. In this case, because nothing was seen on ultrasound and the patient has been only spotting, expectant management is the preferred management.

6-3. B. In a patient with moderate to large free fluid in the pelvis, a cause should be determined. This is even more important in a patient with peritoneal signs, which include rebound tenderness, tenderness to shaking, and cervical motion tenderness on rectal exam. Laparoscopy is adequate because this patient simply may have a collection of fluid or blood from a hemorrhagic corpus luteum that has stabilized or an ectopic pregnancy that can be resected via laparoscope. Because the pregnancy is desired, it probably is best to determine the cause of the moderate free fluid before performing a D&C of what might be a normal pregnancy (Figure 6-2).

6-4. C. The patient in this question most likely has an ectopic pregnancy with a small adnexal mass and an empty uterus. Because she is stable and there is no evidence of fetal cardiac activity in the adnexal mass, it is reasonable to treat her ectopic pregnancy medically with methotrexate. Contraindications for methotrexate use include moderate or large free fluid, baseline liver disease, adnexal

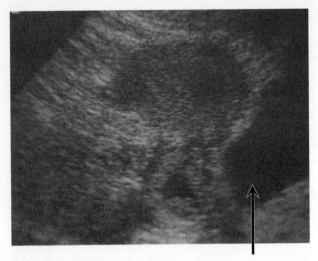

FIGURE 6-2. Free Fluid: In this pelvic ultrasound, you can see free fluid which is consistent with blood in the pelvis. *(Image provided by Departments of Radiology and Obstetrics and Gynecology, University of California, San Francisco).*

mass >3 cm, positive fetal heart rate in the adnexa, or β-hCG >5,000 (occasionally up to 10,000 is used). The latter three findings are suggestive of a gestation that likely is beyond the age where methotrexate would be successful.

 ## SUGGESTED ADDITIONAL READING

Mol BW, Hajenius PJ, Engelsbel S, et al. Serum human chorionic gonadotropin measurement in the diagnosis of ectopic pregnancy when transvaginal sonography is inconclusive. *Fertil Steril.* 1998;70:972–981.

Hajenius PJ, Engelsbel S, Mol BW, et al. Randomised trial of systemic methotrexate versus laparoscopic salpingostomy in tubal pregnancy. *Lancet.* 1997;350:774–779.

Hajenius PJ, Mol BW, Bossuyt PM, et al. Interventions for tubal ectopic pregnancy. *Cochrane Database Syst Rev.* 2000;(2): CD000324.

Heart Palpitations and Fatigue in Pregnancy

 ID/CC: A 30-year-old G_1P_0 woman presents at 8 weeks GA complaining of heart palpitations and fatigue.

HPI: S.C. states that she has not felt well for approximately 3 to 4 months. She states that even before she became pregnant, she noticed occasional heart palpitations, mild shortness of breath with exercise, and excessive fatigue. However, since she became pregnant, she feels these symptoms have grown worse, and now she also has nausea and vomiting that have lasted for the past 3 weeks.

PMHx/PSHx: Appendectomy at age 9

All: NKDA

POb/GynHx: G_1P_0

SHx: Lives with her husband, no domestic violence. No use of ethanol, tobacco, or recreational drugs.

VS: Temp 98.6°F, BP 134/86, HR 110, RR 16

PE: *Gen:* thin-appearing female in NAD. *Neck:* thyroid soft, moderately enlarged without nodules, +bruit. *Lungs:* CTAB. *Cor:* RR, +Flow murmur. *Abdomen:* soft. *Skin*: dry. *Neuro:* mild fine tremor, reflexes 3+ throughout.

THOUGHT QUESTIONS

- What was your differential diagnosis for this patient prior to the exam?
- What aspects of her physical exam are abnormal?
- If you obtained a TSH level and it was found to be low, is that diagnostic for hyperthyroidism?

The differential diagnosis for this patient prior to her exam included nausea and vomiting of pregnancy, hyperemesis gravidarum, hyperthyroidism, and cardiac disease. In addition, all of her symptoms can be seen with a normal pregnancy.

On physical exam, however, you first note a mildly elevated blood pressure and elevated pulse. Her thyroid gland and neurologic exam are abnormal. Besides tachycardia, her cardiac exam is normal with a common flow murmur seen in pregnancy that is secondary to the increased plasma volume experienced in pregnancy.

A low TSH level in early pregnancy is not diagnostic for hyperthyroidism. Interestingly, the hormone human chorionic gonadotropin (hCG), which is secreted in increasing amounts by the placenta in early pregnancy, is structurally similar to TSH, having the exact same α-subunit and some TSH-like activity. Thus, increased amounts of thyroid hormone can be created and a subsequent decrease in TSH level seen. However, this does not cause hyperthyroid disease in an otherwise healthy patient but can create a confusing picture of a low TSH level with a normal or borderline elevated thyroid hormone level in the first trimester.

    ## CASE CONTINUED

You send the patient to the lab for blood work. Her results come back with TSH <0.01 mU/L (low), $fT_4 = 34$ mU/L (high), and thyroid-stimulating immunoglobulin (TSI) 168%. You diagnose her with hyperthyroid disease and instruct her to return for a visit.

QUESTIONS

7-1. What is the most likely diagnosis?
A. Hashimoto thyroiditis
B. Graves disease
C. Hyperemesis gravidarum
D. Toxic multinodular goiter
E. Toxic adenoma

7-2. After confirming the diagnosis, you consult with an endocrinologist and develop a treatment plan. What is the most likely treatment you will choose?
   A. Radioablation with iodine-131
   B. Thyroidectomy
   C. Thionamide therapy with propylthiouracil (PTU)
   D. A β-blocker (i.e., propanolol)
   E. No treatment is necessary at this time

7-3. The patient asks what potential problems could occur to the fetus with this diagnosis and therapy. You inform her which of the following can be seen:
   A. Fetal hypothyroidism
   B. Fetal thyrotoxicosis
   C. Intrauterine growth restriction
   D. All of the above
   E. None of the above

7-4. The patient comes for her next visit. She states she has been looking on the Internet and read that she might need to undergo cordocentesis (sampling of the blood from the umbilical cord prior to delivery). You state the following:
   A. Cordocentesis is never needed during a pregnancy.
   B. Cordocentesis is used only in special circumstances.
   C. Newer treatments and use of ultrasound have replaced the need for cordocentesis.
   D. Cordocentesis is low risk and can be useful during a pregnancy.
   E. None of the above

ANSWERS

7-1. B. Hyperthyroid disease is diagnosed in <1% of pregnant patients. The types of hyperthyroidism generally seen include transient hyperthyroidism due to increased secretion of hCG and Graves disease. Less common etiologies include single toxic adenoma and multinodular toxic goiter. Hashimoto thyroiditis, also called autoimmune thyroiditis, is the most common cause of hypothyroidism in pregnancy. Given her exam findings and laboratory values, the most likely diagnosis in this pregnancy is Graves disease. The most specific test is measurement of TSI level, which is far above the normal range.

7-2. C. Adequate treatment of Graves disease during pregnancy is important for the health of the mother and fetus. Iodine-131 thyroid ablation is contraindicated in pregnancy because radioactive iodine will cross the placenta and concentrate in the fetal thyroid gland. Surgery usually can be avoided during pregnancy but is indicated for hyperthyroid disease refractory to medication therapy. Generally, in the United States, treatment begins with PTU, which inhibits the iodination of thyroglobulin and inhibits conversion of T_4 to T_3. Methimazole works by inhibiting the iodination of thyroglobulin only. It is less commonly used because it has been associated with a reversible scalp defect called fetal aplasia cutis. Adverse effects of thionamide therapy include hepatitis, agranulocytosis, a metallic taste, and nausea. Use of a β-blocker to control adrenergic symptoms is a useful adjunct to thionamide therapy but alone does not suffice for treatment of Graves disease.

7-3. D. The goal of therapy is control of maternal thyrotoxicosis while preventing fetal effects of both hypothyroid and hyperthyroid disease. Graves disease can be associated with fetal thyrotoxicosis with fetal tachycardia, growth restriction, advanced bone age, and craniosynostosis. However, use of thionamide therapy can be associated with fetal hypothyroidism, which is accompanied by fetal goiter, bradycardia, and growth restriction.

7-4. B. The diagnosis and management of fetal hypothyroidism and hyperthyroidism can be challenging. Fetal hypothyroidism and hyperthyroidism are associated with significant adverse effects as discussed in the preceding question/answer. Cordocentesis can play a role in the diagnosis and management of these diseases when less invasive modalities fail. However, the procedure entails significant risk, including preterm labor and delivery, fetal bradycardia, fetal death, and/or the need for emergent cesarean delivery. In addition, cordocentesis is not performed by all obstetricians and is predominately available only at tertiary care centers.

 SUGGESTED ADDITIONAL READING

Laurberg P, Nygaard B, Glinoer D, et al. Guidelines for TSH-receptor antibody measurements in pregnancy: results of an evidence-based symposium organized by the European Thyroid Association. *Eur J Endocrinol.* 1998;139:584–586.

Wing DA, Millar LK, Koonings PP, et al. A comparison of propylthiouracil versus methimazole in the treatment of hyperthyroidism in pregnancy. *Am J Obstet Gynecol.* 1994;170: 90–95.

Low-Risk Aneuploidy Screening

ID/CC: A 31-year-old G_1P_0 woman at 12 weeks GA by dates presents for her initial prenatal visit. She is interested in prenatal diagnosis screening.

HPI: C.S. is a savvy software engineer who has done a fair amount of research regarding prenatal diagnosis screening options. The pregnancy is desired and was spontaneously conceived. A good friend of hers recently had a baby with Down syndrome at age 29 years. She is interested in undergoing the prenatal tests available that will have the highest detection rate of fetal abnormalities but would prefer not to undergo an invasive procedure that may result in miscarriage.

PMHx/PSHx: Noncontributory

FHx: Significant for a 7-year-old paternal male cousin with autistic features and mental retardation.

Meds: PNV

All: NKDA

Labs: Rh negative, antibody screen negative. Her husband also is Rh negative.

THOUGHT QUESTIONS

- What prenatal diagnosis screening tests are reasonable options for this woman? At what GA are these tests performed?
- What are the major differences between a prenatal diagnosis screening test and a diagnostic test?

Based on her age and family history, C.S. is considered to be at low risk for having an offspring with a birth defect or a chromosomal abnormality. However, >70% of Down syndrome children in the United States are born to women younger than 35 years. Consequently, there is a great demand for prenatal diagnosis screening of these women. Table 8-1 lists the different screening tests available, the targeted disorders identified by the tests, the GA at which the tests can be performed, and the sensitivity and specificity for each test. A diagnostic test is always performed on fetal tissue, is invasive, and carries a procedure-related risk of miscarriage. However, it is essentially 100% accurate. Chorionic villus sampling (CVS) and amniocentesis are the two most commonly performed diagnostic prenatal diagnostic tests. Screening tests are meant to identify women at sufficiently high risk of a congenital anomaly to warrant invasive testing. The tests are safe and not invasive. However, no matter how good the test, it will fail to identify all affected pregnancies. This concept of tolerance for risk is essential to convey to patients who are faced with the challenge of opting for one or the other approach.

TABLE 8-1 Summary of First and Second Trimester Screening Approaches

Screening modality	Targeted conditions	Gestational age at screening	Detection rate (%)	False positive rate (%)
Maternal age	DS	10–20 weeks	49	13
Maternal age +NT	DS, T18, T13	11–14	70–75	5
Maternal age +NT+PAPPA +βHCG	DS, T18, T13	11–14	80–86	5
Maternal age + MSAFP + hCG +E3 (triple)	DS, T18, NTD, SLO	15–20	60–70% DS 85% NTD	5
Maternal age +MSAFP + hCG +E3 + INH-A (quad)	DS, T18, NTD, SLO	15–20	70–80	5
Maternal age +NT+PAPPA+ βHCG+(quad)	DS, T18, T13, NTD, SLO	1st + 2nd trimester screening	90–95 DS	5

DS = Down syndrome; T18 = trisomy 18; T13 = trisomy 13; NTD = neural tube defects; NT = nuchal translucency; PAPPA = maternal serum pregnancy-associated plasma protein-A; βHCG = free beta chorionic gonadotrophin; MSAFP = maternal serum alpha-fetoprotein; hCG = human chorionic gonadotropin; E3 = estriol; INH-A = inhibin A; SLO = Smith-Lemli-Opitz syndrome.

CASE CONTINUED

After undergoing genetic counseling, C.S. decided to have a combined first-trimester biochemical screening with nuchal translucency (NT) ultrasound between 11 and 14 weeks, followed by second-trimester maternal serum quad screening and ultrasound between 18 and 20 weeks. Her maternal serum quad screening showed an increased risk for Down syndrome of 1:150, and she elected to have an amniocentesis.

QUESTIONS

8-1. Advantages of NT screening over midtrimester maternal serum screening include:
  A. Detection of neural tube defects (NTDs)
  B. Identification of multiple gestations
  C. Superior quality assurance programs
  D. Screens for trisomy 21, 18, and 13
  E. Both B and D are correct

8-2. After C.S. has her amniocentesis, it is necessary to:
  A. Administer RhoGAM only if she is antibody screen positive.
  B. Give her an IM injection of Rh_0 (D) immune globulin (RhoGAM), postprocedure.
  C. Administer RhoGAM only if the needle went through an anterior placenta.
  D. RhoGAM is not necessary after amniocentesis.
  E. Administer RhoGAM only if the amniotic fluid was bloody (bloody tap).

8-3. What other genetic test should have been offered to this couple?
  A. Screening for cystic fibrosis (CF)
  B. Screening for Tay-Sachs, Canavan, and Gaucher disease if at least one of the two partners is of Ashkenazi Jewish descent
  C. Screen for fragile X in the husband
  D. Review genetic tests performed on the paternal cousin
  E. All of the above are correct

8-4. An increased NT (>3.5 mm) in an 11- to 14-week fetus is associated with:

- A. Bladder outlet obstruction
- B. Structural heart defects
- C. Omphalocele
- D. NTDs
- E. None of the above

 ANSWERS

8-1. E. Although popularity is high, NT screening programs still are not available in many parts of the United States. This test requires extensive operator training to reach acceptable levels of accuracy. Midtrimester maternal serum screening was introduced in the United States in the 1980s, and it is held by stringent quality assurance surveillance. Ultrasound can predict GA with an error of ±4 days up to 16 weeks and diagnose multiple gestations and early pregnancy failure. Anencephaly can be diagnosed reliably during the 11- to 14-week scan, but NT screening has little or no value in the detection of other, more frequent open NTDs. With NT screening, the detection rate of trisomy 13 and 18 is comparable to that of trisomy 21 screening, whereas with second-trimester screening the detection rate of trisomy 18 is <50%, and it has no role in screening for trisomy 13.

8-2. B. C.S. and her husband both are Rh negative; therefore, sensitization is not an issue unless nonpaternity is a factor! In several US studies, nonpaternity may be as high as 15%. Whenever amniocentesis or other invasive procedure is performed in an Rh-negative pregnant woman, the safer approach is to give RhoGAM to prevent potential isoimmunization. Some women may request that RhoGAM not be given if the father of the baby also is Rh negative, which is reasonable if adequate counseling and documentation occurred, but this answer was not given.

8-3. E. All pregnant women and couples who are contemplating pregnancy should be counseled and offer screening for CF. If one or both partners are of Ashkenazi Jewish origin, a panel of three or more serious autosomal recessive genetic disorders can be offered that are more prevalent and can be reliably detected in this ethnic group. The 7-year-old paternal cousin raises the possibility of fragile X. Theoretically, the husband could be a premutation carrier and pass on the premutation to his daughters, who would be unaffected but could have mentally retarded sons.

8-4. B. NT 11- to 14-week scan does not screen for NTDs, with the exception of anencephaly. NTD screening should be offered by either maternal serum screening in the second trimester and/or ultrasound between 18 and 20 weeks. Increased NT between 11 and 14 weeks has been associated with increased risk for chromosomal abnormalities, including Down syndrome, 45X (Turner syndrome), trisomy 13 and 18, and triploidy. The larger the NT, the greater the risk. For those pregnancies with a significantly thick NT but a normal set of chromosomes, other conditions should be excluded. Structural heart defects (40% of fetuses with NTs >3.5 mm will have a heart defect), spinal muscular atrophy, and Noonan syndrome are the best examples, and testing is available for these conditions. Some major structural anomalies such as bladder outlet obstruction and abdominal wall defects, can be seen with sonography as early as 11 to 14 weeks, but these conditions are not necessarily associated with a large NT measurement.

 ## SUGGESTED ADDITIONAL READING

Wapner R, Thom E, Simpson JL, et al. First-trimester screening for trisomies 21 and 18. Trimester Maternal Serum Biochemistry and Fetal Nuchal Translucency Screening (BUN) Study Group. *N Engl J Med.* 2003;349:1405–1413.

ACOG Practice Bulletin. Prenatal diagnosis of fetal chromosomal abnormalities. *Obstet Gynecol.* 2001;97(5 pt 1):suppl 1–12.

ACOG Committee Opinion #296: first-trimester screening for fetal aneuploidy. *Obstet Gynecol.* 2004;104:215–217.

Elevated MSAFP

ID/CC: A 22-year-old G_1P_0 woman at 16 weeks GA by LMP has an elevated level of maternal serum α-fetoprotein (MSAFP).

HPI: N.T. receives a phone call from her obstetrician regarding the results of the triple screen test performed 5 days before. The study showed an MSAFP level of 4.1 MoM (multiples of the median). She initiated prenatal care at 10 weeks gestation and was started on prenatal vitamins. Results of her physical exam 5 days prior was unremarkable, with a fundal height of 13 cm and positive fetal heart tones on Doppler.

PMHx/PSHx: None

Meds: PNV

All: Sulfas

POb/GynHx: Regular menses, every 27 to 29 days.

SHx: Lives with boyfriend who is supportive. No tobacco or ethanol use.

THOUGHT QUESTIONS

- What are the components of the triple screen, and how is it interpreted?
- What are common causes of elevated MSAFP?
- What is the next step in the management of this case?

The triple screen, also known as the expanded AFP test, is a screening test for neural tube defects (NTDs) and fetal aneuploidy. Unlike invasive diagnostic tests, such as amniocentesis and chorionic

TABLE 9-1 Triple Screen Table

	Trisomy 21	Trisomy 18	Trisomy 13	NTDs
MSAFP	Decreased	Decreased	Depends on defects	Increased
Estriol	Decreased	Decreased	Depends on defects	Normal
β-hCG	Elevated	Decreased	Depends on defects	Normal

From Callahan T, Caughey A, Heffner L. *Blueprints Obstetrics and Gynecology*. 4th ed. Baltimore, Md: Lippincott Williams & Wilkins; 2006.

villus sampling, the triple screen is a noninvasive screening test that involves evaluation of maternal serum levels of AFP, unconjugated estriol, and hCG. Because these serum levels depend on GA, the triple screen should be performed between 15 and 20 weeks GA. The levels of the individual markers are altered characteristically depending on the defect (Table 9-1).

α-Fetoprotein is a protein that is structurally similar to albumin and is synthesized by the fetal liver. Elevated MSAFP is used as a screening test primarily for detection of NTDs. A decreased MSAFP is a marker for aneuploidy, including trisomy 21. The more common causes of elevated MSAFP include incorrect dating, fetal demise, multiple gestations, NTDs, ventral abdominal wall defects (gastroschisis and omphalocele), placental abnormalities, and congenital nephrosis. Pregnancies with no explanation for the increased AFP level (unexplained elevated MSAFP) are associated with an increased risk for adverse perinatal outcomes, including intrauterine growth restriction (IUGR) and placental abruption. An ultrasound should be ordered after an abnormal level of MSAFP (screen positive) is detected. Because the serum AFP varies with GA, the risk assessment may need to be recalculated if the ultrasound dates are significantly different than the clinical dates.

 CASE CONTINUED

An obstetric ultrasound revealed a single, live fetus, with biometry consistent with 16 weeks GA (concordant with LMP). A 3-cm lumbosacral myelomeningocele was detected (Figure 9-1A). In addition, the banana sign and the lemon sign were present (Figure 9-1B), but no other fetal anomaly was identified. The patient was counseled and opted to terminate the pregnancy via dilatation and evacuation (D&E). Karyotype of the fetus revealed normal 46,XY.

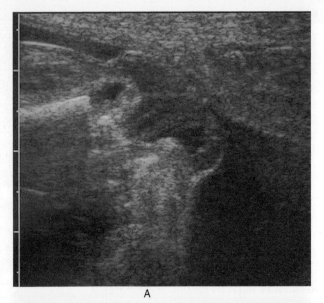

A

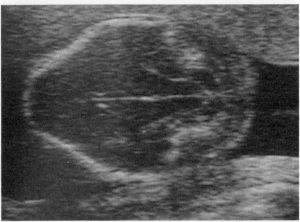

B

FIGURE 9-1. A: Transverse Image of Lower Spine—Note that the skin is open and the membrane of the myelomeningocele is coming through the skin opening. B: Cerebral Findings of Neural Tube Defects—Note the bilateral indentation of the frontal bones (Lemon Sign) and the outward bowing of the cerebellar hemispheres (Banana Sign). *(Image Provided by Departments of Radiology and Obstetrics and Gynecology, University of California, San Francisco).*

QUESTIONS

9-1. The incidence of NTDs is associated with which of the following medications used in pregnancy?

A. Valproic acid
B. Lithium
C. Fluoxetine
D. Prednisone
E. Tylenol

9-2. The recurrence of NTDs can be decreased by administration of:

A. 1 mg folic acid from the time of missed LMP
B. 4 mg folic acid from 1 month prior to conception until 12 weeks GA
C. 0.4 mg folic acid from conception through the end of the pregnancy
D. Diet rich in leafy vegetables periconceptionally
E. Recurrence of NTDs cannot be decreased

9-3. Unexplained elevated MSAFP is associated with which of the following?

A. Abruptio placentae, placenta previa
B. Chronic hypertension
C. Intrauterine growth retardation, preeclampsia
D. Gestational diabetes
E. Decreased perinatal mortality

9-4. A 24-year-old patient is screened as positive for Down syndrome by MSAFP. Which of the following statements is *false?*

A. The risk of trisomy 21 is not increased when a couple has had an affected offspring with trisomy 21 if the affected offspring was conceived prior to a maternal age of 30 years.
B. A normal ultrasound rules out Down syndrome.
C. The likelihood of having a fetus with trisomy 21 on a 16-week amniocentesis is greater than having a liveborn child with trisomy 21.
D. If a child has a firm clinical diagnosis of Down syndrome, obtaining a karyotype is of no further clinical value.
E. Chromosome studies are the only test routinely performed on a midtrimester amniocentesis.

ANSWERS

9-1. A. Use of valproic acid in pregnancy has been associated with a 6% risk of NTDs. Use of lithium during pregnancy is associated with an increased risk for Epstein anomaly, a rare heart defect, but not for NTDs. Fluoxetine is not associated with an increased risk for major malformations. Prednisone does not cross the placenta and is not associated with an increased risk for major anomalies; rather, it increases the risk of PPROM and prematurity. There are no known teratogenic risks associated with use of Tylenol during pregnancy.

9-2. B. Studies have shown that recurrence of NTDs can be reduced from 3.5% to 1.0% by administration of 4 mg folic acid from at least 1 month prior to conception through the end of the first trimester; 0.4 mg folic acid has been shown to be effective in reducing the occurrence of NTDs in women without a prior affected pregnancy. Whether levels of folic acid adequate for NTD prevention can be attained by dietary supplementation is unclear.

9-3. C. Unexplained elevated MSAFP likely is related to the way the placenta acts to transport molecules between the fetal and maternal circulation. These patients are at increased risk for increased perinatal mortality, intrauterine growth retardation, abruptio' placentae, and preeclampsia. Increased maternal and fetal surveillance during the third trimester often is recommended in these pregnancies. Gestational diabetes is not correlated with unexplained elevated MSAFP and, unlike pregestational diabetes, is not associated with increased risk for congenital anomalies.

9-4. C. The likelihood of identifying a fetus with Down syndrome in a 16- to 18-week amniocentesis is higher than having a liveborn with Down syndrome because of the high rate of miscarriage of Down syndrome fetuses (approximately 30%). The risk of recurrence of trisomy 21 is increased over the baseline risk to approximately 1% for women who have had an affected fetus/liveborn with Down syndrome when conceived at a maternal age of 30 years or younger. This higher than expected recurrence rate is thought to result from germline cell mosaicism. Although not currently used for routine screening, several ultrasound findings are associated with Down syndrome, including thickened nuchal fold, mild hydronephrosis, echogenic bowel, and slightly shortened long bones. A normal ultrasound does not rule out Down syndrome because midtrimester ultrasound is normal in at least 50%

of Down syndrome fetuses. Obtaining a karyotype in affected fetuses can yield valuable genetic information that can be used to predict recurrence in future pregnancies. Down syndrome is caused by trisomy 21 in 96% of cases, mosaicism in 1%, and unbalanced translocations in 2% to 3%, with the risk for recurrence much higher in cases of unbalanced translocation in which one of the parents is a balanced translocation carrier. In addition to chromosomes studies, amniotic fluid is routinely tested for AFP levels, which are used as a biochemical screen for detection of open NTDs (sensitivity 98%, specificity 99%).

 ## SUGGESTED ADDITIONAL READING

Canick JA, Macrae AR. Second trimester serum markers. *Semin Perinatol.* 2005;29:203–208.

Impact of folic acid fortification of the US food supply on the occurrence of neural tube defects. *JAMA.* 2001;285:2981–2986.

Nadel AS, Norton ME, Wilkins-Haug L. Cost-effectiveness of strategies used in the evaluation of pregnancies complicated by elevated maternal serum alpha-fetoprotein levels. *Obstet Gynecol.* 1997;89:660–665.

Genetic Sonogram

ID/CC: A 40-year-old G_3P_2 woman at 18 weeks GA presents for genetic sonogram.

HPI: M.A has had an uncomplicated pregnancy. She underwent genetic counseling and first-trimester combined screening at 12 weeks GA. Risk assessment at that time, based on the results of her first-trimester levels of free β-HCG, PAPP-A, and nuchal translucency measurement, put her risk of trisomy 21 at 1:550 and trisomy 18 at 1:10,000.

PMHx/PShx: Appendectomy at age 8

Meds: PNV

All: Penicillin

POb/GynHx: Two term, uncomplicated pregnancies

SHx: Lives with her husband and children. No domestic violence. No use of ethanol, tobacco, or recreational drugs.

FHx: Significant for heart disease in maternal grandmother

Labs: Normal prenatal labs

THOUGHT QUESTIONS

- What is a genetic sonogram? What does it involve?
- What is the difference between a disease-related marker versus an abnormality seen on sonogram?

Although many labels exist, there are essentially two types of sonogram examinations during the second trimester. The first is a *basic* or *standard ultrasound* (often designated a level 1 obstetric ultrasound), which includes the following when feasible: uterus, cervix, ovaries, placenta, amniotic fluid estimate, fetal biometry, and anatomic survey. The second type, called a *targeted* or *specialized sonogram* (often designated a level 2 obstetric ultrasound), is generally a more directed examination geared toward evaluation of a particular organ or set of anomalies. A genetic sonogram is a targeted examination looking for both markers and malformations associated with chromosomal disorders. The difference between a marker and a malformation is important. *Markers* are findings that are associated with a disease but are not a defect. *Malformations* are defects and, even in the face of normal chromosomes, are associated with some degree of illness. Table 10-1 lists some of the sonographic findings of four different genetic syndromes.

TABLE 10-1 Genetic Syndromes and Associated Sonographic Findings

Genetic Syndrome	Sonographic Findings
Trisomy 21 (Down syndrome)	Congenital heart disease, renal pelviectasis, duodenal atresia ("double bubble sign"), thickened nuchal fold, echogenic intracardiac focus, short femur and humerus, cystic hygroma, ventriculomegaly, clinodactyly of fifth digits, widely spaced first and second toes
Trisomy 18 (Edward syndrome)	IUGR, congenital heart disease, clenched hands, clubfoot, strawberry-shaped skull, micrognathia, choroids plexus cysts, omphalocele, hydronephrosis
Trisomy 13 (Patau syndrome)	IUGR, congenital heart disease, holoprosencephaly, agenesis of the corpus callosum, cleft lip/palate, micrognathia, overlapping digits, renal cortical cysts, omphalocele
Turner syndrome (45,X karyotype)	Cystic hygromas, nuchal edema, nonimmune hydrops, renal anomalies, congenital heart disease (predominately coarctation of the aorta)

CASE CONTINUED

The patient undergoes sonogram examination. The uterus, cervix, and ovaries appear normal. The placenta is anterior without evidence of previa. The fetus is in a variable presentation. The sonogram is notable for an echogenic intracardiac focus and mild bilateral fetal hydronephrosis but is otherwise unremarkable.

QUESTIONS

10-1. Which of the following statements regarding an echogenic intracardiac focus (EIF) is true?
- A. A fetal echocardiogram is indicated to evaluate for complex heart disease.
- B. The pediatricians will evaluate the newborn at birth to assess for further cardiac disease.
- C. The presence of an EIF is an indication for invasive diagnostic testing (i.e., amniocentesis).
- D. In the face of a normal karyotype, an EIF is without clinical significance.
- E. None of the above

10-2. Which of the following is the correct definition of hydronephrosis?
- A. Dilation of the renal pelvis
- B. Dilation of the ureter
- C. Dilation of the urethra
- D. Absence of the kidney
- E. Multicystic dilation of the kidney

10-3. The patient from this case states she underwent CVS in the first trimester and had a normal karyotype. Given the above sonogram findings, what is the next step?
- A. Amniocentesis to ensure the CVS karyotype was not falsely normal
- B. Repeat sonogram in 4 to 8 weeks to evaluate the hydronephrosis
- C. No further follow-up needed; provide reassurance only
- D. Antenatal testing to follow amniotic fluid levels
- E. None of the above

10-4. Another common marker seen on sonogram is hyperechoic bowel. Which of the following statements regarding this finding is true?
- A. This finding can be seen in a normal fetus.
- B. This finding can be associated with cystic fibrosis in a fetus.
- C. This finding can be associated with cytomegalovirus infection.
- D. None of the above
- E. All of the above

ANSWERS

10-1. D. EIF is a calcification in the papillary muscle of the heart seen on sonogram as an echogenicity in the four-chamber view of the heart. The finding is seen in approximately 5% of normal fetuses but in 18% of fetuses with trisomy 21. If an EIF is an isolated finding, studies suggest that neither karyotyping nor echocardiogram is indicated. However, if EIF is seen with other markers or malformations, then genetic diagnosis via amniocentesis is commonly offered to the patient.

10-2. A. Hydronephrosis or pyelectasis refers to dilation of the upper urinary tract that can include the renal pelvis and calyces. As an isolated finding, mild disease may be associated with a slightly higher risk for trisomy 21, although this is controversial. However, even in the face of normal chromosomes, more severe dilation can be associated with obstructive diseases of the urinary system, such as ureteropelvic junction obstruction, ureterovesical obstruction, and posterior urethral valves. Therefore, this finding does require follow-up depending on severity.

10-3. B. In the face of a normal karyotype, no further follow-up is required for an EIF. As stated in the answer to question 2, follow-up is required for hydronephrosis, with a sonogram approximately 4 to 8 weeks after the first depending on severity. If the hydronephrosis resolves or remains mild, antenatal testing is not required.

10-4. E. Hyperechoic bowel on sonogram can be associated with poor perinatal outcome, including specifically trisomy 21, cystic fibrosis, in utero cytomegalovirus or toxoplasmosis infection, and growth restriction. However, the finding also can be seen in normal fetuses. As an isolated finding, counseling should be provided and appropriate diagnostic testing provided if desired.

SUGGESTED ADDITIONAL READING

Schluter PJ, Pritchard G. Mid trimester findings for the prediction of Down syndrome in a sonographically screened population. *Am J Obstet Gynecol.* 2005;192:10–16.

Smith-Bindman R, Hosmer W, Feldstein VA, et al. Second-trimester ultrasound to detect fetuses with Down's syndrome: a meta-analysis. *JAMA.* 2001;285:1044–1055.

Bromley B, Lieberman E, Shipp TD, et al. Significance of an echogenic intracardiac focus in fetuses at high and low risk for aneuploidy. *J Ultrasound Med.* 1998;17:127–131.

Bromley B, Lieberman E, Laboda L, et al. Echogenic intracardiac focus: a sonographic sign for fetal Down syndrome. *Obstet Gynecol.* 1995;86:998–1001.

Multiple Gestations

ID/CC: A 37-year-old G_1P_0 woman with a positive urine pregnancy test after ovulation induction.

HPI: D.C. has a history of infertility for 14 months. Infertility workup identified oligo-ovulation/anovulation as a potential cause. During her second cycle with clomiphene citrate, a urine pregnancy test was positive 2 days after her expected menses. An ultrasound at 5.5 weeks gestation depicted two intrauterine gestational sacs, each with a yolk sac and embryonic pole. The intertwin membrane was thick, and two separate distinct placental plates could be distinguished. The embryonic poles each measured 2 mm, consistent with gestational ages of 5 weeks and 5 days. Cardiac activity was not seen. The left ovary has a 2.6-cm corpus luteum cyst. The appearance of the right ovary and uterus was unremarkable.

THOUGHT QUESTIONS

- What type of twin pregnancy is this?
- What are the clinical implications of determining the chorionicity?
- Why is an early ultrasound necessary in this patient?
- When would you schedule the next ultrasound based on the information provided?

A thick intertwin membrane, the twin peak sign, and two separate placental masses are all ultrasonographic features of diamniotic-dichorionic pregnancy. Women who have undergone ovulation induction with pharmacologic agents are at high risk for multiple ovulations and consequently multiple gestations. With clomiphene

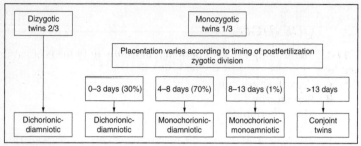

FIGURE 11-1. Classification, frequencies, and placentation type of twin pregnancies.

citrate, the risk of multiple gestations is approximately 8%. Most of these pregnancies are dizygotic; however, these women are also at a slightly higher risk for having monozygotic twin pregnancies. Dizygotic twin pregnancies are always dichorionic-diamniotic, whereas monozygotic twin pregnancies can be dichorionic-diamniotic, monochorionic-diamniotic, or monochorionic-monoamniotic, depending on the moment when division of a single fertilized egg occurred (Figure 11-1). Dichorionic-diamniotic twin pregnancies have the best prognosis overall. Monochorionic-diamniotic pregnancies have a significantly higher risk of complications and birth defects. Monochorionic-monoamniotic pregnancies have a perinatal mortality that is as high as 50% in some series.

Infertility patients have a higher chance of having an ectopic pregnancy, so confirmation of an intrauterine pregnancy is a priority, particularly for patients with a possible tubal factor contributing to their infertility. Once an intrauterine pregnancy is documented, the next question is whether or not the pregnancy is viable. At this stage, the embryo grows at a rate of approximately 1 mm/day, and fetal heart motion must be seen when the crown rump length is ≥5 mm in a normal developing embryo.

CASE CONTINUED

At 31 weeks, D.C. was having symptoms of preterm labor. She was hospitalized and given steroids for fetal lung maturation, tocolysis for 48 hours, and penicillin for GBS prophylaxis until culture results were negative. She had an uncomplicated vaginal delivery of vertex-vertex twin girls 3 days later.

QUESTIONS

11-1. The leading cause of perinatal mortality in twins is attributed to:
  A. Growth restriction
  B. Prematurity
  C. Monochorionicity
  D. Birth defects
  E. Cord accidents

11-2. An ultrasound at 18 weeks shows a monochorionic-diamniotic twin pregnancy complicated by polyhydramnios and cardiomegaly in one twin and oligohydramnios with no visible bladder in the other twin. The best treatment option to attain survival of at least one fetus is:
  A. Amnioinfusion of saline to the sac with no fluid
  B. Indomethacin to reduce the polyhydramnios
  C. Laser separation of the intertwining vessels
  D. Expectant management
  E. Pregnancy termination

11-3. Maternal morbidity and mortality are increased in multiple gestations because of a higher frequency of:
  A. Anemia
  B. Abruption placentae
  C. Urinary tract infections
  D. Pregnancy-induced hypertension
  E. All of the above

11-4. A trial of vaginal delivery in twins is a reasonable option if the following conditions are met:
  A. Nonvertex first twin (A), vertex second twin (B) with an estimated fetal weight (EFW) less than A at 32 weeks gestation
  B. Vertex-breech twin pair of concordant weights at 37 weeks gestation
  C. Vertex-vertex monochorionic-monoamniotic twin pair at 35 weeks gestation
  D. Triplet gestation, all vertex presentations at 34 weeks gestation
  E. Breech-breech twin pair at 38 weeks, concordant growth

ANSWERS

11-1. B. Twin births represent slightly >1% of live births in the United States, yet they account for >14% of the perinatal mortality rate. More than half of these deaths are related to prematurity. The mean gestational age at delivery is 37 weeks for twins, 34 weeks for triplets, and 33 weeks for quadruplet pregnancies. Monochorionic twin pregnancies have a much higher rate of perinatal mortality related to prematurity, growth restriction, twin-to-twin transfusion syndrome, and birth defects compared to dichorionic pregnancies. Growth restriction also affects di-di twin pregnancies more frequently than singletons. Cords accidents are more common in twins than in singletons, but the absolute risk is small.

11-2. C. The clinical vignette depicted represents twin-to-twin transfusion syndrome, which affects 10% to 15% of monochorionic-diamniotic twin pregnancies. Without treatment, the mortality rate approaches 100%. Serial amnioreduction to the recipient (polyhydramnios) has resulted in survival of at least 5% to 20% in some series, but the frequency of neurodevelopmental abnormalities can be high (10% to 20%). More recently, fetoscopic laser separation of the intertwining vessels has shown results similar or superior to conventional amnioreduction procedures, with possible improvement in terms of neurodevelopmental abnormalities, but no randomized controlled trial (RCT) supports this information. Given the poor results overall and the concern for mental handicap, couples should also be offered pregnancy termination as an option. The recurrence of this complication is extremely small.

11-3. E. Although maternal mortality in the developing world is very low, maternal morbidity among pregnancies with multiple gestations is substantially higher than in singleton pregnancies. Preeclampsia and its complications (placental abruption, anemia, urinary tract infections) are all associated with twin pregnancies. Placental previa, placental abruption, and an overdistended uterus all contribute to a high risk for intrapartum and postpartum bleeding complications.

11-4. B. Delivery of twins can be challenging and often tests the skills and resources of a labor and delivery unit. In general, it is advisable to deliver twins in the OR and to use epidural anesthesia because delivery of the second twin may require an emergency cesarean delivery even when vaginal delivery is anticipated. Vertex-vertex is the most common type of presentation and generally is compatible with vaginal delivery. If the presenting twin is vertex and the nonpresenting twin is nonvertex, a trial of vaginal delivery is acceptable provided there is concordant growth and operator experience, among other considerations. A nonvertex-presenting twin in a viable fetus is considered an indication for cesarean delivery. Monochorionic-monoamniotic twins, if viable, should be delivered by cesarean section regardless of the presentation because of the high risk for cord entanglement and intrapartum death. Because of the difficulty in monitoring and potential intrapartum complications, most centers prefer to deliver triplets by cesarean section.

 SUGGESTED ADDITIONAL READING

Ayres A, Johnson TR. Management of multiple pregnancy: prenatal care—part II. *Obstet Gynecol Surv.* 2005;60:538–549.

Robinson C, Chauhan SP. Intrapartum management of twins. *Clin Obstet Gynecol.* 2004;47:248–262.

ACOG Practice Bulletin #56: multiple gestation: complicated twin, triplet, and high-order multifetal pregnancy. *Obstet Gynecol.* 2004;104:869–883.

Rh D-Negative Alloimmunization

ID/CC: A 28-year-old G_4P_2 Caucasian woman at 13 weeks GA by regular LMP presents for her first prenatal care appointment.

HPI: E.H. notes that, in her last pregnancy, she was found to be Rh D-negative with antibodies to Rh D and was followed serially without requiring amniocentesis. At birth, that child was tested and found to be Rh D-negative as well. Both her first child and her husband, who is the father of both children, are Rh D-positive. She wants to know the outlook for this pregnancy.

PMHx: None

Meds: PNV

All: NKDA

POb/GynHx: Two term, normal, spontaneous vaginal deliveries. The first child is Rh positive; the second child is Rh negative; neither child with complications of alloimmunization. One SAB between the two births.

SHx: Lives with Caucasian husband and two children; no domestic violence; social ethanol use; no tobacco or recreational drug use.

VS: Temp 97.8°F, BP 108/64, HR 78, RR 16, Weight 154 lb

PE: *Gen:* NAD. *Abdomen:* soft, nontender, no distension with gravid uterus size = dates. *SSE:* parous cervix, no abnormalities. *BME:* size = dates.

THOUGHT QUESTION

■ Other than her initial prenatal laboratory tests, is there any other testing that should be done for this patient at this point?

As part of the prenatal laboratory tests, an antibody screen is done and a titer if the screen is positive. With this patient's history of being alloimmunized, she is likely to have a positive titer. At 13 weeks, no other particular testing should be done in this patient at this time. However, in many cases it is a good idea to offer genetic counseling about the issue of Rh D alloimmunization to the patient and her partner and to offer blood typing and DNA testing to the partner to determine zygosity. Because of the common occurrence of uncertain paternity, it is a good idea to address this issue in private with the patient.

CASE CONTINUED

Labs: O-negative blood type, anti-D titer 1:8

At the patient's next visit at 16 weeks GA, she asks about the possibility of getting a blood type on the fetus. You discuss with her that, at this point, because the antibody titer is <1:16, there is no reason to risk an invasive procedure. She subsequently has antibody titers drawn at both 16 and 20 weeks GA, which both return values of 1:8. However, at 24 weeks, the antibody titer rises to 1:32.

THOUGHT QUESTION

■ What is the next step in the management of this patient?

At this point, with a titer that is ≥1:16, there is a risk for fetal development of hemolytic anemia. Thus, amniocentesis to assess the amniotic fluid for breakdown products of bilirubin should be performed. At the time of this amniocentesis, if there is even the slightest doubt about the likely blood type of the fetus, fetal cells can be collected and typed. The amniotic fluid is tested using a spectrophotometer, which measures light absorption of the fluid, expressed as Δ OD 450. This measurement is plotted versus gestational age on a graph known as the *Liley curve*. The graph is divided into three sections: zones I, II, and III. Values in zone I and low zone II can be followed every 2 to 3 weeks with repeat amniocentesis. Values in mid zone II or a trend upward should be followed more frequently every week. Values in zone III or a rapid ascension to high zone II warrants direct assessment of fetal hematocrit using percutaneous umbilical blood sampling (PUBS).

Recently, measurement of the peak systolic velocity of the middle cerebral artery of the fetus with Doppler ultrasound has been used to screen for fetal anemia. This method has the advantage of being noninvasive and appears to have a sensitivity for fetal anemia as good as that of amniocentesis and comparison against the Liley curve. Whether this methodology will replace amniocentesis is yet to be seen.

 CASE CONTINUED

Ms. H. undergoes an amniocentesis that shows the Δ OD 450 is in mid zone II. The ultrasound performed at the same time is entirely normal. She is scheduled to return in 1 week for repeat amniocentesis and ultrasound. When she returns at 25 weeks GA, the ultrasound shows some scalp thickening and a small collection of fluid in the abdomen.

 QUESTIONS

12-1. What is the next step in the management of this patient?
A. Repeat amniocentesis
B. PUBS to check fetal hematocrit
C. PUBS for fetal transfusion
D. Emergent delivery
E. Repeat antibody titer

12-2. Which of the following are not signs of fetal hydrops on ultrasound?
A. Scalp thickening
B. Ascites
C. Pericardial effusion
D. Pleural effusion
E. Cystic hygroma

12-3. Based on this patient's history, her husband's Rh status is:

A. Homozygous dominant (DD)
B. Homozygous recessive (—)
C. Heterozygous (D–)
D. 0.5 chance of D–, 0.5 chance of DD
E. 0.33 chance of D–, 0.67 chance of DD

12-4. Given that the gene frequency of the D-negative allele among Caucasians is 0.4, what is the probability that a fetus born to two Caucasian parents will be Rh negative?

A. 0.48
B. 0.16
C. 0.36
D. 0.0256
E. 0.1216

 ANSWERS

12-1. C. In this case, the fetus has now started to show signs of hydrops. In this setting, without another cause for fetal hydrops, it can be assumed to be secondary to fetal anemia from hemolysis. Thus, the fetus needs an intrauterine transfusion (IUT) with Rh D-negative blood that has been crossmatched against the mother's serum. At the initial entry of the needle into the umbilical cord, a sample should be taken to assess fetal hematocrit; this can help guide the volume of transfusion but is not the primary purpose of PUBS. In the setting of a fetus ≥34 weeks, immediate delivery would be an option, but at 25 weeks gestation, the best option is to attempt IUT (Figure 12-1).

12-2. E. Fetal hydrops, in the setting of alloimmunization, is the result of high-output cardiac failure secondary to fetal anemia. The anti-D IgG antibodies cross the placenta and cause hemolysis of the fetal red blood cells carrying the D antigen. Signs of fetal hydrops seen on ultrasound include edema, ascites, and pericardial and pleural effusions. A cystic hygroma, which is collection of fluid at the base of the skull in the neck, is associated with fetal aneuploidy as well as with fetal hydrops. However, its association is more of a precursor to fetal hydrops in a fetus with anomalies rather than an association with fetal anemia and cardiac failure.

68 Early Pregnancy

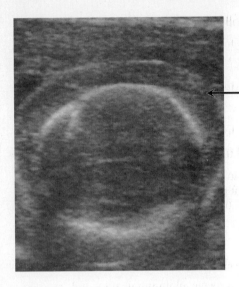

FIGURE 12-1.
Fetal Hydrops—Note
the large amount of scalp
edema. *(Image Provided
by Departments of Radi-
ology and Obstetrics
and Gynecology, Univer-
sity of California,
San Francisco).*

12-3. C. Assuming this patient is being truthful regarding prior paternity, her husband has fathered one Rh D-positive child and one Rh D-negative child. Thus, he must be heterozygous. If he had fathered only Rh D-positive or only Rh D-negative children, his zygosity would be uncertain.

12-4. B. The probability can be calculated in two ways, long and short. The long method involves calculating the probabilities of each of the parents using the Hardy-Weinberg formula:

$$p^2 + 2pq + q^2 = 1$$

where p = probability of dominant allele, and q = probability of recessive allele. Keeping in mind that there is no "d" allele and that being Rh D-negative means the absence of the "D" allele written as "(—)", p = 0.6 and q = 0.4; thus, the parents can each be:

$$DD = p^2 = 0.36, D- = 2pq = 0.48, \text{ and } — = q^2 = 0.16$$

For them to have an Rh-negative child, the following possibilities must occur:

$$D- \times D-; D- \times — ; \text{ or } — \times —$$

This can occur with the following probability:

$$\text{D}- \times \text{D}- \text{ leading to } - = (0.48) * (0.48) * (0.25)$$
$$= 0.0576$$
$$\text{D}- \times - \text{ leading to } - = (0.48) * (0.16) * 2 * (0.5)$$
$$= 0.0768$$
$$- \times - \text{ leading to } - = (0.16) * (0.16) = 0.0256$$
$$0.0576 + 0.0768 + 0.0256 = 0.16$$

The short way is to realize that in a population, the probability of any of the members of that population being homozygous recessive is equal to $q2$, in this case 0.16.

 ## SUGGESTED ADDITIONAL READING

Tran SH, Caughey AB. Erythrocyte alloimmunization and pregnancy. *Emedicine.com Online Journal.* October 2004.

Mari G, Deter RL, Carpenter RL, et al. Noninvasive diagnosis by Doppler ultrasonography of fetal anemia due to maternal red-cell alloimmunization. Collaborative Group for Doppler Assessment of the Blood Velocity in Anemic Fetuses. *N Engl J Med.* 2000;342:9–14.

Cosmi E, Mari G, Delle Chiaie L, et al. Noninvasive diagnosis by Doppler ultrasonography of fetal anemia resulting from parvovirus infection. *Am J Obstet Gynecol.* 2002;187:1290–1293.

II

Third Trimester
of Pregnancy

Elevated Glucose Loading Test

ID/CC: A 32-year-old G_2P_0 woman at 28 weeks GA with glucose level of 157 mg/dL after a 1-hour 50-g oral glucose loading test (GLT).

HPI: This is a desired and uncomplicated pregnancy. G.D. has no complaints and reports normal fetal movements.

PMHx/PSHx: None

Meds: PNV

All: NKDA

SHx: Married. Denies tobacco, alcohol, or recreational drug use.

FHx: Mexican-American origin, no family history of diabetes.

VS: Temp 98.1°F, BP 110/68, HR 88, Weight 164 lb, Height 5 feet 4 inches

PE: *Gen:* 20-lb weight gain since first visit at 10 weeks GA. *Abdomen:* soft, nontender, gravid; fundal height 29 cm. *Doppler:* positive fetal heart tones. *Extremities:* trace edema, left = right.

Labs: Urine dipstick: no proteinuria, positive glucosuria

THOUGHT QUESTIONS

- Who should be screened for diabetes during pregnancy and when?
- What is the appropriate next step in the management of this patient?

Generally, all pregnant women are screened for GDM, whether by the patient's personal and familial risk factors or by laboratory screening. Supporters of universal screening argue that an important percentage of GDM women would be missed if they were screened only with risk factors. One study revealed that although >90% of women with gestational diabetes could be identified using risk factor-based screening, 89% of women would need to undergo the screening, which is essentially universal. Risk factors for GDM include age >30 years, obesity, race/ethnicity (Hispanics, Native Americans, and Pacific Islanders), prior history of GDM, history of large for gestational age (LGA) infant, history of fetal demise of unknown etiology, and first-degree relative with diabetes mellitus. Laboratory screening consists of a 50-g, 1-hour glucose challenge at 24 to 28 weeks in all pregnant women (universal screening approach) or in women who meet at least one high-risk factor criteria (selective screening approach).

Another important issue to consider is what screening threshold to use. Commonly 140 mg/dL 1 hour after the 50-g load has been used. However, studies have suggested this yields a sensitivity of 80% to 85% for all gestational diabetics. Thresholds of 130 mg/dL and 135 mg/dL have been proposed and are used by some. These lower thresholds yield greater sensitivity but increase the screen positive rate (decrease the specificity) to 15% to 20%.

In this patient with an abnormal 1-hour GLT of 157 mg/dL (normal: <140 mg/dL), a 3-hour glucose tolerance test (GTT) with 100 g glucose is indicated. GDM is diagnosed if two or more values are elevated on the GTT (Tables 13-1 and 13-2).

TABLE **13-1** Glucose Screening Tests During Pregnancy

Test	Normal Glucose Level (mg/dL)
Fasting	<95
1 h after 50-g glucose load	<140
2 h after 100-g glucose load	<165

From Callahan T, Caughey A, Heffner L. *Blueprints Obstetrics and Gynecology*. 4th ed. Baltimore: Lippincott Williams & Wilkins; 2006.

TABLE 13-2 Three-Hour Glucose Tolerance Test: Venous and Plasma Criteria for GDM

Timing of Glucose Measurement	Normal Plasma Glucose (mg/dL)
Fasting	95
1 h	180
2 h	155
3 h	140

From Callahan T, Caughey A, Heffner L. *Blueprints Obstetrics and Gynecology.* 4th ed. Baltimore: Lippincott Williams & Wilkins; 2006.

CASE CONTINUED

You order a GTT, which reveals a fasting glucose level of 93 mg/dL, 1-hour level 198 mg/dL, 2-hour level 167 mg/dL, and 3-hour level 134 mg/dL.

THOUGHT QUESTION

■ Based on these test results, you diagnose her as having gestational diabetes. What treatment and follow-up examinations would you recommend?

With confirmation of her diagnosis, dietary treatment should be initiated. More than half of GDM patients are well controlled with diabetic diet alone. In contrast to nonpregnant type 2 diabetic patients, weight loss during pregnancy is not recommended. Daily home monitoring of finger stick blood glucose (FSBG) levels (specifically for fasting and 1-hour postprandial levels) in addition to assessment after 1 week of dietary changes typically are recommended for GDM patients. Targeted glucose levels for GDM patients should be as close as possible to levels of the non-GDM population (fasting <95 mg/dL, 1-hour postprandial <140 mg/dL).

You start her on an ADA diet and instruct her on home glucose monitoring of fasting and 1-hour postprandial FSBG levels. She returns for a follow-up evaluation in 1 week. Her FSBG values the day prior to follow-up are prebreakfast 105 mg/dL, 1-hour post breakfast 154 mg/dL, 1-hour post lunch 171 mg/dL, and 1-hour post dinner

168 mg/dL, all of which are consistent with her values on prior days. The patient states that she has been compliant with her diet.

QUESTIONS

13-1. What would be the most appropriate next step in management?

A. Hospitalize the patient to ensure she follows a strict ADA diet.

B. Continue diabetic teaching and re-evaluate in 1 week.

C. Begin insulin drip.

D. Start insulin subcutaneously and continue FSBG monitoring at home.

E. Hospitalize to begin diabetic teaching and initiation of insulin therapy until metabolic control is obtained.

13-2. Which of the following complications is associated with GDM?

A. Small for gestational age infant

B. Increased risk for shoulder dystocia and brachial plexus injury

C. Neonatal anemia

D. Neonatal hyperglycemia

E. Increased risk for major malformations

13-3. Which of the following is correct with regard to peripartum management and delivery of GDM patients?

A. Antenatal testing should be started between 32 to 34 weeks GA only in diabetic patients taking insulin.

B. Administration of NPH insulin should be continued throughout labor and delivery.

C. Glucosuria is a reliable indicator of poor metabolic control among GDM patients.

D. GDM patients should not be induced prior to 41 weeks, regardless of their glucose control.

E. Insulin is continued during the postpartum period in all insulin-requiring GDM patients.

13-4. She has a term, normal spontaneous vaginal delivery (NSVD) of a 3.9-kg female infant. For her postpartum management you recommend:

    A. Continue ADA diet and follow FSBG for 48 hours.

    B. Continue insulin drip for 48 hours postpartum.

    C. Regular diet, follow-up testing 6 weeks postpartum with a fasting and 75-g glucose loading test.

    D. Regular diet, check fasting glucose once per year starting at age 35.

    E. Continue with ADA diet, decrease insulin to half the antepartum dose.

ANSWERS

13-1. D. If noncompliance is suspected, further diabetic teaching and counseling are reasonable. Hospitalization is not indicated unless glucose levels are extremely poorly controlled. Insulin drip would be used only antepartum unless there is an acute, severe metabolic decompensation such as ketoacidosis. One week of dietary therapy generally is sufficient to evaluate metabolic control and to determine the need to start insulin. For a GDM patient who has inadequate metabolic control, a starting regimen of NPH insulin, 0.5 to 0.7 U/kg/day divided in 2/3 AM and 1/3 PM doses, is a reasonable approach. In addition, a patient who has elevated postprandial values at breakfast and dinner may require regular insulin prior to meals. More recently, providers have begun using fast-acting Lispro or Humalog insulin prior to meals. Home monitoring of FSBG and frequent visits and/or telephone calls by a diabetic nurse specialist have largely prevented the need for routine hospitalization for these patients. Recent trials have shown promising results with the use of glyburide (glibenclamide), an oral hypoglycemic agent that does not cross the placenta, and may become first-line treatment if larger trials confirm the efficacy and safety of the drug.

13-2. B. The complications of GDM are related to the large weight (LGA, macrosomia) and bodily proportions of the fetus (e.g., increased risk of cesarean section, operative delivery, shoulder dystocia, brachial plexus injury) and metabolic complications of the neonate (e.g., hypoglycemia, hypocalcemia, polycythemia, hyperbilirubinemia). Both of these types of complications can be prevented by adequate glucose control during pregnancy. Pre-existing diabetes mellitus is associated with an increased risk of major malformations, which is related to the degree of metabolic control during the time of organogenesis. Unless a patient had pre-existing diabetes that was detected for the first time during pregnancy, GDM is not associated with an increased risk for congenital malformations.

13-3. A. Antenatal testing should be started between 32 to 34 weeks GA in diabetic patients taking insulin to evaluate fetal well-being. Given that NPH insulin is long acting, it should be stopped once the patient is in active labor or on the morning of a planned induction/elective C/S. Pregnant women, irrespective of GDM status, spill glucose in their urine. Therefore, glucosuria should not be used as an indicator of metabolic control. One-hour postprandial FSBG levels provide the best criteria for establishing glucose control in pregnancy. Perinatal mortality is higher among diabetic patients with poor metabolic control. Therefore, GDM patients with poor glycemic control should be delivered after 37 to 38 weeks GA with confirmed fetal lung maturity. Ideally, they should be under adequate metabolic control before delivery to avoid metabolic complications of the neonate. Fetal echocardiogram is generally recommended in pregestational diabetics who are at increased risk for major congenital anomalies, including heart defects, but is not recommended in GDM patients.

13-4. C. After delivery there is a dramatic reduction in insulin requirements because of clearance of placental hormones with anti-insulin action, specifically human placental lactogen (hPL). As a result, GDM patients can be allowed to resume a regular diet after birth. There is a 20% to 30% chance that a GDM patient will develop type 2 diabetes after long-term follow-up. Therefore, screening for early detection should be performed 6 weeks postpartum and annually thereafter.

SUGGESTED ADDITIONAL READING

Crowther CA, Hiller JE, Moss JR, et al. Effect of treatment of gestational diabetes mellitus on pregnancy outcomes. *N Engl J Med.* 2005;352:2477–2486.

Tuffnell DJ, West J, Walkinshaw SA. Treatments for gestational diabetes and impaired glucose tolerance in pregnancy. *Cochrane Database Syst Rev.* 2003;(3):CD003395. Review.

Brody SC, Harris R, Lohr K. Screening for gestational diabetes: a summary of the evidence for the U.S. Preventive Services Task Force. *Obstet Gynecol.* 2003;101:380–392.

Langer O, Conway DL, Berkus MD, et al. A comparison of glyburide and insulin in women with gestational diabetes mellitus. *N Engl J Med.* 2000;343:1134–1138.

Esakoff TF, Cheng YW, Caughey AB. What is the optimal threshold to screen for gestational diabetes among different ethnicities? *Am J Obstet Gynecol.* 2005;193:1040–1044.

Preterm Contractions

ID/CC: A 24-year-old G_3P_2 woman at 28 weeks GA by LMP presents with a complaint of low backache for 3 hours.

HPI: Ms. S works part time at a nursery school and cares for her own two young children. She awoke this morning with mild low back pain and cramping that had grown progressively worse while she went to work. Despite lying down while waiting to be seen by the doctor, she continued to have the pain and felt abdominal tightening approximately every 5 to 10 minutes. She noticed a small amount of vaginal spotting after wiping but had not had any loss of fluid. She confirms normal fetal movement and denies having any dysuria, nausea, vomiting, fever, chills, or any change in bowel movements.

Ms. S notes that this pregnancy has been uncomplicated, although she missed many of her prenatal appointments because of her busy schedule. Her triple marker screen was negative, her 1-hour Glucola test (50-g glucose load) for diabetes was 88 (<140 is within normal limits), and her original urine and cervical cultures were negative.

PMHx/PSHx: None

Meds: PNV

All: NKDA

POb/GynHx: One prior term vaginal delivery, one prior preterm vaginal delivery at 32 weeks GA

SHx: Lives with husband and two children.

VS: Temp 98.0°F, BP 104/64, HR 90, RR 16, Weight 110 lb

PE: *Abdomen:* soft, nontender; contractions palpable. *FHT* (fetal heart tracing): 140s, no decelerations. *Toco:* uterine contractions every 5 minutes. *SVE:* 1-cm dilation, 25% effacement, midposition, soft, –3 station. Group B *Streptococcus* (GBS) culture and vaginal swabs obtained.

Labs: Urine: specific gravity 1.030, nitrite and esterase negative. Wet prep: positive clue cells, no *Trichomonas*

THOUGHT QUESTIONS

- What are this patient's risk factors and possible causes of preterm labor?
- Is this patient in preterm labor?
- What should be done immediately to help stop this patient's contractions?
- What agents are used for stopping contractions and how do they work?

This patient's risk factors/potential causes of preterm labor include bacterial vaginosis (BV), prepregnancy maternal weight <110 lb, and a previous preterm delivery. The latter is her most significant risk factor, increasing her risk threefold over the existing baseline risk of 7% to 8% in the population. In addition, the patient is dehydrated with an elevated urine specific gravity, which can lead to preterm contractions. Theoretically, this is thought to result from elevated levels of antidiuretic hormone (ADH) that arise in response to dehydration and subsequently cross-react with the oxytocin receptor.

Although contractions do occur normally in pregnancy before term, *preterm labor* is defined as contractions causing cervical change that occur before 37 weeks gestation. Given this patient's risk factors for preterm labor and her frequent contractions, intravenous hydration should be initiated. Many practitioners will also consider giving a dose of SQ terbutaline to see whether the contractions can be easily resolved.

Many agents are used for tocolysis. However, only one, ritodrine, is actually FDA approved for this purpose. There are currently five classes of tocolytics: β-mimetics (terbutaline, ritodrine), calcium channel blockers (nifedipine), prostaglandin inhibitors (indomethacin), oxytocin receptor antagonists, and magnesium sulfate. In addition, recent studies have suggested that the hormone progesterone may play a role in the prevention of preterm labor in high-risk patients.

Most tocolytics essentially work by decreasing the availability of intracellular calcium, which is needed to initiate uterine contractions.

CASE CONTINUED

The patient continues to have contractions despite the SQ terbutaline and IV fluids. The repeat cervical exam 1 hour later reveals her cervix is 2 cm dilated with 50% effacement. She is admitted to the hospital and immediately given betamethasone 12 mg IM and a 6-g bolus of magnesium sulfate ($MgSO_4$), followed by a 2 g per hour maintenance rate of $MgSO_4$. As part of her management she is given metronidazole (Flagyl) to treat the BV and IV penicillin. Infusion of magnesium sulfate is stopped after 48 hours. She remains acontractile for the ensuing 24 hours with no further cervical change past 2 cm dilated and 50% effacement. There is much debate about the usefulness of a fetal fibronectin screen in this patient, but in the end a fetal fibronectin test is performed with a negative result.

QUESTIONS

14-1. Why does this patient receive penicillin?
A. To help prevent preterm labor
B. As prophylaxis for chorioamnionitis
C. As treatment for BV
D. To help prevent rupture of membranes
E. As prophylaxis for GBS

14-2. When should she receive her second dose of betamethasone?
A. A second dose is not needed
B. 6 hours later
C. 12 hours later
D. 24 hours later
E. 48 hours later

14-3. What is the mechanism by which magnesium sulfate works to decrease contractions?
A. It is a calcium antagonist and membrane stabilizer.
B. It increases cAMP, thus decreasing free calcium ions.
C. It decreases cAMP, thus decreasing free calcium ions.
D. It blocks calcium channels.
E. It is a prostaglandin inhibitor, decreasing levels of intracellular calcium.

14-4. What is the utility of a fetal fibronectin test in the setting of preterm contractions?

    A. It has a good positive predictive value in helping to determine who will deliver prematurely.

    B. It has a good negative predictive value in helping to determine who will not deliver prematurely.

    C. It has a high specificity in determining who has chorioamnionitis.

    D. It has a high sensitivity in determining who has had premature rupture of membranes.

    E. It has a high sensitivity for determining who has chorioamnionitis.

ANSWERS

14-1. E. Approximately 15% of women are asymptomatic carriers of *GBS,* which historically has been the leading organism causing neonatal sepsis. At the time of admission, most preterm patients have vaginal and anal samples obtained for culture to test for the organism. However, the culture takes a few days to grow, so all preterm labor patients are given antibiotic prophylaxis. The antibiotic of choice is penicillin. GBS is one of many organisms that can cause chorioamnionitis. However, it is particularly virulent, with an associated 25% to 50% mortality rate in preterm neonates with sepsis.

14-2. D. Betamethasone is a corticosteroid that is given to help reduce the incidence of respiratory distress syndrome in preterm neonates between 24 and 34 weeks of gestation. It differs from prednisone in that it crosses the placenta into the fetal circulation. Once there, it is thought to work by increasing the production of surfactant in type 2 pneumocytes in the fetal lung. The neonate benefits optimally from this steroid shot if delivery is delayed at least 48 hours after the first dose. The second dose is given 24 hours after the first.

14-3. A. In addition to being a membrane stabilizer by increasing baseline resting potential, magnesium sulfate acts as an antagonist at calcium channels. This combination of effects thereby decreases smooth muscle contractility of the uterus. Of note, these actions also lead to the side effects of magnesium sulfate. For example, the relaxation of smooth muscle leads to vasodilation and thus the flushing effect experienced by women receiving magnesium sulfate.

14-4. B. Fetal fibronectin detection is one of the latest tests to help determine who is at greatest risk for preterm delivery. Fetal fibronectin is a glycoprotein that helps attach the fetal chorion to the maternal decidua; thus, its presence on a cervical or vaginal swab is abnormal. The test has a 98%–99% negative predictive value. Therefore, a negative test result indicates the likelihood is very low that a patient will deliver in the following week. The test has a poor positive predictive value of approximately 30%; therefore, a positive test does not necessarily mean that a patient is at risk for delivery. False-positive results can be caused by cervical manipulation; therefore, collection of the swab is performed prior to a sterile vaginal exam. Other causes of a false-positive test include amniotic fluid, blood, and semen.

 SUGGESTED ADDITIONAL READINGS

ACOG Committee Opinion. Use of progesterone to reduce preterm birth. *Obstet Gynecol.* 2003;102(5 pt 1):1115–1116.

Meis PJ, Klebanoff M, Thom E, et al. Prevention of recurrent preterm delivery by 17 alpha-hydroxy progesterone caproate. *N Engl J Med.* 2003;348:2379–2385.

Leitich H, Kaiden A. Fetal fibronectin: how useful is it in the prediction of preterm birth? *BJOG.* 2003;110(suppl 20):66–70.

Antepartum Fever

ID/CC: 22-year-old G_1P_0 woman at 28 weeks GA presents with new-onset abdominal pain and fever.

HPI: A.A. reports gradual, progressive pain over the last 12 hours that is localized to the right lateral/flank area without radiation. The pain is now 8/10, constant with occasional exacerbations, and worse with walking. She also notes anorexia and feeling "warm." She denies any nausea or vomiting. Her last bowel movement was 2 days ago. She reports increased urinary frequency over the last month but no dysuria or hematuria. She has felt some "tightening" of the uterus over the last couple of hours.

PMHx/PSHx: None

Meds: PNV

All: NKDA

POb/GynHx: Regular menses. *Chlamydia* infection at age 16 years, no other history of STIs.

SHx: Single, lives with father of baby. Denies tobacco, ethanol, or recreational drug use.

VS: Temp 100.9°F, BP 102/54, HR 110, RR 18, O_2 saturation 99% on room air (RA).

PE: *Gen:* Caucasian female, appears ill. *HEENT:* unremarkable except for mildly dry mouth and lips, neck supple, no lymph adenopathy. *Cor:* unremarkable. *Abdomen:* soft, mildly tender to deep palpation and worse at periumbilical area lateral to the uterus; subtle, localized rebound tenderness, no guarding; bowel sounds present; no costovertebral angle tenderness (CVAT); uterus is soft and nontender, with a fundal height of 26 cm. *Pelvic exam:* long and closed cervix, minimal vaginal discharge, moderate tenderness in the right adnexal region without palpable mass. *Rectal exam:* tender. *Doppler:* fetal heart tones in 150s.

Labs: Stool guaiac negative

THOUGHT QUESTIONS

- What is the differential diagnosis for this patient?
- Which initial studies would you order?
- How should this patient be managed initially?

The differential diagnosis for acute abdominal pain and fever is broad and includes gastrointestinal (GI), obstetric/gynecologic (Ob/Gyn), and genitourinary (GU) sources. With regard to Ob/Gyn causes, torsion of adnexal mass, ruptured ovarian mass, and degenerating fibroid should be considered, but the clinical presentation described is not typical for these conditions. Chorioamnionitis is another obstetric etiology but is very unusual in the absence of rupture of the membranes. GU causes include pyelonephritis and urinary tract stones. Careful physical examination and urinalysis (UA) are important in excluding these diagnoses. GI causes include appendicitis, cholecystitis, and pancreatitis. Of these, appendicitis should be strongly considered given the patient's presentation. In pregnancy, the diagnosis of appendicitis often is delayed, possibly because of the different localization of the appendix secondary to displacement by the gravid uterus and because of the relative decrease in peritoneal signs as compared to nonpregnant patients.

CBC with differential, liver transaminases, amylase, lipase, and UA tests should be obtained for diagnostic purposes. In addition, electrolytes, blood urea nitrogen (BUN), and creatinine (Cr) should be ordered to assess fluid/renal status. Ultrasound of the abdomen and pelvis or spiral CT of the abdomen and pelvis are important tools to narrow the differential diagnosis. A nonstress test (NST) should be obtained upon arrival to assess fetal well-being and to clarify uterine activity. An amniocentesis to rule out chorioamnionitis does not appear indicated at this time. This patient should be admitted for close observation, made NPO, given IV fluids, her pain controlled, and electrolyte abnormalities corrected. A surgical consultation should be obtained.

CASE CONTINUED

You decide to admit the patient. Her initial laboratory studies show a WBC of 16.2 with left shift, Hb 11.7, and platelets 180,000. Liver transaminases are within normal limits; amylase 32. UA shows a specific gravity of 1.020 but is otherwise negative. She is seen by general surgery, who requests a CT of the abdomen and pelvis.

QUESTIONS

15-1. Over the next 2 hours her pain is persistent, and on exam she is tachycardic and has localized rebound tenderness. The next step in management is:
- A. Laparoscopy
- B. Exploratory laparotomy
- C. IV antibiotics
- D. Repeat CT scan of abdomen and pelvis
- E. IV fluid bolus of crystalloids

15-2. If the patient goes to surgery for a possible appendectomy, which of the following would be your recommendation for tocolysis?
- A. Prophylactic IV tocolysis with magnesium sulfate
- B. Tocolytics only for development of regular uterine contractions and/or cervical change
- C. Tocolysis not indicated, given her cervical exam on admission
- D. Prophylactic tocolysis with IV ritodrine (β_2-agonist)
- E. Use of meperidine (Demerol) for painful uterine contractions

15-3. Regarding the use of corticosteroids for fetal lung maturity in this patient, which of the following is the *best* answer?
- A. Should never be used in the setting of an acute infection.
- B. Have little or no effect in reducing respiratory distress syndrome (RDS) at this gestational age and therefore are not indicated.
- C. Should be used if there is concern for premature delivery prior to 34 weeks GA.
- D. Steroids cause WBC elevation and hence would make follow-up of her clinical condition difficult.
- E. The fetus is already "stressed" because of maternal infection, so corticosteroids are not recommended.

15-4. Four days after her surgery, the patient develops painful uterine contractions and progressive cervical change despite tocolytics. Which of the following is correct regarding intrapartum management?
  A. Allow for trial of vaginal delivery if cephalic presentation.
  B. Vaginal delivery is contraindicated because of risk for anterior abdominal wall defect secondary to recent laparotomy.
  C. Early epidural anesthesia should be used.
  D. Encourage vaginal delivery for breech presentation.
  E. Cesarean section is contraindicated because of the risk for wound infection.

 ## ANSWERS

15-1. B. The patient has a surgical abdomen and requires exploration. Laparoscopy is not recommended in pregnancy after 20 weeks GA because of difficult access given the size of the uterus. Although IV antibiotics are indicated, they should not be the primary therapy. Surgery should not be delayed in a patient with worsening status and a surgical abdomen.

15-2. B. Often patients with an acute abdominal process have associated uterine contractions, but they seldom lead to premature delivery. Prophylactic use of tocolytics is not considered standard practice, particularly in this patient who has no cervical change. If uterine contractions are persistent, with a regular pattern, tocolysis may be appropriate. β-mimetics are not a good choice in this already tachycardic patient because of the associated tachycardia.

15-3. C. Steroids are recommended for enhancement of fetal lung maturity between 24 and 34 weeks GA whenever premature delivery is a possibility, as is the case here. A single course is not associated with adverse effects on the fetus. Although maternal side effects can occur with use of steroids in this context, it is unlikely that an acute infectious process will be worsened by its use. A transient elevation of WBC is frequently seen as a result of steroid-induced demargination of leukocytes. However, this should not have a significant impact on assessing her overall clinical response.

15-4. A. Contraindications to vaginal delivery include placenta previa, active genital herpes simplex infection, and history of prior classic cesarean section but do not include recent abdominal laparotomy. Therefore, this patient should be allowed to deliver vaginally if cephalic presentation is confirmed. The risk of abdominal wall defect associated with significant maternal effort, such as pushing in the second stage of labor, is small. In general, breech vaginal deliveries are not attempted for fetuses weighing <1,500 g. The risk of wound infection likely is increased but is not a reason to withhold an indicated procedure. The patient should receive anesthesia as she and the provider believe necessary.

 SUGGESTED ADDITIONAL READING

Cohen-Kerem R, Railton C, Oren D, et al. Pregnancy outcome following non-obstetric surgical intervention. *Am J Surg.* 2005;190:467–473.

Millar LK, Cox SM. Urinary tract infections complicating pregnancy. *Infect Dis Clin North Am.* 1997;11:13–26.

The effect of corticosteroids for fetal maturation on perinatal outcomes. *NIH Consens Statement.* 1994;12:1–24.

Leaking Fluid I

ID/CC: A 32-year-old G_1P_0 woman at 29 weeks GA presents with complaint of leakage of fluid for 2 days.

HPI: A.M. has had an uncomplicated pregnancy until 2 days ago, when she noted a moderate amount of fluid on her underwear. She felt a gush of fluid at that time and has since noted leakage of small amounts of clear fluid. She is uncertain whether the fluid is urine because she has at times had difficulty controlling her bladder, especially during active fetal movement. She has not noticed any contractions, cramps, vaginal bleeding, fevers, or chills. She denies having dysuria but has had urinary frequency.

PMHx: Migraine headaches

PSHx: Appendectomy

Meds: PNV

All: NKDA

POb/GynHx: Unremarkable. No STIs or PID.

SHx: Works as an accountant. Lives with father of baby. No ethanol, tobacco, or recreational drug use.

THOUGHT QUESTIONS

- What type of vaginal exam should you do?
- How can you distinguish between urine and amniotic fluid?
- What is the difference between PROM and PPROM?
- If the bag of water is ruptured, what might be the plan of management?

If this patient has ruptured membranes, you do not want to increase her risk of infection by performing a digital vaginal exam. Therefore, an exam using a sterile speculum is performed. On this exam you look for evidence of rupture—a pool of fluid in the vagina that has a basic pH (a "positive phenaphthazine [Nitrazine] test") and reveals a ferning pattern when dried on a slide. Urine may have a basic pH but will not fern on a slide (other causes of a false-positive Nitrazine test include the presence of blood, semen, and some vaginal infections). *PROM* is premature rupture of membranes ("premature" meaning prior to the onset of labor); *PPROM* is preterm premature rupture of the membranes (preterm meaning prior to 37 weeks gestation). *SROM* is spontaneous rupture of the membranes, which means the membranes rupture of their own accord, as opposed to *AROM* (artificial rupture of the membranes), which means a clinician intentionally ruptures the membranes, usually performed with an amniotomy hook.

Two particularly important neonatal outcomes can result from PPROM: preterm delivery with the risks of prematurity and neonatal infection/sepsis from chorioamnionitis. Therefore, the management of PPROM is a balance, weighing the risk of prematurity with the risk of development of perinatal infection. Thus, at very early GAs (<32 to 34 weeks), if no overt sign of chorioamnionitis is seen, a course of antenatal corticosteroids (ACS), usually betamethasone or dexamethasone, is given to help reduce the incidence of respiratory distress syndrome (RDS) in preterm neonates by enhancing fetal lung maturity. In addition, there is evidence that ACS reduces other morbidities associated with prematurity, including intraventricular hemorrhage and necrotizing enterocolitis. At GAs beyond 34 weeks, the risks of prematurity are less; therefore, ACS is not administered and delivery is allowed to occur and, in certain cases, even is induced. At all GAs, if chorioamnionitis develops, labor is induced or augmented to decrease the risk of neonatal infection/sepsis.

CASE CONTINUED

VS: Temp 98.0°F, BP 100/62, HR 80, RR 16

PE: *Gen:* NAD. *Abdomen:* soft, nontender. Fundal height 28 cm. *SSE:* cervix appears closed, positive pooling of clear yellow fluid, positive Nitrazine, positive ferning. *FHT:* 130s, reactive. *Toco:* uterine contractions every 20 minutes.

Labs: Urine: Specific gravity 1.010; pH 6.0; negative nitrite/esterase/blood; WBC 10.0. Sonogram: vertex presentation, AFI 6.0.

Given the sterile speculum exam findings and the low AFI (a normal AFI at this GA is >8), this patient has ruptured membranes. Her nontender abdominal exam, normal temperature, lack of significant contractions, and normal WBC count suggest that she has not developed chorioamnionitis. She is admitted to the hospital for expectant management of PPROM. She is given 12 mg betamethasone IM, with a repeat dose 24 hours later and is started on ampicillin and erythromycin IV. On hospital day 2 she develops infrequent contractions, uterine tenderness, and a fever to 101.9°F. She is started on oxytocin (Pitocin) and makes rapid progress through labor. She delivers a viable 1,200-g male infant.

QUESTIONS

16-1. What is the primary reason this patient is given ampicillin and erythromycin?
  A. Group B *Streptococcus* prophylaxis
  B. To increase the latency period to the onset of labor
  C. To prevent the development of chorioamnionitis
  D. To treat a bladder infection
  E. To help prevent a bladder infection

16-2. In most cases of PPROM, the cause is:
  A. Preterm contractions
  B. Amniocentesis
  C. Unknown, possibly a subclinical infection
  D. Trauma
  E. Sexually transmitted infections

16-3. Given the early GA of this fetus, why is Pitocin begun rather than a tocolytic?
  A. To help prevent the development of chorioamnionitis
  B. To help prevent neonatal sepsis
  C. To help prevent bleeding
  D. To help prevent abruption
  E. To help prevent fetal distress

16-4. Beyond which GA would PPROM without overt chorioamnionitis be a reason for immediate delivery through induction?
    A. 24 weeks
    B. 26 weeks
    C. 28 weeks
    D. 32 weeks
    E. 35 weeks

 ## ANSWERS

16-1. B. A course of ampicillin and erythromycin has been shown to increase the latency period, the time between rupture of membranes to the onset of labor. Without antibiotics, approximately 50% of patients will go into labor within 24 hours and 75% within 48 hours. In general, the younger the GA, the longer the latency period unless complicated by chorioamnionitis.

16-2. C. Abdominal trauma, procedures such as amniocentesis, preterm labor, and infection are all associated with PPROM; however, in most cases the cause is unknown. Studies suggest that ascending subclinical infection may be the main culprit.

16-3. B. This question exemplifies the difficult and controversial management of PPROM. On initial presentation, this patient lacked any symptoms of chorioamnionitis, such as fever, abdominal tenderness, elevated WBC, maternal tachycardia, fetal tachycardia, or uterine contractions. However, the main cause of PPROM likely is subclinical infection, so she still is at great risk for development of an overt infection. Thus, Pitocin is given because the patient already has developed chorioamnionitis and rapid delivery may help prevent neonatal sepsis.

16-4. E. This is a controversial topic. However, most practitioners agree that at 35 weeks gestation or beyond, the risks of prematurity are low compared to the risk of infection. Some practitioners would consider performing amniocentesis at this GA for fetal lung maturity and giving betamethasone first if the lungs are immature. On the other hand, some practitioners are comfortable at 33 to 35 weeks GA inducing delivery immediately after PPROM. The reason for these different management styles is based in part on the decreasing risk of RDS with increasing GA. At 28 weeks GA, the risk of RDS is 60% to 75%. By 30 weeks GA, the risk is decreased to 40% to 50%. Between 33 to 35 weeks GA, the rate of RDS declines from 20% to 30% to only 6%. Finally, the risk at 36 weeks GA is approximately 3% to 5%.

SUGGESTED ADDITIONAL READING

Mercer BM, Miodovnik M, Thurnau GR, et al. Antibiotic therapy
    for reduction of infant morbidity after preterm premature
    rupture of membranes: a randomized controlled trial. National
    Institute of Child Health and Human Development Maternal-
    Fetal Medicine Units Network. *JAMA.* 1997;278:989–995.
Lieman JM, Brumfield CG, Carlo W, et al. Preterm premature
    rupture of membranes: is there an optimal gestational age for
    delivery? *Obstet Gynecol.* 2005;105:12–17.

Size Less Than Dates

ID/CC: A 34-year-old $G_4P_2S_1$ woman at 28 weeks GA by LMP with size less than dates presents for a scheduled prenatal office visit.

HPI: G.R. denies any symptoms except mild ankle swelling. Her blood pressures have remained in the 130–140/70–90 range since you switched her from benazepril to labetalol at her first prenatal visit (8 weeks GA). She has been charting "kick counts" since you instructed her to begin 3 weeks ago. She has no complaints of headache, visual changes, right upper quadrant pain, or significant edema.

PMHx: Chronic hypertension diagnosed after her last pregnancy 2 years ago.

PSHx: None

Meds: PNV; labetalol 200 mg TID

All: NKDA

POb/GynHx: Two full-term NSVDs resulting in two viable infants, both adequate for GA; pregnancies were complicated by pregnancy-induced hypertension (PIH).

SHx: Lives with husband and two children. No tobacco, ethanol, or recreational drug use.

VS: BP 134/86, HR 92

PE: *Gen:* NAD. *Cor:* RR&R, 1/6 SEM, no S_3, no S_4. *Abdomen:* soft, nontender, no distension, gravid with a fundal height (measured from the pubic symphysis to the top of the uterine fundus) of 24 cm, a 1-cm increment from her prior visit 4 weeks ago. *Extremities:* mild bilateral ankle edema, 2+ deep tendon reflexes (DTR) bilaterally.

Labs: Urine dipstick: negative proteinuria. Normal prenatal labs, Rh positive.

US: Single, living fetus with normal anatomical survey confirmed at 16 weeks GA. Size was equal to dates.

THOUGHT QUESTIONS

- How is uterine fundal height measurement used?
- What are the causes of size less than dates?
- What is the next best step in the management of this case?
- Why was the ACE inhibitor changed to labetalol?

Measuring the uterine height at the fundus and document-ing its continual growth is a very simple method for monitoring fetal growth. In general, the uterus is expected to increase by approxi-mately 1 cm per week. Beyond 20 weeks GA, the fundal height in centimeters should roughly equal the GA in weeks. The most com-mon causes for size less than dates are incorrect dating, small for gestational age (SGA) fetus (estimated fetal weight below the 5th or 10th percentile), transverse fetal lie, and oligohydramnios (from pre-mature rupture of the membranes or decreased/absent fetal produc-tion of urine). Clinical estimation of fetal size is not very accurate and usually cannot differentiate between the above causes.

The next step in management is to obtain an ultrasound for esti-mated fetal weight (EFW). If the EFW is less than the 5th or 10th percentile, the fetus is termed SGA. The differential diagnosis for an SGA fetus includes incorrect dating, constitutionally small size, chromosomal abnormalities, fetal anomalies, maternal/fetal infections, abnormal placentation, and maternal vascular diseases (rheumatologic, cardiovascular, or long-standing diabetes).

Because ACE inhibitors can lead to severe fetal renal dysfunction and death, especially when used in the second and third trimesters, their use is contraindicated during pregnancy. Labetalol, a β-blocker that also offers some α-blockade, is commonly used for blood pressure management in pregnancy. In nonpregnant patients, labetalol is given as a BID medication; however, in pregnancy it is commonly given TID and even QID because of the increased hepatic and renal clearance.

CASE CONTINUED

Ultrasound at 28 2/7 weeks GA (based on dates by 16-week sonogram) shows an active, male, cephalic fetus. The placenta is posterior, with no evidence of previa. The amniotic fluid volume, measured by the amniotic fluid index (AFI), is low–normal at 8.9 (normal AFI: 5 to 20). A detailed survey of fetal anatomy did not reveal any abnormalities. Fetal growth is at the 19th percentile for GA. You discuss these findings with the patient and recommend continuing her current antihypertensive regimen and daily kick counts, with the addition of weekly blood pressure checks and urine dipsticks and weekly antenatal testing with nonstress test (NST) and AFI to begin at 32 weeks GA. You schedule a repeat ultrasound in 3 weeks to check for fetal growth, which subsequently shows no interval fetal growth and a decreased AFI of 3.0. At that time, umbilical cord Doppler flow evaluation shows absent end-diastolic flow.

QUESTIONS

17-1. The most appropriate next step in management is:
A. Hospitalize, continuous FHT monitoring, induction of fetal lung maturity with corticosteroids, and plan for delivery in 48 hours
B. Daily NST and plan delivery at 34 weeks if blood pressures remain stable
C. Continue with pregnancy until 37 weeks if there is no evidence of preeclampsia
D. Optimize blood pressure control and reassess fetal growth in 2 weeks
E. Immediate cesarean delivery

17-2. While the patient is on FHT monitoring, the fetal heart rate drops to 60 bpm. Despite conservative measures (oxygen and changing the patient's position), it remains in the 60s for the next 6 minutes. Her BP is 154/98, and her cervix is 1 cm open and 3 cm long. She is not contracting. The next step in management is:
A. Amnioinfusion
B. Begin oxytocin (Pitocin) induction
C. Emergent cesarean section
D. Hydralazine 5 mg IV
E. Administer betamethasone

17-3. Which of the following is associated with intrauterine growth restriction (IUGR)?
   A. Antiphospholipid antibody syndrome
   B. Turner syndrome
   C. Chronic hypertension
   D. Congenital cytomegalovirus (CMV)
   E. All are correct

17-4. Which of the following is the best predictor of fetal mortality in a high-risk patient at 31 weeks GA?
   A. Nonreactive NST
   B. 6/10 BPP
   C. Reverse diastolic flow in umbilical cord Doppler
   D. Positive oxytocin challenge test (OCT)
   E. Zero kick counts in 1 hour

 ANSWERS

17-1. A.; **17-2.** C. No interval growth is an indication for delivery in a viable pregnancy, as is absent or reversed diastolic flow on umbilical artery Doppler assessment. Induction of fetal lung maturity with steroids is useful when delivery is anticipated between 24 and 34 weeks of gestation. Due to the oligohydramnios and IUGR, this fetus is at risk for fetal death and therefore should be monitored closely until delivery. Amnioinfusion may be used in the setting of repetitive variable decelerations during labor or thick meconium but is contraindicated if fetal compromise is strongly suspected, as in this case. Fetal bradycardia in this already compromised fetus warrants immediate delivery by cesarean section.

17-3. E. Fetal growth restriction is a heterogeneous group of disorders that can be subdivided into two groups of disorders. Decreased growth potential is associated with constitutionally small/small maternal stature, genetic chromosomal abnormalities, intrauterine infections, and teratogenic exposure. IUGR is related to maternal factors such as chronic hypertension, severe anemia, autoimmune disease, severe malnutrition, diabetes with vascular disease, and placental factors such as chronic abruption and multiple gestations.

17-4. C. Reverse diastolic flow on umbilical cord Doppler is the best predictor of adverse perinatal outcome, with a perinatal mortality of 25% to 50% (BPP of 0/10 also has a perinatal mortality of about 50%). NST is a better predictor when reactive or normal (perinatal mortality of 5/1000 within 1 week of the test). In a high-risk population, only 25% of initially non-reactive NSTs have a positive OCT. OCT is also a better predictor when negative or normal (perinatal death of 0.4/1000). A positive OCT (late deceleration in at least 50% of uterine contractions) is associated with fetal compromise but has a false-positive rate of at least 30% to 50%. A normal BPP (10/10) is an excellent predictor of good perinatal outcome (perinatal mortality of 0.8/1000). At 31 weeks, a score of 4/10 should be repeated within 24 hours. Decreased fetal movement warrants antenatal testing but is a poor predictor of adverse perinatal outcome.

SUGGESTED ADDITIONAL READING

Illanes S, Soothill P. Management of fetal growth restriction. *Semin Fetal Neonatal Med.* 2004;9:395–401.

Malcus P. Antenatal fetal surveillance. *Curr Opin Obstet Gynecol.* 2004;16:123–128.

Galan HL, Ferrazzi E, Hobbins JC. Intrauterine growth restriction (IUGR): biometric and Doppler assessment. *Prenat Diagn.* 2002;22:331–337.

Thornton JG, Hornbuckle J, Vail A, et al. GRIT study group. Infant wellbeing at 2 years of age in the Growth Restriction Intervention Trial (GRIT): multicentred randomised controlled trial. *Lancet.* 2004;364:513–520.

Size Greater Than Dates

ID/CC: A 32-year-old G_1P_0 woman at 26 weeks GA by LMP, size greater than dates.

HPI: T.G. is a 32-year-old kindergarten teacher who has had an uncomplicated, planned pregnancy. She prefers to minimize testing and declined the serum screen in the second trimester. She notes rapid breathing but is not short of breath. She reports approximately one to two Braxton-Hicks contractions per hour during the past week. No other complaints.

PMHx/PSHx: None

Meds: None

All: NKDA

SHx: Lives with her husband in a large urban area.

FHx: Noncontributory

VS: BP 110/60, HR 94, RR 24

PE: *Gen:* NAD. *Lungs:* clear to auscultation. *Cor:* RR&R, no murmurs. *Abdomen:* soft, nontender, gravid. Fundal height 31 cm. *Doppler:* positive fetal heart tones. Probable vertex presentation by Leopold maneuvers. *SVE:* closed and long, vertex presentation, −3 station.

Labs: Normal prenatal labs except rubella nonimmune, Hb 11.2, MCV 90

THOUGHT QUESTIONS

- What is the differential diagnosis for size greater than dates (S > D)?

- What is the next best step in management?
- What steps should be taken regarding her rubella non-immune status?

   Incorrect dating, large for gestational age (LGA) fetus (>90%), polyhydramnios, multiple gestations, and large uterine fibroids are the more common causes of S > D. Obesity often is associated with S > D because of the difficulty in palpating the uterine fundus. In addition, obesity is associated with both gestational diabetes (which can lead to polyhydramnios and LGA infants) and LGA infants even in the absence of gestational diabetes.

Ultrasound is helpful for determining GA, multiple gestations, fetal weight, and amniotic fluid volume and for evaluating the uterus and adnexa. In cases where polyhydramnios is identified, a detailed fetal anatomy survey (level II ultrasound) is required to exclude fetal and placental causes of increased amniotic fluid. Prior to the routine use of obstetric ultrasound, 50% of twin pregnancies were not diagnosed until delivery.

The patient is rubella nonimmune. She should be vaccinated immediately postpartum because of the small, theoretical (no cases reported) risk of transmission of this live attenuated virus to the fetus.

CASE CONTINUED

Ultrasound reveals a dichorionic-diamniotic twin pregnancy (Figure 18-1), vertex–vertex presentation, with adequate, concordant growth for both twins at 26 weeks by anthropometrics (fetal measurements such as biparietal diameter, femur length, and abdominal circumference). Amniotic fluid is normal, and the placentas are posterior and fundal.

Two weeks later, she complains of painful uterine contractions every 3 to 4 minutes. She notes no bleeding and no loss of fluid, and the fetuses are active. Her cervical exam is 2-cm dilated, 80% effaced, vertex at −2 station.

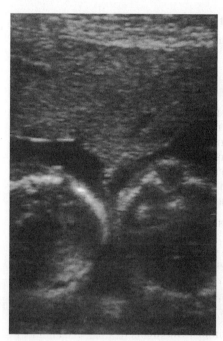

FIGURE 18-1.
Two fetal heads separated
by a thick membrane in
dichorionic-diamniotic twins.
(Image Provided by Depart-
ments of Radiology and
Obstetrics and Gynecology,
University of California,
San Francisco).

QUESTIONS

18-1. The most appropriate management in this case includes
which of the following?

  A. Tocolysis, betamethasone (12 mg, two doses, 24 hours apart),
     ampicillin
  B. Ampicillin, prepare for imminent delivery
  C. Epidural anesthesia, prepare for delivery
  D. Tocolysis, erythromycin
  E. Trendelenburg position, cervical cerclage

18-2. The patient received one of the above therapies and developed gradual onset of shortness of breath and low O_2 saturations. What
is the most likely diagnosis?

  A. Pulmonary embolism
  B. Amniotic fluid embolism
  C. Pulmonary edema
  D. Myocardial infarction
  E. Deep venous thromboembolism

18-3. In the management of twins, which of the following is *correct*?

A. Amniocentesis should only be offered to women older than 35 years carrying twins.

B. The single most important cause of perinatal mortality in twins is related to malformations.

C. Serial ultrasounds are recommended to assess fetal growth.

D. Preeclampsia is less common in twins than singleton gestations.

E. Dichorionic-diamniotic twins are always dizygotic.

18-4. Which of the following statements regarding amniotic fluid disorders is *correct*?

A. Fetal duodenal atresia is frequently associated with oligohydramnios.

B. Maternal diabetes mellitus is associated with polyhydramnios.

C. Therapeutic (reduction) amniocentesis is performed to reduce the chance of preterm labor.

D. Fetal CNS disorders that affect swallowing cause oligohydramnios.

E. Twin-to-twin transfusion syndrome results in polyhydramnios (donor twin) and oligohydramnios (recipient twins).

 ANSWERS

18-1. A. Management of preterm labor involves use of steroids for prevention of RDS and intraventricular hemorrhage (IVH), tocolysis until the desired effect on fetal lung maturity is obtained, and antibiotics for prevention of Group B *Streptococcus* (GBS) sepsis in the neonate. Delivery is not considered imminent in the case presented, and even in cases of advanced cervical dilation, steroids still may have some value if delivery is deferred for just a few hours. Use of tocolysis and antibiotics in the absence of corticosteroid administration is not considered adequate management of preterm labor because the maximal gain from medical intervention is obtained from the latter. Trendelenburg position and emergent cerclage are indicated in cases of incompetent cervix (painless cervical dilation, usually in the midtrimester), not preterm labor.

18-2. C. The combination of twin gestation, corticosteroids, aggressive IV hydration, and IV tocolysis with either magnesium sulfate or β-adrenergic agonists has been associated with pulmonary edema. Physical examination and chest x-ray film should confirm the diagnosis. Pulmonary embolism and amniotic fluid embolism typically present with sudden onset of shortness of breath and low O_2 saturations. Chest x-ray film, electrocardiogram (ECG), arterial blood gas (ABG), spiral CT, or V/Q scan are useful when this diagnosis is suspected.

18-3. C. For dizygotic twin gestations, the risk of aneuploidy in at least one fetus is 1:200 at maternal age 32, which is 3 years earlier than in singleton gestations (risk 1:200 at age 35). Although the rate of malformation in twins is higher than for singletons, prematurity is the number one cause of perinatal mortality in twins. Serial ultrasounds are recommended to assess fetal growth because the fundal height measurements are not well correlated with fetal growth. Furthermore, one fetus may be growing while the other is experiencing intrauterine growth restriction (IUGR). Preeclampsia is more frequent in multiple gestations.

18-4. B. Fetal causes of polyhydramnios include gastrointestinal obstructions and neurologic or mechanical conditions (tracheoesophageal fistulas) that interfere with swallowing. Placental causes include twin-to-twin transfusion syndrome (polyhydramnios in the recipient twin and oligohydramnios in the donor) and placental tumors. Diabetes mellitus with poor glycemic control is a well-known maternal cause of polyhydramnios. Polyhydramnios can be severe enough to lead to maternal respiratory distress, in which case reduction amniocentesis is indicated.

 SUGGESTED ADDITIONAL READING

Senat MV, Deprest J, Boulvain M, et al. Endoscopic laser surgery versus serial amnioreduction for severe twin-to-twin transfusion syndrome. *N Engl J Med.* 2004;351:136–144.

Monteagudo A, Roman AS. Ultrasound in multiple gestations: twins and other multifetal pregnancies. *Clin Perinatol.* 2005;32:329–354.

Marino T. Ultrasound abnormalities of the amniotic fluid, membranes, umbilical cord, and placenta. *Obstet Gynecol Clin North Am.* 2004;31:177–200.

Ott WJ. Reevaluation of the relationship between amniotic fluid volume and perinatal outcome. *Am J Obstet Gynecol.* 2005;192:1803–1809.

Decreased Fetal Movement

ID/CC: A 26-year-old G_2P_1 Hispanic woman at 33 weeks GA presents complaining of a decrease in her baby's movements.

HPI: M.T. states that her baby usually is quite active in the mornings and evenings. Last evening she noticed a few movements before she fell asleep, but this morning she felt no movement after awakening. She ate breakfast and then laid down on her couch to concentrate on the movements. During the following hour she felt the baby move only twice. She states that she has otherwise been feeling well. She denies having any contractions, loss of fluid, or vaginal bleeding. Ms. T presented late for prenatal care at 24 weeks gestation but has otherwise had an uncomplicated pregnancy. She was dated by 24-week ultrasound because her LMP was uncertain.

PMHx: Migraine headaches

PSHx: None

Meds: PNV

All: NKDA

POb/GynHx: One uncomplicated NSVD at 36 weeks GA, 5 lb 8 oz. Menarche age 12, regular menses every 28 days. Denies STIs, PID. Normal Pap smears.

SHx: Lives with father of baby and her daughter. Denies use of tobacco, ethanol, or recreational drugs.

THOUGHT QUESTIONS

- What is the differential diagnosis for decreased fetal movement? Which diagnosis is most common?
- What is a normal amount for a fetus to move? Should the fetus be moving all the time?
- What are some ways to test for fetal well-being?

The differential diagnosis for decreased fetal movement includes fetal sleep cycle, oligohydramnios, fetal effects of maternal drug use (e.g., opiates, steroids), fetal distress or lack of well-being (e.g., uteroplacental insufficiency), and fetal demise. In addition, perhaps the most common reason for decreased movement is simply that the mother is unaware that movement is occurring. For example, the baby may move into a particular position that makes sensation of fetal movement difficult.

Regarding normal fetal movement, it is difficult to give a specific answer because each fetus and mother are different. Generally, in the middle to late third trimester, a mother should feel two periods of good fetal activity each day. During these periods of activity, the fetus should move or kick at least four to six times in 1 hour. Women often are instructed to do "kick counts" to ensure fetal well-being. To accomplish this, the patient is instructed to sit quietly once or twice per day after a meal and count fetal movements. If fewer than four to six movements are felt in 1 hour, she should contact her care provider.

There are many ways to test for fetal well-being. They may include (1) kick counts; (2) nonstress test (NST) of the FHR; (3) modified biophysical profile (BPP), which includes NST and calculation of amniotic fluid volume; (4) formal BPP to examine fetal movement, tone, breathing, amniotic fluid, and NST; and (5) an oxytocin challenge test (OCT), also known as a contraction stress test (CST). Of note, the CST can also be initiated using nipple stimulation, which increases circulating levels of oxytocin in the patient. However, because oxytocin levels cannot be controlled with this method, there is a greater risk for having uncontrolled, prolonged, or tetanic contractions.

CASE CONTINUED

VS: Temp 98.0°F, BP 110/64, HR 90, RR 18

PE: *Abdomen:* soft, nontender. Fundal height 32 cm. *FHT:* 130s, nonreactive without decelerations. *Toco:* no contractions.

Labs: Urine dipstick: SG 1.010, negative nitrites/esterase, negative ketones, negative glucose. Sonogram: AFI 16.2, vertex presentation.

Because the NST is not reactive, vibroacoustic stimulation (VAS) is performed. A VAS unit is placed against the maternal abdomen and emits a noise meant to stimulate the baby. The fetus responds to the VAS with one small heart rate acceleration, which is only a minimally reassuring response. Thus, a BPP is performed. The fetus is evaluated by sonogram for 30 minutes, which in this case reveals a cephalic fetus with several pockets of amniotic fluid each measuring >4 cm. During this observation period, the fetus, which has its hips and knees flexed, extends an arm and a leg several times and has three large discrete body movements. One episode of breathing >30 seconds is noted. After the BPP, the patient is placed back on the monitor and now has a reactive NST.

QUESTIONS

19-1. What score does the fetus receive for the BPP?
   A. 2/10
   B. 4/10
   C. 6/10
   D. 8/10
   E. 10/10

19-2. What is the most appropriate next step for this patient?
   A. Repeat the NST in 1 week
   B. Repeat the NST in 24 hours
   C. Observation for 24 hours
   D. Immediate delivery
   E. No further testing

19-3. What is the definition of a reactive FHR tracing for a fetus in the late third trimester?
   A. One acceleration >10 bpm lasting at least 10 seconds in 10 minutes
   B. Two accelerations >15 bpm lasting at least 15 seconds in 10 minutes
   C. Two accelerations >15 bpm lasting at least 15 seconds in 20 minutes
   D. Two accelerations >15 bpm lasting at least 15 seconds in 30 minutes
   E. Two accelerations >20 bpm lasting at least 20 seconds in 30 minutes

19-4. What is the criteria for a completed CST or OCT?
   A. Two contractions in 10 minutes
   B. Three contractions in 10 minutes
   C. Two contractions in 20 minutes
   D. Three contractions in 20 minutes
   E. Three contractions in 30 minutes

ANSWERS

19-1. D. The BPP is an evaluation completed over approximately 30 minutes by ultrasound. The following variables are evaluated for a total of ten points possible: two points for a reactive FHR tracing; two points for at least one episode of fetal breathing movements (or hiccoughs) lasting at least 30 seconds; two points for at least three discrete body or limb movements; two points for at least one episode of active extension with return to flexion of a limb, hand, or trunk; and two points for an amniotic fluid index >5 or at least one pocket measuring 2—2 cm or greater. Variables that are not met completely are given zero points rather than one because there is no partial scoring in this test. Based on these criteria, this patient's BPP score is 8/10, with two points taken off for a nonreactive FHR tracing.

19-2. E. A score of 8/10 or 10/10 is considered "reassuring"; therefore, the patient can be followed expectantly but should return if further episodes of decreased fetal movement occur. Depending on the clinical situation and GA, a score ≤4 consideration of delivery.

19-3. C. Interpretation of an FHR tracing involves the evaluation of four factors. The first is the baseline heart rate, which normally is between 110 and 160 bpm. The second factor is a determination of heart rate variability, which is represented by the fluctuations in the amplitude of the baseline heart rate. Put more simply, it is the appearance of the heart rate (i.e., does it look like a straight line and lack variability, or is it jagged?). The third factor is the absence or presence of decelerations and their relationship, if present, to a contraction. The fourth factor is the presence of accelerations in the baseline heart rate. A "reactive" tracing for a fetus >32 weeks EGA by definition is a 20-minute continuous tracing that has two accelerations >15 beats above baseline heart rate lasting at least 15 seconds. A "reactive" tracing for a fetus <32 weeks EGA is a 20-minute continuous tracing that has two accelerations >10 beats above baseline lasting at least 10 seconds. A *reactive tracing* is a term used for a tracing that is considered normal or reassuring.

19-4. B. CST or OCT is defined as three contractions within a 10-minute period. A CST can occur spontaneously if the patient is contracting on her own, or it can be achieved via oxytocin (Pitocin) or nipple stimulation. A negative or reassuring CST is a tracing without decelerations; a positive or abnormal CST is one with decelerations. Although there is some disagreement among obstetricians, a CST with decelerations associated with less than half of the contractions is generally considered "indeterminate." Again, a CST is used as another measure of fetal well-being. A positive CST warrants consideration of immediate delivery or continuous observation. A negative CST is reassuring, and the patient can be scheduled for outpatient testing in the future depending on the situation for which the test was performed.

SUGGESTED ADDITIONAL READING

Tan KH, Smyth R. Fetal vibroacoustic stimulation for facilitation of tests of fetal wellbeing. *Cochrane Database Syst Rev.* 2001;(1):CD002963.

Abdominal Pain Associated with High Blood Pressure in Pregnancy

ID/CC: A 27-year-old G_1P_0 woman at 35 weeks GA presents with complaint of 6 hours of worsening right upper quadrant (RUQ) pain.

HPI: K.S. has had an entirely normal antepartum course until she woke up this morning with mild RUQ pain. She ate a normal breakfast that neither aggravated nor alleviated the pain. The pain increased over the morning, and this brought her to the labor ward. She also complains of increased swelling of her feet, such that her shoes no longer fit. She has no headache, visual symptoms, nausea, vomiting, or other GI complaints. On review of systems she notes that her rings no longer fit on her fingers.

PMHx/PSHx: None

Meds: PNV

All: NKDA

POb/GynHx: Regular menses every 28 days.

SHx: Lives with father of baby; no domestic violence. No use of ethanol, tobacco, or recreational drugs.

VS: Temp 98.3°F, BP 156/93, HR 72, RR 16

PE: *Gen:* NAD. *Lungs:* CTAB. *Abdomen:* mild RUQ tenderness, otherwise soft, no distension, with gravid uterus size = dates. *Lower extremity:* 3+ pitting edema. *Reflexes:* 3+ bilateral lower extremities, 2+ bilateral upper extremities, no clonus. *SVE:* cervix is long, closed, −3 station. *FHT:* 140s, reactive, moderate variability, no decelerations.

109

Labs: Urine 2+ protein; Hct 38.9; WBC 9.4; Plts 92,000;
ALT 94; AST 107; LDH 786; Cr 0.4; Tbili 0.2; uric acid 7.4.

THOUGHT QUESTIONS

- Prior to the physical exam, what was the patient's differential diagnosis?
- Prior to the lab results, what was the patient's differential diagnosis?
- What is the most likely diagnosis after obtaining lab results?
- What is the next step in the management of this patient?

By history, the patient had RUQ pain, which can be caused by inflammation of the liver or gallbladder, gastritis, musculoskeletal, HELLP (hemolysis, elevated liver enzymes, low platelets) syndrome, hepatitis, or even a right lower lobe pneumonia. However, with no exacerbation or alleviation by eating, gallbladder disease and gastritis are unlikely. Furthermore, with no symptoms of upper respiratory infection, pneumonia is unlikely. HELLP syndrome is a variant of severe preeclampsia. The patient's elevated blood pressure, proteinuria, nondependent edema of her hands, and brisk reflexes on physical exam support this diagnosis. Furthermore, the lab results are all consistent with a diagnosis of hemolysis (increased LDH), elevated liver enzymes (increased ALT and AST), and low platelets (<150,000). Hepatitis is less likely with normal bilirubin and relatively mild LFT elevations.

Preeclampsia is the triad of elevated blood pressure, proteinuria, and nondependent (facial and hand) edema. It is differentiated into mild and severe preeclampsia, with mild preeclampsia being the classic triad in the absence of any of the features of severe preeclampsia. The diagnosis of severe preeclampsia is made if the patient develops any of the following: headache, RUQ pain, scotomata, blood pressures >160/110 for two readings at least 6 hours apart, oliguria (<30 cc/hr for several hours), pulmonary edema, proteinuria >5 g in 24 hours, and HELLP syndrome. The only treatment for preeclampsia is stabilization of any acute issues and delivery of the fetus. The management of preeclampsia depends on the severity of illness plus the GA at diagnosis. If expectant management

TABLE 20-1 Management of Mild and Severe Preeclampsia Based on Gestational Age

Gestational Age	Mild Preeclampsia	Severe Preeclampsia
<24 wk	Expectant management vs. TAB	TAB is recommended
24–34 wk	Expectant management with ACS	Expectant management with ACS*
34–36 wk	Expectant management	Induction of labor
36 wk to term	Expectant management vs. IOL	Induction of labor

*Expectant Management in Severe Preeclamptics is Reasonable Only Until the Development of Symptoms Such As Headache, Right Upper Quadrant Pain, Visual Symptoms, LFT More Than Twice Normal, Plts <100,000, Blood Pressures That Cannot be Controlled with Two Agents, Pulmonary Edema, Oliguria, or Seizure.

is used between 24 and 34 weeks GA, antenatal corticosteroids (ACS), generally betamethasone, are given to accelerate fetal lung maturity. The general management guidelines for different gestational ages are given in Table 20-1.

CASE CONTINUED

Because of her diagnosis of HELLP syndrome, the patient is begun on magnesium sulfate, and prostaglandin gel is placed intravaginally for cervical ripening for induction of labor.

Laboratory results are rechecked after 6 hours and reveal that LFTs have increased further to ALT/AST = 112/134 and platelets have decreased to 76. On exam, the cervix now is 1.5 cm dilated and 60% effaced, and the patient is begun on oxytocin (Pitocin). She contracts regularly with Pitocin and delivers vaginally 12 hours later. Samples for lab tests are drawn 20 minutes prior to birth.

QUESTIONS

20-1. What are the most likely results from the lab tests drawn 20 minutes prior to birth?
   A. ALT/AST 76/84; Plts 54
   B. ALT/AST 134/146; Plts 132
   C. ALT/AST 76/84; Plts 132
   D. ALT/AST 134/146; Plts 54
   E. ALT/AST 276/292; Plts 18

20-2. Magnesium sulfate, which is given for seizure prophylaxis, is continued for:
  A. 6 hours postpartum
  B. 24 hours postpartum
  C. 48 hours postpartum
  D. Until blood pressures normalize
  E. Until patient is discharged

20-3. Exacerbation of what systemic disease most resembles severe preeclampsia?
  A. Rheumatoid arthritis
  B. Ulcerative colitis
  C. Scleroderma
  D. Diabetes
  E. Lupus

20-4. A patient presents 72 hours after delivery to the emergency department having had a seizure at home. She should be begun on:
  A. Phenytoin
  B. Tegretol
  C. Magnesium sulfate
  D. Valium
  E. Phenobarbital

ANSWERS

20-1. D. Test result abnormalities in preeclampsia will not improve until delivery and often not for hours to days after delivery. One exception is an often transient improvement in test result abnormalities when steroids are given, particularly in the setting of betamethasone (ACS) given for probable preterm delivery. Choices A, B, and C all show some lab improvement. However, this is not expected in this patient who did not receive ACS. The values in choice E are possible, but lab values tend to follow a trend, so one would expect the next set of results to be closer to those in choice D. Lab tests should be followed closely postpartum, watching for the nadir of the platelets. If laboratory results plummet, ACS have been used postpartum, leading to more rapid resolution of platelet and LFT abnormalities.

20-2. B. In patients with preeclampsia, magnesium sulfate is often given for seizure prophylaxis. This is commonly continued for 24 hours after birth. The basis for this treatment is that the bulk of eclamptic seizures occur antepartum, intrapartum, and in the first 24 hours postpartum. Thus, with this therapy most eclamptic seizures will be prevented. Some physicians treat with magnesium sulfate beyond 24 hours if the lab values continue to worsen, blood pressures are poorly controlled, or severe headache continues. However, this management style has never been studied and is based on risk aversion rather than clinical evidence.

20-3. E. Patients with systemic lupus erythematosus (SLE) can have symptoms and lab test abnormalities very similar to patients with severe preeclampsia. Furthermore, all of the diagnostic criteria for severe preeclampsia, including pulmonary edema, oliguria, and even seizures, can be seen in these patients. To determine which is the more likely cause, two lab tests have been used. Patients having a lupus flare usually will have a decreased total complement level, and patients with severe preeclampsia usually have an elevated uric acid level. Other than these values, careful discussion with the patient and her rheumatologist is important and may help in the differential diagnosis. Class RF diabetics (refer to the White classification of gestational diabetics) have the elevated blood pressures and proteinuria of preeclampsia, but they usually do not have the lab test abnormalities and symptoms of preeclampsia.

20-4. C. Even with postpartum seizures, magnesium sulfate has been shown to be as efficacious or more so than other commonly used antiseizure medications in patients with eclampsia. In patients who are admitted with postpartum eclampsia, a set of lab tests, including electrolytes and Ca^{2+}, and preeclamptic tests (LFTs, Cr, LDH, and CBC) should be ordered. Usually these patients warrant a neurology consultation as well as a head CT. The usual finding in eclampsia is some cerebral edema in the occipital cortex. As long as the lab results and blood pressures are stable, the magnesium sulfate is continued IV for 24 to 48 hours and then stopped. Usually the patient is watched for an additional 24 hours and then discharged home without further antiseizure medications unless such drugs are recommended by the neurologist.

 ## SUGGESTED ADDITIONAL READING

Chames MC, Haddad B, Barton JR, et al. Subsequent pregnancy outcome in women with a history of HELLP syndrome at < or = 28 weeks of gestation. *Am J Obstet Gynecol.* 2003;188:1504–1507; discussion 1507–1508.

Altman D, Carroli G, Duley L, et al., Magpie Trial Collaboration Group. Do women with pre-eclampsia, and their babies, benefit from magnesium sulphate? The Magpie Trial: a randomised placebo-controlled trial. *Lancet.* 2002;359:1877–1890.

Sibai BM, Mercer BM, Schiff E, et al. Aggressive versus expectant management of severe preeclampsia at 28 to 32 weeks' gestation: a randomized controlled trial. *Am J Obstet Gynecol.* 1994;171:818–822.

Martin JN Jr, Perry KG Jr, Blake PG, et al. Better maternal outcomes are achieved with dexamethasone therapy for postpartum HELLP (hemolysis, elevated liver enzymes, and thrombocytopenia) syndrome. *Am J Obstet Gynecol.* 1997;177:1011–1017.

Itch in the Third Trimester

ID/CC: A 22-year-old G_2P_0 Central-American woman at 33 weeks GA by LMP presents with generalized itching.

HPI: C.P. began itching on her palms and soles 3 days ago. The pruritus mainly is nocturnal. It now is generalized but predominantly occurs over her abdomen, palms, and soles; her face is spared. She now has difficulty sleeping. She has not noticed any skin changes or lesions. She reports she has not changed detergents or soaps and has not worn any new clothing or jewelry. She denies use of any medications.

PMHx: Transient cholestasis associated with use of oral contraceptives. Hepatitis as a child in Nicaragua.

PSHx: D&C

Meds: None

All: NKDA

POb/GynHx: Regular menses, first trimester SAB 1 year ago.

SHx: Single, father of baby supportive. Denies use of tobacco, ethanol, or recreational drugs.

FHx: Noncontributory

VS: Temp 98.2°F, BP 120/72, HR 88

PE: *Gen:* NAD. No skin lesions except for a few excoriations on arms and abdomen secondary to scratching. No lymphadenopathy. *HEENT:* no icterus, unremarkable. *Abdomen:* soft, nontender, gravid. Unable to assess hepatic border or spleen because of gravid uterus. No uterine contractions, normal fetal movements.

THOUGHT QUESTIONS

- What is the differential diagnosis?
- What diagnostic studies would you recommend?

The clinical case presented is most compatible with intra-hepatic cholestasis of pregnancy (IHCP). The presentation of pruritus with no associated skin lesions is typical. Liver function tests usually are normal or show mild elevation of AST and alkaline phosphatase (Alk Phos). Approximately 10% to 30% of patients with IHCP have jaundice. Pruritic urticarial papules and plaques of pregnancy (PUPPP) can also cause intense itching but are accompanied by erythematous papules and plaques that usually arise first on the abdomen. Cholestasis from either intrahepatic or extrahepatic obstruction produces pruritus similar to the pattern of IHCP. Multiple skin disorders, parasitoses, and malignancies can be associated with pruritus.

In a patient with these classic presenting symptoms of IHCP, initial studies should include CBC with differential, liver function tests, and serum bile acids. If icterus is present, viral hepatitis studies and abdominal ultrasound should be ordered to exclude cholelithiasis and pancreatic abnormalities. In the setting of no other source of the pruritus, the diagnosis of IHCP can be made clinically. In addition, elevated levels of bile acids are also diagnostic.

CASE CONTINUED

Two weeks later the patient has persistent pruritus despite treatment with diphenhydramine (Benadryl). Her physical exam is unchanged except for a few excoriations secondary to scratching.

Labs: WBC 7.9; Hct 34; Plts 234,000; AST 44; Alk Phos 430; cholic acid 66 μM; Tbili 0.8; PT 1.1; hepatitis A IgG (+); IgM (−); hepatitis B and C (−).

US: Abdominal: normal, single, live, vertex, intrauterine pregnancy, size equals dates.

QUESTIONS

21-1. Based on the data provided, you recommend which of the following?
- A. Treat pruritus and continue with pregnancy until term
- B. Begin antenatal testing, therapy for pruritus, and deliver after confirmation of fetal lung maturity after 36 weeks GA
- C. Liver biopsy
- D. Administer *S*-adenosyl-L-methionine and repeat liver panel
- E. Administer vitamin K and repeat liver panel

21-2. IHCP is associated with which of the following?
- A. 10% chance of major malformations in the offspring
- B. Negligible risk of recurrence in subsequent pregnancies
- C. Pruritus and jaundice may not resolve after delivery
- D. Potential cholestasis triggered by antibiotic use in patients with a history of IHCP
- E. Increased risk for preterm delivery and perinatal mortality

21-3. One week later the patient complains of malaise, anorexia, and intractable vomiting. Lab studies indicate liver failure and hypoglycemia. Of the following, the most likely diagnosis and treatment plan are:
- A. HELLP syndrome, steroids
- B. Acute fatty liver of pregnancy (AFLP), supportive measures and prompt delivery
- C. Severe IHCP, ursodeoxycholic acid therapy
- D. AFLP, plasmapheresis
- E. HELLP syndrome, induction of labor

21-4. Which of the following is a characteristic of PUPPP?
- A. Recurrence in subsequent pregnancies is common.
- B. High-potency topical corticosteroids usually are effective in relieving pruritus.
- C. It usually appears in first trimester and the lesions begin on the abdomen.
- D. It is associated with late intrauterine fetal death.
- E. It does not resolve unless treated.

ANSWERS

21-1. B.; **21-2.** E. IHCP is associated with an increase in perinatal mortality and prematurity but is not associated with congenital malformations. The recurrence risk is 1:3 in subsequent pregnancies, and approximately 50% of patients have a positive family history, suggesting a genetic basis. Treatment of pruritus is important for comfort care but does not improve perinatal outcome. Recommended practice is delivery between 36 to 38 weeks GA in an attempt to prevent late intrauterine demise. Many clinicians also check fetal lung maturity prior to induction of labor to ensure that they are not causing iatrogenic morbidity such as RDS. Antenatal testing is generally started at 32 to 34 weeks gestation, although its benefit has not been proven. Liver biopsy is almost never indicated because IHCP typically is a benign maternal condition that resolves postpartum. S-adenosyl-L-methionine is among one of many therapies used in the treatment of itching in IHCP, with doubtful symptomatic relief and no change in the perinatal outcome. Few cases of IHCP are complicated by a prolonged PT, which can be reverted by the administration of vitamin K. Women with prior history of IHCP should be alerted that cholestasis might develop when taking OCPs, which resolves after discontinuation of its use. However, an association between cholestasis and antibiotic use in patients with a history of IHCP has not been reported.

21-3. B. The clinical scenario described strongly suggests AFLP, a rare complication of pregnancy that carries a high mortality if unrecognized. Management includes supportive care and delivery without delay. Plasmapheresis for treatment of AFLP has been proposed but has not been shown to affect outcomes. Fifty percent of AFLP cases are associated with severe preeclampsia or the HELLP syndrome, neither of which is evident in this patient. Steroids may be helpful for treatment of HELLP syndrome, particularly when it occurs postpartum. IHCP can cause mild jaundice and mild elevations of liver enzymes and rarely elevations of PT, but it has an otherwise benign maternal course. Ursodeoxycholic acid has been used for treatment of IHCP but has no role in AFLP.

21-4. B. PUPPP is a common, benign dermatitis of pregnancy that typically presents in the third trimesters with 1- to 2-mm erythematous papules that quickly coalesce to form urticarial plaques that first arise on the abdomen. The face is uniformly spared, and pruritus is the major complaint. High-dose topical steroids usually are effective, with use of oral steroids reserved for only the more severe cases. PUPPP is not associated with poor pregnancy outcome and resolves spontaneously during the pregnancy or postpartum. Recurrence in subsequent pregnancies is rare. Histologic examination shows a mild nonspecific lymphohistiocytic perivasculitis. The cause is unknown.

 SUGGESTED ADDITIONAL READING

Brites D. Intrahepatic cholestasis of pregnancy: changes in maternal-fetal bile acid balance and improvement by ursodeoxycholic acid. *Ann Hepatol.* 2002;1:20–28.

Glantz A, Marschall HU, Mattsson LA. Intrahepatic cholestasis of pregnancy: relationships between bile acid levels and fetal complication rates. *Hepatology.* 2004;40:467–474.

Kroumpouzos G, Cohen LM. Specific dermatoses of pregnancy: an evidence-based systematic review. *Am J Obstet Gynecol.* 2003;188:1083–1092.

Aronson IK, Bond S, Fiedler VC, et al. Pruritic urticarial papules and plaques of pregnancy: clinical and immunopathologic observations in 57 patients. *J Am Acad Dermatol.* 1998;39:933–939.

Vaginal Bleeding in Pregnancy III—Third Trimester

ID/CC: A 27-year-old G_3P_1 woman at 28 weeks GA brought in by ambulance complains of vaginal bleeding more than her period.

HPI: M.P. was at home playing with her 3-year-old son when she felt liquid trickle from her vagina. Thinking it likely was urine but concerned about amniotic fluid, she went to the bathroom, where she was shocked to discover that she was bleeding and had passed several golf ball-sized blood clots. She immediately called 911 and was brought to the hospital. She notes that she had no contractions at home but has experienced some mild cramping since she arrived at the hospital. The fetus has been active throughout. She is not lightheaded and has no other complaints. Her antepartum course has been entirely normal. She had normal labs in the first trimester, a normal serum triple screen, and, by her report, a normal ultrasound at 19 weeks.

PMHx/PSHx: None

Meds: PNV

All: NKDA

POb/GynHx: Term cesarean section (C/S) for breech fetus 3 years ago, SAB 4 years ago

SHx: Lives with husband; no domestic violence. No ethanol, tobacco, or recreational drug use.

VS: Temp 98.0°F, BP 116/73, HR 94, RR 20

PE: *Gen:* NAD. *Lungs:* CTAB. *Abdomen:* soft, nontender, no distension with gravid uterus, size = dates. *SSE:* approx 50 cc of old blood and clots in vault; no active bleeding from cervix. *FHT:*

140s, reactive, moderate reactivity, no decelerations. *Toco:* contractions on monitor every 3 to 4 minutes.

Labs: WBC 7.6; Hct 33.4; Plts 249,000; Kleihauer-Betke: pending

THOUGHT QUESTIONS

- What is your differential diagnosis at this point?
- What further history and physical exam would you like?
- What is the significance of the Kleihauer-Betke test?
- How would an obstetric ultrasound help with the possible diagnoses?

The differential diagnosis of third-trimester vaginal bleeding includes placental abruption, placenta previa, vasa previa, cervical bleeding (trauma, polyp, cancer), vaginal bleeding (trauma), and rectal bleeding (hemorrhoids, anal fissure). History and physical exam can be used to differentiate between uterine and nonuterine causes of bleeding. On history, recent intercourse may be the cause for cervical bleeding. On physical exam, a site of bleeding may be seen on the cervix, vaginal wall, or in the perirectal region with associated hemorrhoids. The Kleihauer-Betke test is used to determine the presence of fetal blood in the maternal circulation. A positive test result is suggestive of a fetomaternal hemorrhage, which is consistent with placental abruption.

Uterine sources of bleeding sometimes can be identified on ultrasound. During ultrasound examination, the site of placentation should be identified and a diagnosis of previa given if the placenta inserts over the internal os of the cervix. Although a fresh retroplacental clot of ≥300 cc usually can be recognized on ultrasound as a sonolucent region behind the placenta, ultrasound is not particularly sensitive for detection of placental abruption. Finally, vasa previa, a blood vessel in the membranes near or over the cervix, is a difficult diagnosis to make. Concern for vasa previa should be raised if there is a succenturiate lobe (an accessory placenta with a vascular connection to the main placenta) on one side of the cervix and the rest of the placenta on the other, because the vascular connection may traverse the internal os. The diagnosis can only be made prior to labor using Doppler flow to identify a blood vessel next to the cervix.

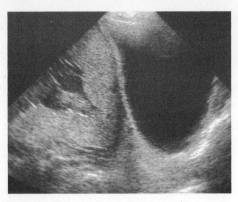

FIGURE 22-1.
Complete Placenta
Previa—Note that the
placenta previa is central,
completely covering the
internal os of the cervix.
*(Image Provided by
Departments of Radiology
and Obstetrics and Gyne-
cology, University of
California, San Francisco).*

CASE CONTINUED

Ms. P. has not had intercourse in the past several days and has had
no problems with constipation or hemorrhoids. On physical exam,
she has no evidence of cervical, vaginal, or rectal bleeding. She
continues with mild contractions, and the ultrasonographer arrives
to perform an obstetric ultrasound.

US: Posterior placenta that inserts just past the internal os of the
cervix. Otherwise, normal fetus, normal amniotic fluid, no evidence
of abruption (Figure 22-1).

QUESTIONS

22-1. Which of the following is part of the initial care for a
patient with a known placenta previa who presents with bleeding
and contractions at 28 weeks GA?
  A. Magnesium sulfate and betamethasone
  B. Terbutaline and betamethasone
  C. Betamethasone and immediate cesarean delivery
  D. Betamethasone and glucose loading test (GLT)
  E. Magnesium sulfate, betamethasone, GLT

22-2. Which of the following is not a risk factor for placenta previa?
  A. Multiple fundal fibroids
  B. Prior C/S
  C. Bicornuate uterus
  D. Fetal macrosomia
  E. Multiple gestations

22-3. Placenta previa, particularly with a history of a prior cesarean delivery, is associated with an increase in:

A. Placental abruption

B. Placenta accreta

C. Uterine rupture

D. Successful vaginal birth after cesarean (VBAC)

E. Female fetus

22-4. Which of the following is a likely reason the placenta previa was not seen on the initial scan?

A. No previa at the time, and it since has grown over the cervix.

B. The bladder was full, which pushed the placenta up during the ultrasound.

C. Fetal movement.

D. Sonographer error.

E. It usually is not seen so early in pregnancy.

 ANSWERS

22-1. A. In any preterm patient between 24 and 34 weeks of gestation who presents at risk for imminent delivery, a course of betamethasone should be given. In a patient with a placenta previa who is contracting and bleeding, a tocolytic also is indicated. The tocolytic of choice in this setting usually is magnesium sulfate because both terbutaline and nifedipine can cause maternal tachycardia, which could mask a sign of further bleeding. If the well-being of either the patient or the fetus becomes worrisome, cesarean delivery may be necessary. At this GA, however, judicious use of tocolytics to delay delivery long enough to achieve fetal benefit from a course of betamethasone is important to decrease the rate of respiratory distress syndrome. Finally, although the GLT usually is done at the beginning of the third trimester to screen for gestational diabetes and is an important part of prenatal screening, appropriate management of this patient requires stabilization of her bleeding and contractions prior to performing routine prenatal labs. In addition, the GLT would be inaccurate in the setting of antenatal corticosteroid administration and should not be performed until at least 96 hours after the patient has received betamethasone.

22-2. D. Risk factors for placenta previa include history of prior placenta previa, uterine anomalies (e.g., bicornuate uterus), uterine scarring (e.g., prior cesarean delivery), multiple gestations, multiparity, increasing maternal age, and smoking. Fetal macrosomia, which occurs from growth in the second half of pregnancy, is not related to placentation.

22-3. B. Abnormal placentation of placenta previa is associated with placenta accreta in approximately 5% of cases. In patients with a prior C/S, this rate increases to 25%; with three or more C/S, the rate is ≥50%. Placenta accreta is invasion of the placenta beyond the uterine endometrium and even into the myometrium or beyond. In particular, a placenta increta extends into the myometrium and a placenta percreta extends outside of the uterine serosa. This extension/ invasion can occur into the bowel, bladder, or rarely the pelvic vasculature. There is no association of placenta previa with uterine rupture, placental abruption, or a female fetus. There is no association with a successful trial of labor after C/S because all patients with placenta previa deliver via C/S.

22-4. D. A routine aspect of any obstetric ultrasound is placentation. If the lower aspect of the placenta is difficult to see transabdominally, it can be examined more closely using a translabial or transvaginal probe. The placenta implants early in pregnancy and does not grow to cover more surface of the uterine cavity. However, it is possible for portions of it to infarct and thus seemingly shrink. Finally, if the bladder is full during the obstetric ultrasound, it can compress the lower uterine segments together and make a lowlying placenta look like a previa. However, the opposite is not true.

SUGGESTED ADDITIONAL READING

Taipale P, Orden MR, Berg M, et al. Prenatal diagnosis of placenta accreta and percreta with ultrasonography, color Doppler, and magnetic resonance imaging. *Obstet Gynecol.* 2004;104:537–540.

Ananth CV, Smulian JC, Vintzileos AM. The effect of placenta previa on neonatal mortality: a population-based study in the United States, 1989 through 1997. *Am J Obstet Gynecol.* 2003;188:1299–1304.

Faiz AS, Ananth CV. Etiology and risk factors for placenta previa: an overview and meta-analysis of observational studies. *J Matern Fetal Neonatal Med.* 2003;13:175–190.

III

Labor and
Delivery

Leaking Fluid II—Epidemiology and Biostatistics

ID/CC: A 32-year-old G_1P_0 woman at 39 weeks GA presents with complaint of fluid leakage occurring 2 hours ago.

HPI: M.R. has had an uncomplicated pregnancy. Two hours ago, she felt a gush of fluid that soaked her pants and dining room chair seat. Since then, she has noted continued leakage of small amounts of clear fluid. She has noticed mild cramping over the past hour, but no vaginal bleeding, fevers, or chills. She also notes normal fetal movement.

PMHx/PSHx: Mild asthma

Meds: PNV, albuterol inhaler PRN

All: Penicillin

POb/GynHx: Unremarkable.

SHx: M.R. is a senior medical resident; her husband is a molecular biologist. No ethanol, tobacco, or illicit drug use.

THOUGHT QUESTIONS

- What type of vaginal exam should you do?
- What are the tests for amniotic fluid?
- If the bag of water is ruptured, what might be the plan of management?

If this patient has ruptured membranes, you do not want to increase her risk for infection by performing a digital vaginal exam. Therefore, an exam using a sterile speculum is performed. On this exam, you look for evidence of rupture. The three "tests" for amniotic fluid are pooling (pool of fluid in the vagina or generated with patient Valsalva), the phenaphthazine (Nitrazine) test (Nitrazine paper is yellow and turns blue when exposed to the basic pH of amniotic fluid), and the fern test (amniotic fluid reveals a ferning pattern when dried on a slide).

In the setting of rupture of membranes prior to onset of labor known as premature rupture of membranes (PROM), most commonly the management is to effect the onset of labor in this setting known as induction or augmentation of labor.

     ### CASE CONTINUED

VS: Temp 98.0°F. BP 120/74, HR 80, RR 16

PE: *Gen:* NAD. *Abdomen:* soft, nontender. *SSE:* cervix appears closed, positive pooling of clear yellow fluid, positive Nitrazine, positive ferning. *FHT:* 130s, reactive, no decelerations. *Toco:* no uterine contractions.

Sonogram: vertex presentation, AFI 6.0.

Given the setting of PROM, you offer to admit Dr. R. for induction of labor with oxytocin. She balks at the idea of intervention and wants to know about other options. In particular, she is interested in minimal intervention and is concerned that such intervention will increase her risk for cesarean delivery or harm to her baby. Her husband inquires whether you have any epidemiologic evidence to support the plan you have made for management.

THOUGHT QUESTIONS

- What types of epidemiologic studies are performed to answer clinical questions?
- What types of biostatistical tests are used to compare proportions? means?

■ If a study finds no difference between two management plans, what is the measure of certainty that no difference actually exists?

Epidemiologic studies are undertaken to ascertain disease frequency, distributions, and determinants within populations of subjects, to identify risk factors for disease, and to examine whether different treatments are effective. Many types of studies can be performed, each having different strengths and weaknesses.

Case-control studies begin with collecting a group with the disease (cases) and a group without the disease (controls). Other data about these patients, particularly concerning exposure to a particular factor of interest, then can be collected and compared. These designs are useful when studying relatively rare diseases. Case-control studies are more commonly retrospective in nature because the outcome of interest has already occurred and can be identified.

In *cohort studies*, subjects initially are classified according to the presence of an exposure and then followed for a length of time to ascertain the development of a particular disease. This design is best for investigating relatively common diseases or the risks associated with rare exposures because sufficient data can be gathered in a relatively short time. These types of studies may be retrospective or prospective in nature. In *retrospective studies,* the study can be started after both the exposure and the disease have occurred, whereas in *prospective studies* exposed and nonexposed subjects are identified and then followed over time to ascertain disease development. Prospective studies are by their nature more complex, time consuming, and expensive to perform but are very useful for identifying possible risk factors.

In *interventional studies,* the investigator purposely intervenes. The study may entail the allocation of a particular exposure but more commonly examines the efficacy of a particular treatment. Patients then are followed prospectively, and their outcomes are measured, noted, and analyzed. An interventional study may involve just the treatment of all patients with a particular disease to determine how they respond; however, these studies often are randomized so that some patients are treated and others are not. This allows the results of the study to show that the efficacy of treatment is related to the treatment itself rather than to confounding factors.

The "gold standard" of these types of studies is the prospective, double-blind, *randomized, placebo-controlled trial*. In this study design, the subjects are randomized to either an exposed (treatment) group or a nonexposed (placebo) group, which allows these types of studies to provide reliable evidence of causation or prevention. A placebo should be identical to the treatment pill in shape, size, and color. Randomization allows for control of other factors that may affect investigation except the specific exposure under investigation. These factors are controlled for whether or not the investigator can identify them. The differences in survival rates between the two treatment groups then are compared. The *double-blind* description refers to the concept that neither the patient nor the physicians running the study know who received the treatment. This can be difficult to achieve when there are obvious side effects from medications or particularly involved surgeries. The blinding of a study is important because it has been shown that simply being told you will be receiving a treatment has been shown to have an effect on outcomes. Although randomized, placebo-controlled trials (RCTs) are the best scientific approach to many questions, they often are prohibitive in terms of both time and cost.

One of the fundamental purposes of biostatistics is to be able to compare the summary statistics of two or more groups and determine the likelihood that the two groups are different. When measuring the central tendency of a distribution of a variable, often means and medians are used. With a normal distribution, the two are the same, and usually the means are compared. In order to compare two means, usually the Student *t*-test is used. Another way to analyze outcomes is to compare the proportion of a population that has achieved some outcome or threshold. In this setting, the common comparator is the chi-square test.

Finally, when considering studies, it is important to think of the results not as absolute but of possibly making one of two types of errors. Results essentially can fall into one of four categories: true positive, true negative, false positive, or false negative. The first two mean that the results indicated by the study are correct. A false-positive result is known as a *type I error*. This is what researchers attempt to avoid by having the null hypothesis rejected only if it falls outside of a 95% confidence interval or using a $p < 0.05$ standard in statistical tests. A false-negative result is known as *type II error*. Unfortunately, the standards used to examine type II error are poorer. Many studies with negative results do not report the probability of a type II error. The probability of not making a type II error is known as *power*. Compared to the <5% chance of making a type I error, commonly the standard for making a type II error is <20%, or only 80% power. One of the reasons for this is that many times to ensure a negative finding it is not worth the cost of increasing the sample size to ensure greater power. For the purposes of clinicians, it is important to understand these issues and the statistical tests used to compare outcomes.

CASE CONTINUED

You discuss the existing literature with Dr. R. and her husband. The best study on the topic is a randomized controlled trial of several thousand women with PROM who were randomized to induction versus watchful waiting. This study found that the length of labor and rate of cesarean delivery were the same between the two groups; however, the rate of chorioamnionitis was higher in the expectant management group. Many other cohort studies suggest that length of ROM longer than 16 to 18 hours predisposes to higher risk for infection. Given these results, Dr. R. decides to proceed with induction of labor.

QUESTIONS

23-1. Which of the following is increased in the setting of SROM as compared to patients with spontaneous labor?
   A. Cesarean delivery
   B. Length of labor
   C. Chorioamnionitis
   D. Placental abruption
   E. Operative vaginal delivery

23-2. Which of the following will lead to the longest ROM to delivery interval in the setting of PROM?
   A. Oxytocin
   B. Misoprostol
   C. Dinoprostone (Cervidil)
   D. PGE$_2$ gel
   E. Expectant management

23-3. You want to examine whether acupuncture can be used to induce labor. You know that 5% of the women who deliver at your hospital use acupuncture in pregnancy. Given your lack of funding and limited research time, what would be the first type of study you might perform to examine this question?

    A. Case-control study

    B. Cohort study of all pregnant women

    C. Prospective RCT

    D. Descriptive study of women receiving acupuncture

    E. Descriptive study of all women in labor

23-4. Your preliminary study found some intriguing results, and you applied for and received a large RO1 grant from the National Institutes of Health (NIH). In your study design of the intervention, you wanted to rule out the effect of physician bias and treating the experimental and control groups differently. What type of study would best accomplish this?

    A. Cohort study of all pregnant women and use of multivariate analyses

    B. Randomized, double-blind trial

    C. Randomized, placebo-controlled trial

    D. Randomized, single-blind trial with sham acupuncture

    E. Cohort study of pregnant women with a placebo control group

ANSWERS

23-1. C. Women with SROM are more likely to have prolonged ROM and therefore have slightly higher rates of chorioamnionitis overall. Given that length of labor is measured from the beginning of regular uterine contractions, these women have similar length of labor to those without SROM, although they will have a longer ROM to delivery time. The rates of cesarean delivery, placental abruption, and operative vaginal delivery have not been demonstrated to differ between the two groups.

23-2. E. Women with induction or augmentation in the setting of PROM have the same length of labor as those with expectant management, as the length of labor is measured from the onset of regular uterine contractions. Women with expectant management have a longer time interval to the onset of uterine contractions and therefore have a longer ROM to delivery time interval. This likely is a component of the etiology for the higher rate of chorioamnionitis.

Whether these patients are treated with oxytocin or prostaglandin agents, no difference in the length of labor has been demonstrated.

23-3. A. To best examine an exposure that occurs to a small minority of the population in an inexpensive fashion, case-control studies often are the study design used. In this case of 5% of your population receiving acupuncture, even if you obtained five controls for every case examined, you would only need 30% of the patients who would be examined in a cohort study, thus requiring less time for chart review and data collection and analysis. Although an RCT is the gold standard of study designs, it would be much too expensive as the initial pilot study to examine this question. Descriptive studies are fine for determining rates of complications but do not examine differences between interventions or exposures.

23-4. B. In order to remove physician bias from an RCT, a double-blind study design must be used. Generally, *single blind* means that the patient is unaware of what group they are assigned to, whereas *double blind* means that both the patient and clinician are unaware. In the setting of trials using drugs, this is readily accomplished using placebo pills or solutions. However, in the setting of procedures this is more difficult. In the study described, sham acupuncture, which involves a treatment that is not designed to induce labor, would be the best way to accomplish patient blinding. The best way to accomplish physician blinding would be to have a clinician who is not providing the obstetric care provide the acupuncture treatment. Multivariate analysis can control for potential confounding factors, particularly those that are readily measured, such as patient age, race, or medical history. However, it is difficult to control for physician bias, which cannot be easily measured.

 ### SUGGESTED ADDITIONAL READING

Glantz SA. *Primer of Biostatistics* (Paperback). McGraw-Hill Medical; 6th ed, 2005.

Cummings SR, Browner WS, Grady D, Hearst N, Newman TB, Hulley SB. *Designing Clinical Research: An Epidemiologic Approach* (Paperback). Lippincott Williams & Wilkins; 2nd ed, 2001.

Postterm Pregnancy

ID/CC: A 27-year-old G_1P_0 woman at 41 3/7 weeks GA presents for antenatal testing.

HPI: L.O. has had an uncomplicated pregnancy except for nausea and vomiting that lasted until 18 weeks gestation. Since then she has been fine and has gained 28 lb during the pregnancy. When she was seen most recently 4 days earlier for antenatal testing, she had a reactive nonstress test (NST) with no decelerations and an amniotic fluid index (AFI) of 11. Today she presents with occasional contractions that occur more at night, normal fetal movement, and no complaints of vaginal bleeding or leaking fluid.

PMHx: Mild asthma

Meds: PNV, albuterol metered-dose inhaler (MDI)

All: NKDA

POb/GynHx: G_1P_0

SHx: Lives with husband; no domestic violence. No ethanol, tobacco, or recreational drug use.

VS: Temp 98.4°F, BP 122/74, HR 84, RR 16

PE: *Abdomen:* soft, nontender, no distension with gravid uterus, fundal height = 40 cm. *SVE:* 1 cm long, −2 station, midposition, firm. *FHT:* 140s, reactive, no decelerations. *Toco:* one contraction seen.

US: AFI 3.2.

THOUGHT QUESTIONS

- Is her testing reassuring or nonreassuring?
- As far as the cervix is concerned, is it inducible? What is the Bishop score?

Ms. O. has presented for antenatal testing at 41 3/7 weeks gestation. A variety of regimens are used for antenatal testing around the country, but most involve one or more of the following:

1. *Nonstress test* (NST). This is an FHT assessment that is considered reactive (reassuring) if it has two accelerations ≥15 bpm over the baseline lasting for at least 15 seconds over a 20-minute period.
2. *Biophysical profile* (BPP). Can be considered with or without the NST. The ultrasound component of the BPP consists of evaluation of fetal movement, fetal tone, fetal breathing movements, and amniotic fluid. Each component is worth two points each, and no partial credit is given.
3. *Modified BPP.* An NST plus a check of the amniotic fluid usually is done as an AFI, which is the sum of four measurements, one taken in each quadrant of the patient's abdomen of the largest vertical pocket of fluid (measured in centimeters) in that quadrant. Normal AFI ranges from 5 to 20. An index <5 is considered oligohydramnios and >20 is considered polyhydramnios.
4. *Oxytocin challenge test* (OCT) or *contraction stress test* (CST). This test involves giving the patient intravenous oxytocin until she experiences three contractions in 10 minutes and then observing the FHT for fetal heart rate decelerations associated with contractions. A negative/reassuring test has no decelerations and is indicative of a fetus that presumably can tolerate labor.

Ms. O. has a reactive NST, which is reassuring. However, she has oligohydramnios, which is nonreassuring, and she should be delivered. Her cervix is unfavorable, defined as a cervix that has a low probability of successful induction and therefore may require agents to effect preinduction cervical ripening. One scale that is used to assess the cervix is the Bishop scoring system (Table 24-1). If the Bishop score is ≤4, the cervix is considered unfavorable; a score of 5 to 9 is moderately favorable; and ≥10 is very favorable. Using Table 24-1, Ms. O.'s Bishop score is 1 for dilation, 1 for station, and 1 for position, for a total score of 3.

TABLE 24-1 Determining the Bishop Score

Points Given	0	1	2	3
Dilation (cm)	Closed	1–2	3–4	≥5
Effacement (%)	0–30	40–50	60–70	≥80
Station	−3	−2	−1 or 0	≥1
Position	Posterior	Mid	Anterior	
Consistency	Firm	Medium	Soft	

Note: The Bishop score is the sum of the five categories.

CASE CONTINUED

Because of oligohydramnios, you counsel Ms. O. to undergo an induction of labor. Because of her unfavorable cervix, you discuss the possibility of using a prostaglandin for cervical ripening, to which she agrees. A prostaglandin gel is placed in the vagina two times, 4 hours apart, during which time the fetus is monitored and has a reassuring heart tracing. Her cervix changes to 1 cm, 50%, −2 station, midposition, soft consistency. Her Bishop score now is 6, and Ms. O is begun on IV oxytocin (Pitocin) and achieves a contraction pattern of every 2 to 3 minutes upon reaching a continuous infusion of 12 mu/min. Two hours later, her exam reveals she is 3 cm dilated, and you perform an artificial rupture of the membranes (AROM) to further augment her labor, which reveals moderately thick meconium-stained fluid.

QUESTIONS

24-1. Which of the following is not associated with meconium-stained fluid?
   A. Endomyometritis
   B. Meconium aspiration syndrome
   C. Oligohydramnios
   D. Preterm labor
   E. Postterm pregnancy

24-2. Which of the following point deductions from the BPP is most consistent with a long-standing issue?
   A. Absent fetal movement
   B. Absent fetal tone
   C. Fetal breathing movement
   D. Amniotic fluid
   E. Nonreactive NST

24-3. Which of the following prostaglandin preparations is not used for cervical ripening?
   A. PGE_2 gel
   B. $PGF_{2\alpha}$
   C. PGE_{1M} (misoprostol) vaginally
   D. PGE_2 suppository
   E. PGE_{1M} orally

24-4. During the labor of this patient with oligohydramnios and meconium, which of the following would not be an indication for use of an intrauterine pressure catheter (IUPC)?
   A. Amnioinfusion for recurrent variable decelerations
   B. Amnioinfusion for moderate meconium
   C. Amnioinfusion for recurrent late decelerations
   D. Difficulty measuring contractions because of maternal obesity
   E. To assess strength of contractions

ANSWERS

24-1. D. Meconium, the fetus's first bowel movement, can cause meconium aspiration syndrome when the meconium travels to the neonate's lungs as a result of aspiration in utero or at birth. It also has been associated with higher rates of infection during and after delivery of the uterus. Meconium is more commonly seen in pregnancies complicated by events that lead to fetal stress, such as cocaine use, infection, or chronic hypertension. It also is seen more with post-dates pregnancies and with oligohydramnios. It is not commonly associated with preterm labor or delivery.

24-2. D. All of the other findings on the BPP speak to the current status of the fetus. If the mother has taken an opioid minutes before the BPP, there likely will be reduced fetal movement, fetal tone, fetal breathing motion, and a nonreactive NST, but the amniotic fluid will be normal. Alternatively, in a fetus with a placenta whose function is diminishing over time, the fetus may acutely look good on the ultrasound, but the amniotic fluid will be low. Using the modified BPP (NST plus AFI), both the acute and the chronic issues are examined. Remember that two points are assigned for each of the five categories of the BPP, so scores range from 0/10 to 10/10 and include only the even numbers. Management based upon the BPP often is situation dependent. However, in a term pregnancy, scores from 0 to 4 usually are managed by delivery. A score of 0 or 2 may require immediate delivery, again depending on the clinical situation. A score of 6/10 usually is managed by repeat testing in a shorter interval than would normally be used for testing. For example, if on labour and delivery (L&D), then repeat in 6 hours. If antepartum testing, then consider repeat in the next 24 hours. Scores of 8/10 and 10/10 are considered reassuring results.

24-3. B. Until recently, only PGE_2 was used for cervical ripening. Its most common application was in gel form, placed intravaginally every 4 to 6 hours. The next preparation brought into use was dinoprostone (Cervidil), an intravaginal suppository also containing PGE_2. This preparation was placed intravaginally and could be left in for up to 12 hours. The suppository was attached to netting and a string for easy removal. More recently, misoprostol (PGE_{1M} [Cytotec]) has been studied for use as a cervical ripening agent. Case reports and small trials have demonstrated that misoprostol at higher doses increased rates of uterine hyperstimulation. However, this effect has not been seen with the 25-μg dose. $PGF_{2\alpha}$ (Prostin) is not used for cervical ripening but rather is used postpartum in patients with uterine atony and hemorrhage.

24-4. C. An IUPC is placed into the uterus via the vagina for two essential purposes: (1) to measure and time contractions and (2) to be used as a conduit for infusion of normal saline into the amniotic cavity. The first use is important for a patient who is not making adequate cervical progress during the active phase of labor. The differential diagnosis in this situation includes the three Ps. Either the fetus (Passenger) will not fit through the pelvis (Passage), or the contractions are not strong enough (Power). In the latter case, the strength of the uterine contractions must be quantified via calculation of Montevideo units and, if determined to be inadequate, uterine contraction augmentation with oxytocin should be considered. The second use of amnioinfusion is to dilute meconium, which decreases the rate of meconium aspiration leading to meconium seen below the vocal chords upon intubation in randomized trials.

Amnioinfusion also is used in the presence of repetitive variable decelerations, indicative of umbilical cord compression, particularly in the setting of known oligohydramnios. However, infusing fluid into the uterine cavity is unlikely to help in the setting of late decelerations, which are caused by uteroplacental insufficiency.

 ### SUGGESTED ADDITIONAL READING

Hannah ME, Hannah WJ, Hellmann J, et al. Induction of labor as compared with serial antenatal monitoring in post-term pregnancy. A randomized controlled trial. The Canadian Multicenter Post-term Pregnancy Trial Group. *N Engl J Med.* 1992;326:1587–1592.

Sanchez-Ramos L, Olivier F, Delke I, et al. Labor induction versus expectant management for postterm pregnancies: a systematic review with meta-analysis. *Obstet Gynecol.* 2003;101:1312–1318.

Ghey AB, Washington AE, Laros RK Jr. Neonatal complications of term pregnancy: rates by gestational age increase in a continuous, not threshold, fashion. *Am J Obstet Gynecol.* 2005;192:185–190.

Tran SH, Caughey AB, Musci TJ. Meconium-stained amniotic fluid is associated with puerperal infections. *Am J Obstet Gynecol.* 2003;189:746–750.

Poor Progress During Labor

ID/CC: A 38-year-old G_1P_0 woman at 41 weeks GA in active labor with no cervical change in 2 hours.

HPI: B.D. presented to labor and delivery at 5-cm dilation, 100% effacement, and −2 station. Her contractions were 3 minutes apart and painful. At the time of admission, she was ruled in for rupture of membranes and stated that she had been leaking fluid for approximately 2 days. She also stated that she had been having contractions every 10 to 15 minutes during the previous 24 hours. In the hospital, she progressed normally to 8-cm dilation and −1 station but remained there for 2 hours. During this time she developed a fever of 101.0°F and was diagnosed with chorioamnionitis. Ms. D is discouraged about the last two exams being the same and asks, "Doctor, am I going to need a C/S?"

PMHx: Moderate obesity

PSHx: Appendectomy

Meds: PNV

All: NKDA

POb/GynHx: Gestational diabetes mellitus (GDM), class A2 (insulin controlled). The patient was found to be diabetic at 28 weeks gestation. She was poorly controlled by diet and was started on insulin at 34 weeks.

SHx: Lives with father of baby. Denies use of tobacco; occasional use of ethanol.

VS: Temp 101.4°F, BP 100/60, HR 100, RR 16

PE: *Finger stick blood sugar:* 78. *FHT:* 170s, moderate variability, no decelerations. *Toco:* contractions every 3 minutes. *Abdomen:* estimated fetal weight (EFW) by Leopold maneuvers = 3,900 g. *SVE:* 8-cm dilation, 100% effacement, −1 station. The position, left occiput transverse (LOT), based on the location of the sagittal suture and fontanelles, is depicted in Figure 25-1.

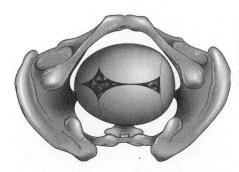

FIGURE 25-1.
Left occiput transverse position, with the posterior fontanelle to the **left** and the anterior fontanelle to the **right.**

THOUGHT QUESTIONS

- What is "normal" labor for a nulliparous versus a multiparous patient?
- What are at least three reasons to explain this patient's lack of progress?
- How could you evaluate the origins of this patient's labor pattern?
- Does she need a cesarean delivery?

      Labor is divided into several stages: the first stage is from the onset of contractions until full dilation; the second stage is from full dilation until delivery of the fetus; and the third stage is from delivery of the fetus until delivery of the placenta. Some have called the first hour after delivery of the placenta the fourth stage. The first stage of labor is further divided into latent and active phases, which are demarcated by an increase in the rate of dilation that usually occurs when the cervix is dilated between 3 and 4 cm.

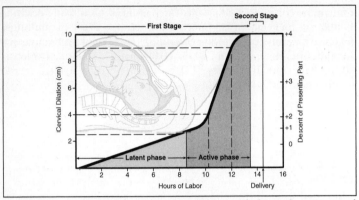

FIGURE 25-2. Friedman labor curve (created in 1961) shows the progress of labor, with cervical dilation plotted versus time.

Abnormal or protracted labor in a nulliparous patient without an epidural is defined as follows: latent phase lasting >20 hours, active phase with <1.2-cm dilation each hour or descent <1 cm per hour, or second stage >2 hours (3 hours with an epidural). In a multiparous patient, prolonged latent phase is defined as >14-hour duration, active phase with <1.5-cm dilation each hour or <2 cm descent per hour, or second stage >1 hour (2 hours with an epidural). These are the values for the 5th percentile; thus, 95% of patients will have a labor course faster than these values. The Friedman curve describes this in graphical form (Figure 25-2).

This patient's current protracted labor course may be explained by large fetal weight (her risk factors for this include maternal obesity and GDM), chorioamnionitis leading to inadequate forces, and malpresentation. To evaluate the etiology, an intrauterine pressure catheter (IUPC) should be placed to measure the force of the contractions. An external tocometer only indicates the timing and length of contractions; it does not quantify the strength. More than 70% of patients who stop making cervical change for 2 hours with inadequate forces measured by an IUPC and who then are started on oxytocin (Pitocin) will go on to have a vaginal delivery.

 CASE CONTINUED

An IUPC is placed revealing uterine forces of 120 Montevideo (MV) units (the sum of the pressures due to contractions over 10 minutes). Because contractions generally need to be more than 180 to 200 MV units to be considered adequate, the patient is started on Pitocin to help her achieve adequate forces. After 2 hours of adequate forces, she is rechecked and found to be completely dilated and –1 station. In addition, the fetal head now is in the occiput anterior position.

 QUESTIONS

25-1. What is the correct order of the cardinal movements of labor?
A. Flexion, descent, engagement, internal rotation, extension, external rotation
B. Flexion, engagement, internal rotation, descent, extension, external rotation
C. Descent, engagement, flexion, internal rotation, external rotation, extension
D. Engagement, flexion, descent, external rotation, extension, internal rotation
E. Engagement, flexion, descent, internal rotation, extension, external rotation

25-2. What is the diagnosis for this patient if she failed to dilate despite adequate forces?
A. Arrest of dilation
B. Arrest of descent
C. Protracted labor
D. Malpresentation
E. Slow slope active

25-3. After pushing for 3 hours in the second stage, the fetus does not descend beyond –1 station. The patient is exhausted and requests assistance. What is the most appropriate next step?
A. Continue pushing
B. Vacuum-assisted vaginal delivery
C. Forceps-assisted vaginal delivery
D. Forceps-assisted rotation to the occiput posterior position
E. Cesarean delivery

25-4. Consider instead that after pushing for 3 hours with epidural anesthesia, the fetus descends from −1 to +1 station but not beyond that. EFW is 4,800 g by Leopold's maneuvers and ultrasound. The fetal position is left occiput anterior, and the patient has epidural anesthesia. What is the most appropriate next step?

A. Continue pushing
B. Vacuum-assisted vaginal delivery
C. Forceps-assisted vaginal delivery
D. Forceps-assisted rotation to the occiput posterior position
E. Cesarean delivery

ANSWERS

25-1. E. The cardinal movements of labor begin with engagement as the fetal head enters the pelvis. As the head flexes, the smallest diameter of the head presents and descent is accomplished. The head is in the occiput transverse position until it undergoes internal rotation to the occiput anterior or posterior (the former is ideal) position. As the fetal head is pushed through the birth canal it extends to pass beneath and around the symphysis pubis. Once the head is pushed out, restitution or external rotation occurs and the head can be seen to shift to face laterally.

25-2. A. Arrest of dilation is defined as no dilation despite 2 hours of adequate forces. Adequate forces are considered 180 to 200 MV units. MV units are measured as the sum of the pressure differences during contractions from the baseline resting uterine tone to the peak of a contraction measured in mm Hg over a 10-minute period (as measured by an IUPC). Similarly, arrest of descent refers to no descent of the fetus in the pelvis despite adequate forces. The descent of the fetus is measured by station, where station is defined as the number of centimeters above (−) or below (+) the ischial spines. Protracted labor is nonspecific, that is, slow or arrest of progress without a description of adequate forces. Slow slope active course applies to an active phase that is protracted but again is nonspecific and does not specify forces. Malpresentation refers to an abnormal presentation of the fetus, for example, in the transverse presentation.

25-3. E.

25-4. E. Cesarean delivery is the recommended mode for both of these scenarios. Very specific criteria should be met before an assisted delivery with vacuum or forceps is performed. First, the fetal station must be +2 or lower to be a low operative delivery or 0 to +2 for a midpelvic delivery. Poor neonatal outcomes have been associated with deliveries of the fetus from above 0 station. Most practitioners prefer the station to be lower than 0 to +1 before offering an operative vaginal delivery. In addition, the practitioner must know the fetal position to correctly apply the assisting device, the bladder must be emptied to avoid trauma, and the patient must have adequate anesthesia. Finally, EFW should not be greater than 4,000 to 4,500 g unless the patient has previously delivered a baby of comparable size without injury (this is somewhat controversial). In Question 25-3, the indication for cesarean delivery is the high station. Even if the patient wishes to achieve vaginal birth via operative vaginal delivery, in the United States, high operative deliveries are rarely, if ever, performed other than in an extreme emergency. In Question 25-4, the indication for cesarean delivery is the high EFW in conjunction with failure to progress beyond +1 station. In the second scenario, shoulder dystocia is the main risk of attempting an assisted delivery of a baby this size in a mother with diabetes. Shoulder dystocia, the inability of the shoulders to be delivered secondary to fetopelvic disproportion, can be a catastrophic event causing great morbidity to the neonate. Rotation to the occiput posterior position is not an option as the occiput anterior position is preferred.

 ## SUGGESTED ADDITIONAL READING

Vahratian A, Zhang J, Hasling J, et al. The effect of early epidural versus early intravenous analgesia use on labor progression: a natural experiment. *Am J Obstet Gynecol.* 2004;191:259–265.

Zhang J, Troendle JF, Yancey MK. Reassessing the labor curve in nulliparous women. *Am J Obstet Gynecol.* 2002;187:824–828.

Nonreassuring Fetal Testing—Fetal Heart Rate Decelerations

ID/CC: A 23-year-old G_6P_2 woman at 36 weeks GA is brought in by ambulance with complaints of vaginal bleeding and contractions.

HPI: H.A. began experiencing contractions approximately 4 hours ago. The contractions increased in intensity over the ensuing 1 to 2 hours, and at that time she noticed in the toilet some bright red blood that kept passing out of her vagina for the next 2 hours. At that point, she called the ambulance. She notes no leaking of clear fluid and notices that the fetus has been overly active. She has been to prenatal care appointments only occasionally. Her first appointment was at 22 weeks, when she had normal lab results. She had one other appointment at 29 weeks, when she had a normal 1-hour glucose loading test. She is an active user of crack cocaine and, upon further questioning, admits to using the drug approximately 6 hours ago.

PMHx/PSHx: Substance abuse, primarily cocaine

Meds: PNVs

All: NKDA

POb/GynHx: Two prior term NSVDs, three prior TABs

SHx: Father of baby not involved; she lives on the streets and both of her children have been placed into foster care; she occasionally trades sex for money or drugs. Occasional ethanol and tobacco use; frequent crack cocaine use (at least daily).

VS: Temp 98.0°F, BP 166/83, HR 92, RR 20

PE: *Gen:* NAD. *Lungs:* CTAB. *Abdomen:* soft, nontender, no distension with gravid uterus, size = dates, palpable contractions. *SSE:* old blood and clots in vault, no active bleeding from cervix. *SVE:* cervix 1 cm dilated, 50% effaced, −2 station. *FHT:* 140s, nonreactive, moderate variability, occasional decelerations after contractions. *Toco:* contractions every 1 to 2 minutes.

THOUGHT QUESTIONS

- What are the primary issues of concern in this patient?
- What unifying diagnosis encompasses all of the concerning issues?
- What laboratory tests should be ordered?

          In this patient, the issues that are of most concern are (1) her vaginal bleeding, (2) fetal heart rate decelerations, (3) blood pressure of 166/83, and (4) history of crack cocaine use. Each of the first three issues should bring several conditions to mind. For example, vaginal bleeding in the third trimester can be related to placenta previa, placental abruption, or labor. However, cocaine abuse leading to uterine contractions and placental abruption brings all of these findings into one etiology.

Although Ms. A.'s cocaine use likely is the cause of her elevated blood pressure, preeclampsia still should be ruled out by ordering lab tests that include CBC, LFTs (AST, ALT), LDH (for hemolysis), and a creatinine level. Because of her vaginal bleeding and the concern for abruption, a set of coagulation factors in addition to the CBC should be ordered. Also, a Kleihauer-Betke test for fetal blood in the maternal circulation is a good idea. Her urine should be sent for protein and toxicology screens.

CASE CONTINUED

The patient's initial lab results return.

Labs: Hct 32.1; WBC 9.7; Plts 189,000; AST/ALT 18/22; LDH 476; PT/PTT/INR 12.3/33.6/1.1; Cr 0.5; Kleihauer-Betke: pending; urine dipstick: trace protein; tox: pending

The lab results do not suggest preeclampsia. However, because of the patient's elevated blood pressure, you begin a 24-hour urine collection to quantitate the proteinuria. Over the next hour, the patient's contractions become less frequent, every 2 to 3 minutes, but stronger in intensity. The patient asks for pain medicine, and you check the cervix. It now is 3 cm dilated, 80% effaced, and −1 station, and you notice more vaginal bleeding. The fetal heart tracing is shown in Figure 26-1.

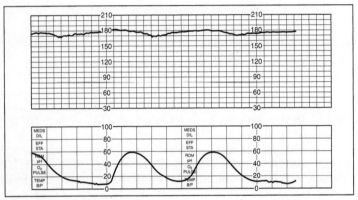

FIGURE 26-1. Fetal heart tracing.

 QUESTIONS

26-1. Describe the fetal heart tracing:
A. Bradycardia with intermittent accelerations, moderate variability
B. Bradycardia with intermittent accelerations, minimal variability
C. Normal fetal heart rate with minimal variability and late decelerations
D. Fetal tachycardia with minimal variability and late decelerations
E. Fetal tachycardia with minimal variability and early decelerations

26-2. Which of the following is the best next step in management?
A. Urgent cesarean section
B. Elective cesarean section
C. Forceps delivery
D. Augmentation of labor
E. Begin magnesium sulfate for seizure prophylaxis

26-3. When the fetus is delivered, what do you expect to see regarding the placenta?
A. Placenta previa
B. Vasa previa
C. Adherent clot on the posterior placental surface
D. Placenta adherent to the uterus
E. Placenta accreta

26-4. Which of the following substances has not been associated with fetal abnormalities including developmental delay?
A. Cocaine
B. Alcohol
C. Marijuana
D. Benzodiazepines
E. Phenobarbital

 ANSWERS

26-1. D. A fetal heart rate tracing (FHT) is best read systematically, with specific attention paid to the baseline heart rate, variability, accelerations, decelerations, and timing of the decelerations with contractions. The normal fetal heart rate is between 110 and 160 bpm. Variability historically has been categorized as short-term and long-term variability. Now, many providers tend to examine only short-term variability and refer to it simply as variability, which is indicative of fetal ability to withstand insults. FHT then is evaluated for the presence of accelerations in fetal heart rate and whether FHT is formally reactive (the presence of two accelerations of at least 15 bpm over the baseline lasting at least 15 seconds in a 20-minute period). Decelerations, if present, are described in terms of their length and how low they descend. Their timing is associated with contractions. If the deceleration begins and ends with the contraction, it is designated an *early deceleration* and is associated with fetal head compression. If the deceleration begins at or beyond the midpoint of the contraction and does not begin to resolve until after the contraction ends, it is designated a *late deceleration*. This is a sign of poor placental perfusion during the contraction, which can be related to maternal hypotension, increased placental resistance, or decreased placenta–uterine interface. Variable decelerations, not mentioned in this question, are recognizable from their "V" shape. Any deceleration that reaches its nadir within 30 seconds of beginning is considered a *variable deceleration,* regardless of timing. These are commonly caused by compression of the umbilical cord. This FHT should be interpreted as tachycardic with a baseline in the 170s, with minimal variability and recurrent late decelerations. In Figure 26-1, FHR >160s baseline is worrisome, particularly in the setting of late decelerations.

26-2. A. This is a nonreassuring FHT with evidence of fetal tachycardia, minimal variability, and recurrent late decelerations. This patient is likely having an abruption, which is leading to decreased fetal oxygenation, particularly during the contractions. Because she is remote from vaginal delivery (cervix dilated only 3 cm), an urgent or emergent cesarean delivery should be performed. If she was fully dilated, an operative vaginal delivery would be another option.

26-3. C. This patient most likely has a placental abruption, which commonly manifests as a placenta that separates easily and has an adherent retroplacental clot. She is unlikely to have a placenta previa because there was no evidence on examination, although a marginal previa is always possible in these situations. A vasa previa, fetal blood vessel lying over the cervix, is unlikely, as the fetus would not have been likely to be viable given the amount of blood loss experienced by the patient. A placenta accreta, attachment of the placenta deeper than the endometrium and into the myometrium or beyond, is unlikely and inconsistent with this patient's history.

26-4. C. There is no systematic evidence that marijuana or its active ingredient tetrahydrocannabinol (THC) leads to fetal anomalies. Cocaine has been associated with developmental delay. Benzodiazepines and alcohol have been associated with fetal anomalies, specifically fetal alcohol syndrome. Phenobarbital use in patients with seizure disorders has been associated with both fetal anomalies and developmental delay.

SUGGESTED ADDITIONAL READING

Sameshima H, Ikenoue T, Ikeda T, et al. Unselected low-risk pregnancies and the effect of continuous intrapartum fetal heart rate monitoring on umbilical blood gases and cerebral palsy. *Am J Obstet Gynecol.* 2004;190:118–123.

Fox M, Kilpatrick S, King T, et al. Fetal heart rate monitoring: interpretation and collaborative management. *J Midwifery Womens Health.* 2000;45:498–507.

Siira SM, Ojala TH, Vahlberg TJ, et al. Marked fetal acidosis and specific changes in power spectrum analysis of fetal heart rate variability recorded during the last hour of labour. *BJOG.* 2005;112:418–423.

Klauser CK, Christensen EE, Chauhan SP, et al. Use of fetal pulse oximetry among high-risk women in labor: a randomized clinical trial. *Am J Obstet Gynecol.* 2005;192:1810–1817; discussion 1817–1819.

Prior Cesarean Section in Labor

ID/CC: A 29-year-old G_4P_1 woman at 38 weeks GA presents with frequent contractions.

HPI: K.R. presents with complaints of contractions that occur every 3 to 4 minutes and began 1 hour ago. She has not noticed any frank vaginal bleeding but did pass a brown clump from her vagina yesterday. She has not had any leak of clear fluid, and her fetus is very active. She has had an uncomplicated antepartum course and signed a consent form to undergo a trial of labor after cesarean (TOLAC) 2 weeks ago. She underwent a cesarean delivery in her last pregnancy because she failed to dilate past 7 cm.

PMHx/PSHx: C/S

Meds: PNV

All: NKDA

POb/GynHx: Term C/S for failure to progress (FTP) of 3,800-g infant 4 years ago, TAB 9 years ago, SAB 2 years ago

SHx: Lives with husband and 4-year-old daughter; no domestic violence. No ethanol, tobacco, or recreational drug use.

VS: Temp 97.6°F, BP 114/68, HR 74, RR 16

PE: *Gen:* NAD. *Lungs:* CTAB. *Abdomen:* soft, nontender, no distension with gravid uterus, size = dates. *SVE:* cervix 4 cm dilated, 90% effaced, +1 station, *Leopold maneuvers:* cephalic, 3,700 g. *FHT:* 140s, reactive, occasional variable deceleration to the 110s. *Toco:* contractions on monitor every 3 to 4 minutes.

Labs: Hct 36

THOUGHT QUESTIONS

- What is the biggest risk faced by this patient with a history of prior C/S?
- What is her approximate chance for successful vaginal delivery?
- How are patients with a prior C/S managed in labor?

The biggest risk Ms. R. faces is uterine rupture. Uterine rupture is reported to occur in 0.5% to 1% of patients undergoing a TOLAC. It is increased in patients who are induced, receive prostaglandin agents, and have more than one uterine scar. The risk of uterine rupture is decreased in patients who have had a prior vaginal delivery and who present in active labor.

On average, the overall probability of a patient achieving a vaginal birth after cesarean (VBAC) is approximately 70%. This probability is increased in patients who have a nonrecurring indication for their first cesarean (e.g., breech, herpes, previa) and in patients who have had a vaginal birth either prior or subsequent to cesarean delivery. Conversely, it is decreased in patients with a prior delivery for failure to progress and in patients who are being induced. Based on data from several recent case series associating prostaglandin agents with increased risk for uterine rupture, most clinicians will not use misoprostol as a cervical ripening agent in patients with a prior cesarean, and some clinicians will not use any prostaglandins at all. Oxytocin, although not conclusively associated with uterine rupture, usually is used with caution in these patients.

CASE CONTINUED

While in labor and delivery, Ms. R. makes reasonable progress, changing to 6 cm over the next 2 hours. At this point she requests an epidural, which is placed without complication. Two hours later, she is 8 cm dilated, +2 station, and her fetal heart tracing has recurrent variable decelerations. You place an intrauterine pressure catheter (IUPC) and begin an amnioinfusion. The fetal heart rate tracing improves and then, 30 minutes later, looks like Figure 27-1.

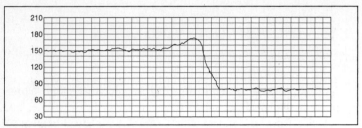

FIGURE 27-1. Fetal heart rate tracing.

 QUESTIONS

27-1. The next step in management is:
A. Adjust the IUPC
B. Immediate delivery
C. Augment with oxytocin (Pitocin)
D. Give terbutaline
E. Increase O_2 by face mask

27-2. The most worrisome finding on physical exam at this point would be:
A. Compound presentation
B. Complete cervical dilation
C. Fetal head no longer palpable
D. Contracted pelvis
E. Breech presentation

27-3. Which of the following is not an indication for C/S?
A. Previous C/S
B. Breech
C. No cervical change for 4 hours at 2 cm dilated
D. Fetal bradycardia
E. Placenta previa

27-4. The amnioinfusion was begun:
A. To decrease the recurrent variable decelerations
B. To dilute meconium
C. To cool the fetus down
D. To increase the strength of the contractions
E. To help measure the strength of the contractions

ANSWERS

27-1. B.

27-2. C. The patient's fetal heart tracing is not reassuring and actually quite worrisome. There is a prolonged deceleration that lasts for 6 minutes. The fetal heart rate variability is diminished, which indicates decreased fetal ability to withstand hypoxic insults. Either the decelerations must be stopped or the fetus must be delivered. If there was evidence of uterine hyperstimulation or a tetanic contraction, an SC shot of terbutaline could help relax the uterus. However, there is no evidence of either phenomenon by IUPC. To accomplish the delivery, an examination should be performed to assess cervical dilation, determine the most appropriate route of delivery, and assess for any evidence of uterine rupture. Signs and symptoms suggestive of uterine rupture include a previously palpable fetal head that now is floating or nonpalpable, vaginal bleeding, or maternal sensation of "popping" or abdominal pain. If the cervix is fully dilated, the fetus can be delivered via an operative delivery more quickly than via emergent C/S. However, if the patient is not fully dilated, an emergent C/S is indicated because uterine rupture carries significant morbidity and mortality for both the mother and the baby.

27-3. C. Indications for C/S include malpresentation (e.g., breech or transverse), nonreassuring fetal status (e.g., recurrent late decelerations, bradycardia), outbreak of genital herpes, failure to progress in the active phase of labor, fetal macrosomia, and having had a prior C/S or full-thickness myomectomy. A patient at 2 cm dilated has not yet entered the active phase of labor and may remain unchanged in the latent phase for many hours.

27-4. A. In general, amnioinfusions have been best studied with regard to their effect on reducing fetal meconium aspiration. In small studies, it has been shown that infusing 500 cc of normal saline into the uterine cavity in the setting of moderate or thick meconium presumably can dilute the meconium and reduce the amount of meconium seen below the vocal cords after delivery (i.e., reduce the amount/occurrence of meconium aspiration). Amnioinfusion also has been used in the setting of recurrent variable decelerations to help cushion the compromised cord by increasing the amount of fluid in the intrauterine environment, which is the situation in the present case. Amnioinfusion has never been used or studied to cool down the fetus, to measure the contractions, or to increase contractions.

 ## SUGGESTED ADDITIONAL READING

Landon MB, Hauth JC, Leveno KJ, et al. Maternal and perinatal outcomes associated with a trial of labor after prior cesarean delivery. *N Engl J Med.* 2004;351:2581–2589.

Zelop CM, Shipp TD, Repke JT, et al. Uterine rupture during induced or augmented labor in gravid women with one prior cesarean delivery. *Am J Obstet Gynecol.* 1999;181:882–886.

Sheiner E, Levy A, Ofir K, et al. Changes in fetal heart rate and uterine patterns associated with uterine rupture. *J Reprod Med.* 2004;49:373–378.

IV

Postpartum Period

Case 28

Postpartum Vaginal
Bleeding

Postpartum Vaginal Bleeding

ID/CC: A 34-year-old G_5P_5 woman presents with vaginal bleeding 3 hours after a vaginal delivery.

HPI: L.H. delivered a 4,000-g baby over a third-degree perineal laceration (tear into the anal sphincter) with a right vaginal sulcus tear (tear high into the posterolateral vaginal wall). Both lacerations were repaired, with use of local anesthesia. The labor was complicated by premature rupture of membranes and chorioamnionitis, but the labor course was normal. Estimated blood loss (EBL) was 400 cc.

Ms. H. was well until 3 hours after delivery, when she noted passage of several large clots and was found to be sitting in a pool of blood. She currently is complaining of moderate pelvic cramping and mild vaginal discomfort at the site of the repairs. She denies having rectal pain. She has been able to void 500 cc of urine since the delivery. You estimate that she has lost approximately 500 cc of blood in addition to the 400 cc she lost at the delivery.

PMHx/PSHx: None

Meds: Currently receiving IV oxytocin (Pitocin)

All: NKDA

POb/GynHx: Four prior term NSVDs

THOUGHT QUESTIONS

- What are the main causes of postpartum hemorrhage?
- How do you distinguish between each cause?
- For which conditions is this patient at particular risk?

Postpartum hemorrhage (PPH) is defined as blood loss of ≥500 cc after a vaginal delivery and ≥1,000 cc after a cesarean delivery. Common causes of immediate (within minutes of delivery) PPH include uterine atony, retained products of conception, vaginal laceration, and cervical laceration. Less common causes include placenta accreta, uterine inversion, uterine rupture, and coagulopathy. PPH that occurs more remote from delivery (1 hour to several weeks) may be caused by retained products of conception (POC), vaginal or retroperitoneal hematomas (although these result in concealed hemorrhage), and placental site subinvolution.

Distinguishing between each cause is achieved by careful examination and consideration of the patient's risk factors. Feeling the uterine fundus abdominally or doing a bimanual exam will help identify uterine atony. Inspection of the placenta will reveal whether a lobe or pieces of the placenta are missing. Examination of the vaginal walls and cervix can be difficult but is important. (Adequate exposure of the cervix requires appropriate retractors to retract the vaginal walls. A ring forceps then is used to grasp the anterior lip of the cervix. Using a second ring forceps, further cervical tissue is grasped and inspection of the cervix accomplished by "walking" along the cervix.) Inversion of the uterus occurs as the placenta delivers, dragging the attached uterus through the vagina. Placenta accreta is a diagnosis of exclusion, and women with a previous cesarean section scar and an anterior placenta are at high risk. Risk factors for atony include grand multiparity, macrosomia, and chorioamnionitis. Chorioamnionitis places this patient at risk for both immediate and delayed PPH because it can complicate the delivery of an intact placenta, placing the patient at risk for retained POC.

CASE CONTINUED

VS: Temp 99.8°F, BP 100/60, HR 115, RR 16

PE: *Gen:* pale, anxious. *Abdomen:* soft. Fundus 3 cm above the umbilicus and moderately tender. *GU:* perineal laceration appears intact. Sulcus tear cannot be evaluated secondary to patient discomfort.

Labs: (Prior to delivery) Hgb 10; Hct 33.2

The patient is taken back to the operating room. Repeat CBC is sent. Using conscious sedation, a careful examination is performed. The sulcus tear appears intact and hemostatic. The uterus is explored manually; 800 cc of clot and retained placental products are expressed. Under ultrasound guidance, gentle sharp curettage is performed to remove remaining placental products. Exam of the placenta expressed at delivery reveals a missing lobe. Final Hgb is 6.8, Hct 20.0.

QUESTIONS

28-1. Two hours after an NSVD, a patient complains of rectal pain. This is a potential presentation of which of the following?
   A. Nerve injury
   B. Cervical laceration
   C. Vaginal hematoma
   D. Breakdown of a perineal laceration
   E. Infection of a perineal laceration

28-2. Immediately after NSVD of a 4,000-g infant and delivery of an intact placenta, a patient is noted to have significant continued blood loss up to 700 cc. Her uterus is firm. What is the next source of bleeding to rule out?
   A. Retained POC
   B. Uterine inversion
   C. Cervical laceration
   D. Vaginal laceration
   E. Uterine atony

28-3. What is the most common cause of PPH?
A. Vaginal laceration
B. Perineal laceration
C. Uterine atony
D. Cervical laceration
E. Retained placental products

28-4. A preeclamptic (BP 168/102) patient delivers a 3,800-g infant. Immediately after delivery of the placenta, Pitocin is begun. Despite Pitocin and uterine massage, the uterus remains boggy and the patient continues to bleed. What medication should be given next to stop the bleeding?
A. Magnesium sulfate
B. Penicillin
C. Methylergonovine (Methergine)
D. Prostaglandin $F_{2\alpha}$ (Hemabate)
E. Pitocin IM

ANSWERS

28-1. C. Injury of a blood vessel without disruption of the overlying epithelium during delivery can lead to a contained (often concealed) bleed called a vaginal hematoma. As blood fills the adjacent space, pressure builds, causing vaginal or rectal pain. This is an important diagnosis because the condition can lead to significant and even life-threatening blood loss.

28-2. C. A cervical laceration should be suspected when bleeding is noted after delivery despite a firm uterus. A very small laceration or an exposed vessel may be repaired simply with 15 minutes of pressure to the area using a ring forceps. Larger lacerations should be repaired with suture. Of particular importance for larger lacerations is identification of the apex, because these lacerations may extend into the lower uterine segment and be hidden.

28-3. C. The most common cause of PPH is uterine atony. Risk factors include prolonged labor with Pitocin augmentation, macrosomia, multiple gestations, multiparity, chorioamnionitis, exposure to magnesium sulfate, and a previous history of atony. After delivery of the placenta, IV Pitocin is generally begun as prophylaxis for atony along with abdominal massage of the uterus. If the uterus remains boggy (and inspection of the placenta reveals it to be intact), bimanual massage is performed. If the patient continues to bleed and the uterus remains boggy, use of other medications should be considered. Uterotonic agents include oxytocin (Pitocin), methylergonovine (Methergine), 15-methyl-prostaglandin $F_{2\alpha}$ (Hemabate, Prostin), and misoprostol.

28-4. D. Methergine is contraindicated in hypertensive patients, and Hemabate is contraindicated in asthmatics. Therefore, the next medication to use in this patient is Hemabate. Side effects of the medication include nausea and diarrhea.

 SUGGESTED ADDITIONAL READING

Jackson KW Jr, Albert JR, Schemmer GK, et al. A randomized controlled trial comparing oxytocin administration before and after placental delivery in the prevention of postpartum hemorrhage. *Am J Obstet Gynecol.* 2001;185:873–877.

Gerstenfeld TS, Wing DA. Rectal misoprostol versus intravenous oxytocin for the prevention of postpartum hemorrhage after vaginal delivery. *Am J Obstet Gynecol.* 2001;185:878–882.

CASE 29

Postpartum Fever

ID/CC: A 28-year-old G_1P_1 woman status post C/S presents with a fever of 101.4°F.

HPI: C.M. delivered a 3,400-g baby 5 days prior to presentation. Her labor course was significant for premature rupture of membranes that required induction of labor. She had a slow slope active course and developed chorioamnionitis. She underwent a primary low transverse C/S for arrest of descent at 0 station. She had a Foley catheter in place for the majority of her labor until 12 hours postpartum. After the catheter was removed, she was unable to void and again had the Foley catheter in place for an additional 24 hours. She received cefotetan for chorioamnionitis and continued receiving the antibiotic until 48 hours postpartum. Her fever intrapartum declined and normalized within 6 hours after delivery.

Ms. M. now presents with complaint of fever for 12 hours. She has lower abdominal cramps and back pain. She is breastfeeding, and her breasts are mildly tender. She has some pain with voiding. Her lochia has been mild and appears light reddish-orange. She has noticed a foul smell.

PMHx:	Frequent UTIs
PSHx:	C/S only
Meds: (Vicodin)	PNV, ibuprofen, hydrocodone and acetaminophen
All:	NKDA
POb/GynHx:	No STDs or PID.
SHx:	Lives with father of baby; denies ethanol, tobacco, or recreational drug use.

THOUGHT QUESTIONS

- What is your differential diagnosis for this patient's postpartum fever?
- What risk factors does she have for each of these diagnoses?
- What is endomyometritis?

The differential diagnosis includes both complications from surgery as well as postpartum conditions. Her differential includes endomyometritis, pyelonephritis, breast engorgement, mastitis, wound infection, and septic pelvic thrombophlebitis.

Her risk factors for endomyometritis are stated below. Risk factors for pyelonephritis include history of frequent UTIs and need for catheterization. Surgery and the postpartum period place her at risk for wound infection and septic pelvic thrombophlebitis. Breast-feeding, breast engorgement, and previous mastitis are risk factors for mastitis; this patient lacks the latter.

Endomyometritis or endometritis is an infection of the uterine lining and/or the wall of the uterus. It is a not uncommon complication of cesarean delivery. Other risk factors for endomyometritis include length of labor, duration of membrane rupture and chorioamnionitis, number of internal exams, retained placental products, internal fetal monitoring, and lower socioeconomic status. Presentation usually includes abdominal pain, fever, and foul-smelling lochia. Management includes a careful D&C if retained POC is suspected, in addition to antibiotic coverage. A mild case of endomyometritis after vaginal delivery may not require IV antibiotics, but generally infection after a cesarean section does.

CASE CONTINUED

VS: Temp 102.0°F, BP 112/52, HR 110, RR 14

PE: *Gen:* mild distress, shivering. *Breasts:* mildly erythematous nipples without cracks. Soft to palpation without tenderness or masses. No axillary lymphadenopathy noted. *Lungs:* CTAB. *Cor:* tachy, regular rate, no murmurs. *Abdomen:* Bowel sounds soft. Fundus

6 cm below umbilicus and moderately tender to palpation. No CVAT appreciated. *GU:* lochia has tomato souplike appearance and is foul smelling. *Extremities:* no calf pain or swelling noted.

Labs: Urine: SG 1.010; trace blood; negative nitrite/esterase; WBC 14.4

A diagnosis of endomyometritis is made based on the patient's fever, elevated WBC, tender uterus, and foul-smelling lochia. The patient is started on ampicillin, gentamicin, and clindamycin for broad-spectrum coverage of a likely mixed microbial infection (some hospitals use only a second-generation cephalosporin). She responds within 24 hours with decreasing abdominal tenderness and defervesces. Once she has been afebrile for 48 hours and without abdominal tenderness, she is discharged to home.

QUESTIONS

29-1. What antibiotic regimen should she receive at home?
A. Cephalexin (Keflex) 500 PO QID for 10 days
B. Keflex 500 PO QID for 14 days
C. Ofloxacin 400 mg PO BID and metronidazole (Flagyl) 500 mg PO BID for 14 days
D. Dicloxacillin 500 mg PO BID for 14 days
E. No antibiotics needed

29-2. The same patient does not respond within 48 hours to the antibiotic regimen. She is started on heparin and defervesces in 24 hours. What is her most likely diagnosis?
A. Septic pelvic thrombophlebitis
B. Deep venous thromboembolism
C. Endomyometritis with retained placental products
D. Pulmonary embolism
E. Pelvic abscess

29-3. Assume this patient presented instead with right breast pain and right axillary lymphadenopathy consistent with mastitis. What is the treatment?
A. Avoid breastfeeding on the right. No antibiotics needed.
B. Encourage continuation of breastfeeding from both breasts. No antibiotics needed.
C. Encourage continuation of breastfeeding from both breasts and start intravenous antibiotics.
D. Avoid breastfeeding on the right and start oral antibiotics.
E. Encourage continuation of breastfeeding from both breasts and start oral antibiotics.

29-4. What is the most common organism associated with mastitis?
- A. Group B *Streptococcus*
- B. *Staphylococcus aureus*
- C. *Streptococcus viridans*
- D. *Escherichia coli*
- E. *Enterococcus*

ANSWERS

29-1. E. There is no evidence supporting the use of PO antibiotics after clinical improvement on intravenous antibiotics (generally a 2- to 4-day course). Indicators of clinical improvement include no fever for 48 hours, absent uterine tenderness, and normal WBC count.

29-2. A. Septic pelvic thrombophlebitis is an uncommon cause of postpartum fever. Its pathogenesis likely is as follows: infection of the placenta leads to congestion and thrombosis of the myometrial then the ovarian veins. The presentation often is similar to that of endomyometritis but with spiking fevers despite 48 to 72 hours of antibiotics. Therapy requires treatment with heparin, although length of therapy is controversial.

29-3. E. See answer to question 29-4 below.

29-4. B. Mastitis has an incidence of approximately 2% of postpartum patients. Presentation includes history of engorgement followed by unilateral breast pain, erythema, fevers, and chills. This is a similar presentation for engorgement in the absence of mastitis, which can cause fever, but pain usually is bilateral and resolves with feeding. The most common organism involved is *S. aureus*, spread from the neonate's nose and throat to the breast. Treatment usually is dicloxacillin 500 mg PO QID for 7 to 10 days (or erythromycin if penicillin allergic). Continued breastfeeding is an important part of therapy, although pain medications or pumping may be required given the level of discomfort this can cause the mother. Fever beyond 48 to 72 hours or a palpable mass suggests abscess formation, which requires surgical drainage.

SUGGESTED ADDITIONAL READING

French LM, Smaill FM. Antibiotic regimens for endometritis after delivery. *Cochrane Database Syst Rev.* 2004;(4):CD001067.

CASE **30**

Desires Contraception

CC/ID: A 29-year-old G_4P_2 is 2 days postpartum after a normal vaginal delivery. She is due to be discharged from the hospital today and would like to discuss contraception options.

HPI: She is breastfeeding without problems and intends to do so for 1 year. She and her husband have used condoms in the past. She briefly used the "minipill" many years ago but stopped taking the pills because she did not like how "they made her feel." This pregnancy was unintended. She breastfed her older child, who is now 18 months old, for approximately 1 year. She and her husband have been married for 4 years, and both are monogamous. He is 34 years old and healthy.

PMHx: Migraines with visual symptoms since childhood

PSHx: None

Meds: Sumatriptan (Imitrex)

POb/GynHx: D&C twice, two NSVDs. Regular cycles, chlamydia infection 10 years ago, normal pap smears.

All: NKDA

THOUGHT QUESTIONS

- What additional information would be useful in identifying appropriate contraception?
- Does this patient's history of migraines or the fact that this patient is breastfeeding affect your recommendations for contraception?

Desire for future fertility will help determine if she and her husband are candidates for permanent sterilization. If she is sure she wants no more children, she may consider a tubal ligation. This involves surgically occluding the fallopian tubes with bands, clips, suture, or coagulation. The failure rate is 0.2% to 0.4%. Vasectomy involves surgical ligation of the vas deferens. Because this procedure is less invasive, it is safer than tubal ligation. The failure rate is <0.5%, the majority of which is due to intercourse too soon after vasectomy when viable sperm are still present distal to the occlusion.

Severe headaches are a relative contraindication to combined oral contraceptive use and should be considered on a case-by-case basis. In this patient who has classic migraines, combined oral contraceptives are contraindicated. Studies of the older high-dose pills indicated that users with migraine headache had a higher risk of stroke. Studies of low-dose formulations are equivocal, but some studies have found a fourfold increased risk for ischemic stroke. If this patient had common migraines (no associated aura), low-dose formulations could be used with careful surveillance and discontinued at the first sign of visual symptoms.

Regarding this patient's plan to breastfeed:
1. Progestin-only contraceptive methods do not diminish milk production.
2. Lactation amenorrhea should not be used to delay the use of other contraceptives. With perfect use, which requires that the infant be younger than 6 months, the breast milk be the exclusive form of nutrition, and the mother be amenorrheic, the failure rate can be as low as 2%. However, the actual failure rate of 15% to 55%, making it a poor primary form of birth control (Table 30-1).

TABLE 30-1 Contraceptive Options in Breastfeeding Women

Method	When to Start in Lactating Women	Effect on Breast Milk
Condoms, sponge	Immediately after lochia stops; (counsel against intercourse prior to this time because as it carries a risk for of infection)	No effect
Cervical cap, diaphragm	4–6 weeks post-partum, after the cervix and vagina have returned to a non-pregnant state	No effect

TABLE 30-1 Contraceptive Options in Breastfeeding Women (*continued*)

Progestin-only methods	Initiate immediately post-partum	No significant impact on milk production
Combined methods	Wait 3—6 weeks post-partum to initiate	Quantity and quality of breast milk diminished if started before lactation established
IUD	4—6 weeks, once uterus involuted; is used immediately post-partum some countries.	No effect
Tubal ligation	Usually done within first 24 hours post-partum	No effect

CASE CONTINUED

PE: Postpartum exam is normal.

After further discussion, she states that her husband does not want more children, but she herself is not sure. She is not sure whether her husband would consider a vasectomy. She agrees that she would do better with a long-acting form of contraception. She has heard about the IUD and thinks she may want to try it.

THOUGHT QUESTIONS

- How does her history of chlamydia infection affect your recommendation?
- In a postpartum patient such as this, when would be an appropriate time to insert an IUD?

Although a history of sexually transmitted infections (STIs) is a relative contraindication to IUD use, the physician should weigh current risk for STI more heavily in assessing whether a patient is a good candidate for an IUD. This patient is in a monogamous relationship and therefore is at low risk for STIs.

In a postpartum patient, you should wait until 6 weeks after delivery before placing an IUD. Prior to this time the uterus may not have reverted to its prepregnancy size, and the cervix may still be open, leading to high expulsion rates. Two types of IUDs currently are available on the U.S. market: the copper IUD (no hormone reservoir) and the levonorgestrel IUD (with a progestin reservoir).

QUESTIONS

30-1. You are seeing another postpartum patient whose history and exam are similar to those of the patient above except that she does not have any history of headaches. An appropriate contraceptive plan is:
   A. Postpartum tubal ligation.
   B. Prescription for combined OCPs starting now.
   C. A 3.5-mg injection of leuprolide given in 6 weeks.
   D. Prescription for transdermal combined contraceptive patch starting in 6 weeks.

30-2. A 30-year-old G_1P_1 woman comes to your office requesting contraception. She is single and currently is sexually active with two partners. She was using the diaphragm without problem but now would like to use OCPs. She has no medical problems. Her cycles are regular. She denies a history of STDs or abnormal pap smears. She smokes one pack of cigarettes per day. Her physical exam is normal. You correctly advise her that:
   A. Her smoking history is an absolute contraindication to OCP use.
   B. DMPA will induce amenorrhea in most women after the third injection.
   C. She is a good candidate for an IUD.
   D. OCPs do not decrease the risk of STDs.

30-3. A 22-year-old G_0 woman calls your office stating that the condom broke during intercourse 2 days ago. Her LMP began 12 days ago, and her cycles are regular and occur every 28 to 30 days. She wants to know if there is anything she can do to prevent pregnancy. You correctly advise her that:
   A. You can prescribe low-dose combined OCPs that she should start taking immediately.
   B. You can prescribe two doses of combined OCPs, with each dose containing 100 µg ethinyl estradiol and either 1 mg norgestrel or 0.5 mg levonorgestrel. She should take the first dose immediately and the second dose in 12 hours.
   C. She is too late for the "morning after" (Yuzpe) regimen because intercourse occurred 2 days ago.
   D. She is not likely to become pregnant because her last menses was only 10 days prior to intercourse.

30-4. A 29-year-old G_3P_3 woman would like to use long-acting contraception and asks you about the IUD. She is not using contraception now and is in a mutually monogamous relationship. Her gynecologic history is only notable for persistent LGSIL for which she underwent cryotherapy. You correctly advise her that:

A. The copper IUD must be changed every 2 years to maintain effectiveness.

B. She is not a candidate for the IUD given her history of LGSIL and the fact that she had cryotherapy.

C. The IUD increases her risk for ectopic pregnancy from her current baseline risk.

D. Common side effects of the IUD are metrorrhagia and dysmenorrhea.

 ANSWERS

30-1. D. The estrogen component in combined OCPs will decrease the quantity and quality of lactation if started before milk production has been established (by 4 to 6 weeks). This is mediated by the negative effect of estrogen on prolactin secretion. The transdermal contraceptive patch delivers a combination dose of both an estrogen and progestin and is similar to combined OCPs except for the mechanism of delivery. There is no contraindication to its use once breast milk supply is established. However, if a lactating woman reports a decrease in milk production after starting combined contraception, you should consider changing her prescription to a progesterone-only form of contraception. In a patient who is uncertain about permanent sterilization, tubal ligation is contraindicated. Leuprolide acetate is a GnRH agonist and is not used for birth control.

Neither barrier methods nor progestin-only methods, including medroxyprogesterone acetate (Depo-Provera), affect lactation. Progestin-only contraceptives act primarily by thickening cervical mucus and making the endometrium unsuitable for implantation. They are less reliable in suppressing ovulation. Depo-Provera is an intramuscular injection of progesterone that is administered every 3 months and has a failure rate of 0.3%. Like progesterone-only pills, it can be given in the immediate postpartum period.

30-2. B. In addition to thickening the cervical mucus and altering endometrium, circulating levels of progestin with DMPA are sufficiently high to block the LH surge and, therefore, ovulation. The levels also are sufficiently high to support the endometrial lining, hence menstrual flow does not occur. Cigarette smoking plus age 35+

is a contraindication to OCP use. This patient is 30 years old. OCPs have been shown to decrease the risk of STDs. This is thought to be due to alterations in cervical mucus. A history of multiple sexual partners makes this patient a poor candidate for the IUD.

30-3. B. Two regimens are commonly used for emergency contraception. The Yuzpe method (combined OCPs) uses two doses of at least 100 μg ethinyl estradiol and either 1 mg progesterone or 0.5 mg levonorgestrel taken 12 hours apart. The progestin-only method uses 0.75 mg levonorgestrel or 1.5 mg norgestrel taken 12 hours apart. Nausea and vomiting are common, especially with the Yuzpe method, so antiemetics are often prescribed. Both regimens are effective up to 72 hours after intercourse and cause a 75% to 85% reduction in the pregnancy rate.

30-4. D. Average monthly blood loss with menses increases approximately 35% with the IUD. Dysmenorrhea occurs in up to 20% of women. Removal rates for pain and bleeding in the first year are 12%. Otherwise, the copper IUD can stay in place for up to 10 years. A history of dysplasia is not a contraindication to IUD use. However, you should establish that her pap smear is negative prior to insertion. Finally, IUDs are so effective in preventing pregnancy that a woman's overall risk for ectopic pregnancy actually is reduced. However, if she does become pregnant with an IUD in place, her ectopic risk becomes 5% to 8%.

 ### *SUGGESTED ADDITIONAL READING*

Truitt ST, Fraser AB, Grimes DA, et al. Combined hormonal versus nonhormonal versus progestin-only contraception in lactation *Cochrane Database Syst Rev.* 2003;(2):CD003988.

ACOG Practice Bulletin. The use of hormonal contraception in women with coexisting conditions. obstetrics and gynecology. Number 18, July 2000. *Int J Gynaecol Obstet.* 2001;75:93–106.

Kaunitz AM. Beyond the pill: new data and options in hormonal and intrauterine contraception. *Am J Obstet Gynecol.* 2005; 192:998–1004.

V

General
Gynecology

Acute Abdominal Pain

Acute Abdominal Pain

CC/ID: A 21-year-old woman presents to the emergency room complaining of 3 hours of worsening RLQ pain.

HPI: She reports a dull pain that started earlier in the day and has intensified to the point that she can barely move. She became nauseated shortly after the pain began and vomited twice before arriving at the emergency department. She had two similar episodes of pain in the last few days, but the episodes were less intense and had resolved after approximately 1 hour. She denies fever or chills. Further ROS is negative.

PMHx: Mild asthma

PSHx: LEEP procedure 4 years prior

Meds: Albuterol (Ventolin) PRN

PGynHx: LMP 4.5 weeks ago, irregular menses every 4 to 8 wks, no STDs, sexually active, uses condoms, cervical dysplasia 4 years ago

PObHx: Never pregnant

All: NKDA

THOUGHT QUESTIONS

- What is included in the differential diagnosis?
- What single lab test would be most helpful?

Based on the history, this patient's differential diagnosis is broad and includes

177

- Appendicitis
- Ectopic pregnancy
- Ovarian torsion
- Cervical stenosis due to scarring or anatomic abnormalities
- Ruptured ovarian cyst
- Degenerating uterine fibroid
- PID
- Gastroenteritis
- Bowel obstruction

Of these conditions, ruptured ovarian cyst is less likely because the associated pain typically does not wax and wane. PID typically presents with gradually increasing diffuse pelvic pain. Bowel obstruction is unlikely in a young patient with no prior surgery, and gastroenteritis usually is associated with nausea and vomiting followed by abdominal pain and then diarrhea. Cervical stenosis can cause painful uterine cramps as the uterus tries to push out menstrual blood against an obstructed cervical os. This is an unlikely diagnosis for this patient because she has had normal menses since her LEEP procedure. Pain from a degenerating fibroid usually is constant and lasts for several days.

The most helpful test is a urine pregnancy test. If the patient is pregnant, ectopic pregnancy is high on the differential.

CASE CONTINUED

VS: Temp 99.5°F, BP 114/68, HR 96, RR 16

PE: Uncomfortable appearing. *Abd:* soft, ND. Diffusely tender, worse in RLQ. Moderate rebound to RLQ. Normal BS. *Pelvic:* Normal-appearing vagina and cervix. *BME:* Uterus normal size AV/AF. Tenderness in RLQ with manipulation of cervix and uterus. Right adnexal mass, 7 to 8 cm and tender to palpation.

Labs: WBC: 8.1, Hct: 38.6, urine pregnancy test: negative, stool guaiac: negative

THOUGHT QUESTIONS

- Now what is your most likely diagnosis?
- What imaging study (if any) would be most helpful now?
- What is your treatment plan?

After the physical exam, ovarian torsion is most likely given the finding of a tender adnexal mass. We can exclude an ectopic pregnancy based on the negative pregnancy test. PID less likely because she is afebrile, has a normal WBC, and the finding of a mass, although a tubo-ovarian abscess (TOA) is possible. A large adnexal mass also is unlikely for a ruptured ovarian cyst. Appendicitis usually is associated with an elevated WBC count and fever. One other possibility is a pedunculated fibroid that has outgrown its blood supply and is infarcting, although this is less likely in a young woman.

A pelvic ultrasound would the most helpful at this time. For our most likely diagnoses, the findings would be as follows

Ovarian torsion: Ovarian mass, typically neoplasm or a large functional cyst. No ovarian artery flow may be seen if the ovarian blood supply is compromised.

Ruptured cyst: Usually free fluid found in the cul-de-sac. An ovarian cyst may be seen.

Appendicitis: Often normal because US is only 50% sensitive for appendicitis (CT is the better study).

PID: Normal ultrasound exam (unless a pelvic abscess is present).

Degenerating/infracting pedunculated fibroid: Solid pelvic mass with normal ovaries visualized.

Ovarian torsion is a gynecologic surgical emergency, and the treatment is laparoscopy or laparotomy. The cyst must be removed and the torsion relieved before the ovary itself is compromised.

CASE CONTINUED

A pelvic ultrasound is obtained (Figure 31-1).

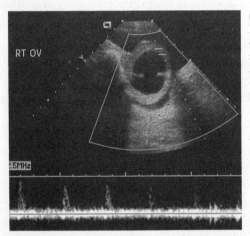

FIGURE 31-1.
Large simple cyst in the ovary. Note the Doppler signal from the ovarian artery is diminished, as only brief arterial flow is allowed during systole. *(Image Provided by Department of Radiology and Obstetrics and Gynecology, University of California, San Francisco).*

QUESTIONS

31-1. What type of ovarian cyst does this patient most likely have?
A. Corpus lutein cyst
B. Cystic teratoma
C. Follicular cyst
D. Theca lutein cyst

31-2. On routine physical exam of a 28-year-old woman, you palpate a 5-cm left ovary. After obtaining an ultrasound that reveals a simple 4.2-cm cyst, the best management is to:
A. Obtain a CA-125 test
B. Observe for 6 weeks and repeat the ultrasound
C. Obtain a CT scan
D. Exploratory surgery and removal of the ovary and/or cyst

31-3. The most common ovarian neoplasm to undergo torsion is:
A. Endometrioid tumor
B. Benign cystic teratoma
C. Cystadenocarcinoma
D. Granulosa cell tumor

31-4. A woman presents with sudden acute pelvic pain, tachycardia, and hypotension. A urine pregnancy test is negative. The most likely cause is a:
A. Ruptured endometrioma
B. Ruptured cystic teratoma
C. Ruptured corpus luteum cyst
D. Ruptured uterine cornua

ANSWERS

31-1. C. Functional cysts result from normal physiologic functioning of the ovary. Follicular cysts, the most common form of functional cysts among women of reproductive age, arise from failure of mature follicles to rupture. Corpus lutein cysts, also a type of functional cyst, are formed when the corpus luteum becomes enlarged and hemorrhagic. Rupture of these cysts can cause acute pelvic pain and hemoperitoneum. Theca lutein cysts arise form high levels of β-HCG and usually are bilateral. A cystic teratoma is the most common benign neoplasm of women of reproductive age.

31-2. B. Most follicular cysts resolve within 60 days. For reproductive-age women with cysts <6 cm, observation for 6 weeks with a follow-up ultrasound is appropriate. Cysts >6 cm that persist for more than 60 days or appear solid or complex on ultrasound probably are not functional cysts. In this case, exploratory surgery often is warranted. Of note, ultrasound is better than CT scan for imaging the pelvic organs, especially the ovaries.

31-3. B. Malignant ovarian neoplasms usually involve adhesions and hence rarely undergo torsion. Teratomas are benign and can be large and irregularly shape. They are the most likely ovarian neoplasm to undergo torsion. Endometrioid tumors, cystadenocarcinoma, and granulosa cell tumors are all malignant ovarian neoplasms.

31-4. C. All ruptured ovarian cysts cause acute pelvic pain. Endometriomas and cystic teratomas rarely grow quickly enough to undergo acute rupture. Rupture of the uterine cornua may occur in the case of a cornual (interstitial) ectopic pregnancy. This patient has a negative pregnancy test. Only a corpus luteum cyst can cause sufficient hemoperitoneum leading to hypovolemia. This occurs when a lacerated vessel on the ovary (usually an artery) continues to bleed after rupture of the cyst wall.

SUGGESTED ADDITIONAL READING

Quan M. Diagnosis of acute pelvic pain. *J Fam Pract*. 1992;35:422–432.

Webb EM, Green GE, Scott LM. Adnexal mass with pelvic pain. *Radiol Clin North Am*. 2004;42:329–348.

Porpora MG, Gomel V. The role of laparoscopy in the management of pelvic pain in women of reproductive age. *Fertil Steril*. 1997;68:765–779.

CASE **32**

Acute Pelvic Pain I

CC/ID: A 28-year-old $G_3P_0S_2$ woman 8 weeks GA by LMP presents with severe right-sided abdominal pain.

HPI: The pain started gradually 2 days ago. It is constant, dull, and not worsened by movement or eating. She reports mild fevers and denies nausea or emesis. Her bowel movements are normal. She denies vaginal bleeding or an abnormal vaginal discharge now, but she did have some spotting 4 days ago. This is a desired pregnancy.

PMHx: Anemia

PSHx: Appendectomy

Meds: PNV

PGynHx: Regular cycles, heavy menses lasting 7 to 8 days, no STDs

PObHx: Two first-trimester losses

All: NKDA

THOUGHT QUESTION

- What would be the common causes of this patient's pain?

In a pregnant patient with acute pelvic pain, ruling out ectopic pregnancy should be the first consideration. Ectopic pregnancy usually presents with unilateral pelvic pain and can be accompanied with vaginal bleeding or spotting. Other likely causes of this patient's pain include appendicitis, ovarian torsion, ruptured ovarian cyst, and a degenerating uterine fibroid. Given the patient's history, gastroenteritis, bowel obstruction, and nephrolithiasis are

183

less likely. A pelvic infection or PID is possible but less likely because the pregnancy provides a barrier to ascending cervical infections.

CASE CONTINUED

VS: Temp 98.2°F, BP 116/78, HR 84, RR 16

PE: Uncomfortable appearing. *Abd:* soft, ND. Marked tenderness over palpable mass in right mid quadrant. Mild rebound to right side. No guarding. Normal BS. *Pelvic:* Normal-appearing vagina and cervix. *BME:* uterus 14-week size and irregular; tender to palpation, especially on right. Adnexa nontender and without masses.

THOUGHT QUESTION

- On physical exam, the uterus is larger than expected based upon the patient's last menstrual period. What likely possibilities could account for this finding?

During early pregnancy, the most common cause of a size > dates finding on physical exam is that the pregnancy is further along than the patient's recollection of her last menstrual period. Often this happens because the patient has an episode of bleeding that she perceives as her period. A fibroid uterus also can cause a size > dates finding. A less likely reason for this finding is multiple gestations.

CASE CONTINUED

Labs: WBC: 8.9, Hct: 30.6, UA: negative, β-HCG: 26,769

Ultrasound: Intrauterine pregnancy measuring 8 weeks and 5 days with cardiac motion. Diffusely myomatous uterus with 5-cm right fundal fibroid.

THOUGHT QUESTIONS

■ How is this patient's pregnancy related to her acute pain?

■ How does the ultrasound exam help with management of this patient's pain?

Fibroids are responsive to estrogen. They tend to enlarge during pregnancy and regress during menopause. When they enlarge rapidly, they can outstrip their blood supply, undergo degeneration, and consequently cause bouts of acute pain. The time course for resolution of symptoms varies from several days to 2 weeks. The ultrasound demonstrates a viable pregnancy. Because the pregnancy is desired, termination or even surgical treatments are not desirable options. Management is limited to treatment with pain medications.

QUESTIONS

32-1. The ethnicity most highly associated with fibroids is:
A. Asian
B. African American
C. Hispanic
D. Caucasian

32-2. The cause of this patient's anemia is:
A. Rupture of a degenerating fibroid
B. Polymenorrhea
C. Metrorrhagia
D. Menorrhagia

32-3. Fibroids are associated with:
A. Recurrent acute cystitis
B. Recurrent pregnancy loss
C. Endometrial hyperplasia
D. Endometritis

32-4. As this patient's pregnancy approaches term, she is at risk for:
- A. Precipitous vaginal delivery
- B. Polyhydramnios
- C. Cesarean section
- D. Fetal macrosomia

 ANSWERS

32-1. B. Uterine fibroids are the most common tumor of the female pelvis. They are estimated to occur in 20% to 25% of women of reproductive age. The incidence of fibroids is three to nine times higher among black women compared to Asian, Hispanic, and white women.

32-2. D. The most common symptom of fibroids is abnormal uterine bleeding. The typical pattern is heavy periods of longer duration (menorrhagia), which result in iron deficiency anemia. According to the postulated mechanism, fibroids alter the endometrial microvasculature and consequently impair normal endometrial hemostatic functions. Metrorrhagia is characterized by bleeding between cycles, with flow usually less than menses. Polymenorrhea occurs if similar periods occur at intervals <21 days.

32-3. B. Fibroids may distort the endometrial cavity and fallopian tubes and thus interfere with implantation. If sufficiently large, the fibroid uterus can compress a ureter and cause hydronephrosis, but fibroids rarely cause bladder infections. Endometrial hyperplasia occurs when the lining is not shed regularly. Endometritis is an infection of the endometrium and is not a complication of fibroids. However, in rare cases, a prolapsing cervical fibroid can cause ulceration and secondary infection.

32-4. C. Fibroids have the potential for excessive growth during pregnancy. This may lead to intrauterine growth restriction, malpresentation, premature labor, and dystocia. If the fibroid blocks the presenting part, cesarean section may be necessary. Polyhydramnios is commonly due to fetal structural and chromosomal abnormalities.

SUGGESTED ADDITIONAL READING

Wallach EE, Vlahos NF. Uterine myomas: an overview of development, clinical features, and management. *Obstet Gynecol.* 2004;104:393–406.

Myers ER, Barber MD, Gustil-Ashby T, et al. Management of uterine leiomyomata: what do we really know? *Obstet Gynecol.* 2002;100:8–17.

Qidwai GI, Caughey AB, Jacoby A. Obstetric Outcomes in Women with Sonographically Identified Uterine Myomas. *Obstet Gynecol.* 2006;107:376–382.

Vaginal Discharge

ID/CC: A 25-year-old G$_0$ woman presents with complaint of a new vaginal discharge.

HPI: F.H. states that she recently became involved with a new sexual partner. They have been sexually active for the past month, and she is using oral contraceptive pills (OCPs) for birth control. She noticed a whitish-gray vaginal discharge approximately 1 week ago and now has significant pruritus as well. She recently was treated for bronchitis but does not recall the course of antibiotic she completed. She has had yeast infections before and wonders whether this episode is another one. Ms. H. denies a history of sexually transmitted infections (STIs) or PID but does not know her partner's sexual history. She denies having fever or chills, or abdominal or pelvic pain. She denies having dysuria, dyspareunia, or abnormal bleeding.

PMHx/PSHx: Tonsillectomy as a child

Meds: OCPs

All: NKDA

POb/GynHx: Last Pap smear 6 months ago. No history of abnormal Pap smears. Menarche at age 13; regular 28-day cycles when not on OCPs, bleeds for 4 days. LMP 2 weeks ago. First became sexually active at age 17 and has had two partners in the past 6 months.

SHx: Lives alone. No use of tobacco; occasional use of marijuana; social use of ethanol.

THOUGHT QUESTIONS

- What is your differential diagnosis?
- What will you look for in the physical examination to distinguish among these diagnoses?

■ How can you distinguish between a vaginal infection and a pelvic infection, and why is it important to do so?

Your differential diagnosis for vaginal discharge should include both sexually transmitted and nonsexually transmitted infections: gonorrhea, chlamydia, trichomonas vaginalis, vaginal candidiasis, and bacterial vaginosis. On examination, any evidence of pruritus, the type of vaginal discharge, and the appearance of the cervix are helpful for determining the diagnosis. On bimanual examination, the presence of cervical, uterine, or adnexal tenderness can help clarify the presence of a pelvic infection. You should have a good idea of the diagnosis after taking the history and performing physical examination, with the wet mount and KOH confirming your diagnosis.

Distinguishing between a vaginal infection and a pelvic infection is important because pelvic infections can lead to infertility and, if left untreated, significant morbidity. Pelvic inflammatory disease (PID) can present in many ways, but its three cardinal symptoms are pelvic pain, uterine tenderness, and adnexal tenderness.

CASE CONTINUED

VS: Temp 98.6°F, BP 98/64, HR 72, RR 16

PE: *Gen:* thin female, NAD. *Lungs:* CTAB. *Cor:* RR&R. *Abdomen:* soft, nontender, no distension with normal BS. *EGBUS:* normal female genitalia with mild erythema on labia minora. *SSE:* white-gray thin discharge, foul smelling. Normal-appearing cervix. Cervical cultures obtained. *BME:* Small anteverted uterus, nontender. No adnexal masses. No CMT.

Labs: Wet prep: no clue cells; motile protozoa seen, many WBCs seen. KOH: no pseudohyphae seen. Vaginal pH 6.0. Urine dipstick: SG 1.020, negative nitrates/negative leukocyte esterase, negative RBC/WBCs

You diagnose Ms. H. with *Trichomonas* vaginalis (Figure 33-1). You discuss this diagnosis with her and explain how the disease is transmitted and the need to treat her partner as well. As part of a full discussion of STIs, you instruct the patient to follow up on the results

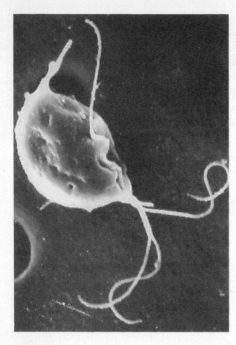

FIGURE 33-1.
Trichomonad at high
resolution. *(From Cox FEG.
Modern Parasitology: a Textbook of Parasitology. 2nd ed.
Oxford: Blackwell Science;
1993:9, with permission.)*

of her cervical cultures taken today and you discuss whether the
patient wishes to be tested for hepatitis C, hepatitis B, and HIV. Lastly,
you discuss the need for condom use to help prevent STIs.

QUESTIONS

33-1. What is the medication and dosage you prescribe for this
patient and her partner?
  - A. Metronidazole 2 g orally one time only
  - B. Metronidazole 5 g as 0.75% gel intravaginally, every
    night for 5 days
  - C. Azithromycin 1 g orally one time only
  - D. Ofloxacin 400 mg PO BID for 7 days
  - E. Fluconazole, 150 mg orally only

33-2. If this patient had presented with increased malodorous discharge without pruritus, what diagnosis would be more likely and what would you see on wet mount/KOH?
- A. *Chlamydia*—clue cells
- B. *Chlamydia*—WBCs
- C. Vaginal candidiasis—pseudohyphae
- D. Bacterial vaginosis—clue cells
- E. Bacterial vaginosis—WBCs

33-3. Use of broad-spectrum antibiotics can contribute to the development of which infection?
- A. Bacterial vaginosis
- B. *Chlamydia*
- C. Vaginal candidiasis
- D. Gonorrhea
- E. None of the above

33-4. If this patient had also presented with dysuria, which three infections listed below could cause urethritis?
- A. Gonorrhea, *Chlamydia*, and *Trichomonas*
- B. Gonorrhea, *Chlamydia*, and candidiasis
- C. Gonorrhea, *Trichomonas*, and bacterial vaginosis
- D. *Chlamydia*, *Trichomonas*, and candidiasis
- E. None of the above

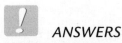 *ANSWERS*

33-1. A. The recommended treatment with a cure rate of 90% to 95% is metronidazole 2 g PO for both the patient and partner. A regimen of 500 mg PO BID for 7 days can be given to those who do not respond to the one-time dosage. In addition, it is recommended that the patient and partner abstain from sex or that they use condoms for 2 weeks following therapy to avoid reinfection. Patients must be informed that alcohol should be avoided when taking metronidazole because significant nausea and emesis will occur in a reaction similar to that caused by disulfiram (Antabuse).

33-2. D. The most likely diagnosis is bacterial vaginosis in which clue cells are seen on a wet mount. However, chlamydia can be asymptomatic and present similarly (in this case, WBCs would be seen on wet mount). Bacterial vaginosis is an interesting infection that, at one time, was considered sexually transmitted. We now know this is not true. As evidenced by its name, *vaginosis*, the condition usually is a nonirritating entity, and many women remain asymptomatic. These women do not require treatment for asymptomatic infections (although this is controversial). The diagnosis is made by the presence of a malodorous discharge, clue cells (epithelial cells stippled with bacteria) on wet mount, a basic vaginal pH, and the presence of a fishy odor with addition of KOH ("whiff test").

33-3. C. Taking broad-spectrum antibiotics predisposes the patient to the development of vaginal candidiasis. Other predisposing factors include use of oral contraceptives or steroids and the presence of diabetes.

33-4. A. Gonorrhea and *Chlamydia* can cause cervicitis, urethritis, and PID. *Trichomonas* infection can cause vaginitis and urethritis. Although candidiasis can cause dysuria, this generally is due to irritation rather than an actual infection of the urethra. Note that the most common cause of urethritis is a urinary tract infection, which is associated with a very different group of microorganisms.

 ### *SUGGESTED ADDITIONAL READING*

Swygard H, Sena AC, Hobbs MM, et al. Trichomonas: clinical manifestations, diagnosis and management. *Sex Transm Infect.* 2004;80:91–95.

CASE **34**

Sexual Assault

 ID/CC: A 21-year-old G_0 woman presents to the emergency room after being sexually assaulted.

HPI: E.C. was on her way home from a campus library at approximately 11:00 PM. Just a few hundred feet from the library, she was grabbed by an unidentified man and raped at knifepoint. At first she had struggled and was struck several times in the face and abdomen. After the assailant left, Ms. C. was able to make her way back to the library where campus security was called, and she was brought to the local university hospital.

PMHx/PSHx: Appendectomy at age 7

Meds: None

All: Penicillin, anaphylaxis

POb/GynHx: G_0; menarche age 13; regular menses. Sexually active, currently monogamous with male partner; using OCPs.

SHx: College senior; lives with two other women three blocks from campus. Denies use of tobacco, ethanol, or recreational drugs.

THOUGHT QUESTIONS

- What further history should be obtained from this patient?
- What do you need to consider during the physical examination?

Although questioning may feel intrusive, obtaining additional information will help guide your medical management of this patient. In addition, because you may be called as a witness to this crime, it is important to get a clear, detailed story as soon as possible. Additional history regarding the event itself should include any information regarding identification of the assailant, particularly if he or she was known to the victim; how long ago the attack occurred; what specific physical and sexual assault took place, specifically whether oral, vaginal, or anal penetration occurred; whether the victim believes there was ejaculation; whether the victim has any history of STIs; and what the victim's physical complaints are. Often, the police will be involved before the physician. However, if they have not yet been involved, they need to be called to report the crime.

The physical examination of a victim of sexual assault must be performed in a systematic manner. Often there will be a "rape kit," a collection of instructions on how to proceed with evidence collection, which includes shaking out the victim's clothing, collecting tissue from under the fingernails, and combing the pubic hair to collect foreign hair or other material. In addition to evidence collection, cultures of any possible exposure should be collected. If the patient has been physically assaulted, photographic evidence should be collected as well.

CASE CONTINUED

Upon further review with the patient, she reports that the attack was 1 hour ago. Currently what hurts the most is the left side of her face. Vaginal penetration occurred, but she is unsure about ejaculation. She did not recognize the perpetrator and cannot describe him because it was quite dark. She has no history of STIs, but she is concerned about her risk for contracting an STI as a result of this assault.

VS: Temp 97.2°F, BP 118/66, HR 98, RR 24

PE: *Gen:* in moderate emotional distress, tear-stained face, dirt on lower extremities (LEs), bruises and scrapes on face and LEs. *HEENT:* ecchymoses on left side of face and around left eye. *Back:* nontender, no CVAT. *Chest:* RR&R, tender beneath the left breast, ecchymoses. *Abd:* soft, nontender, no distension. *Pelvic:* normal external genitalia, no obvious bruising or evidence of trauma. Pubic hair combed out to collect samples. *SSE:* swabs of vagina and cervix are taken for cultures and for the rape kit. *BME:* patient is apprehensive about exam, but no evidence of CMT, no adnexal masses or tenderness; uterus is midline, normal in size.

THOUGHT QUESTION

- At this point, what laboratory tests should be sent in addition to the cultures collected?

     In this patient who has been exposed to an unknown assailant, there is no test that can be performed immediately to determine whether she has been exposed to or infected with an STI. It is common to offer baseline testing on the off-chance that she is infected in order to establish causality. Thus, baseline serum testing for hepatitis B, hepatitis C, HIV, and RPR are commonly performed. A serum pregnancy test is also sent to establish a baseline.

CASE CONTINUED

You offer the patient the additional baseline testing and she agrees. She also wants to know whether she is at risk for getting pregnant. She has been using OCPs for 2 years and rarely misses a pill. The last time she missed a pill was 3 months ago. You reassure her that the possibility is remote, given that she is so compliant with her OCP use. You then offer her prophylactic treatment for her possible exposure to STIs.

QUESTIONS

34-1. If this patient had not been taking OCPs, which of the following would be an appropriate form of emergency contraception?
- A. IUD placement
- B. Lo/Ovral, two-pill dose, given twice
- C. Depo-Provera IM
- D. Vaginal misoprostol
- E. Alesse, five-pill dose, given twice

34-2. Your offered treatment of STI prophylaxis should include which of the following?
- A. Ceftriaxone 250 mg IM × 1
- B. Azithromycin 1 g PO × 1 + doxycycline 100 mg PO BID × 1 week
- C. Azithromycin 2 g PO × 1
- D. Ofloxacin 400 mg PO × 1 + ceftriaxone 250 mg IM × 1
- E. Ciprofloxacin 500 mg PO × 1 + ceftriaxone 250 mg IM × 1

34-3. Which of the following is unnecessary at this point in her management?
- A. X-ray films of the face
- B. Social services consultation
- C. Prophylaxis for HIV
- D. Psychiatry consultation
- E. Chest x-ray film

34-4. No prophylaxis can be given to prevent which of the following?
- A. *Chlamydia trachomatis* infection
- B. *Neisseria gonorrhoeae* infection
- C. HIV infection
- D. Human papilloma virus (HPV) infection
- E. Hepatitis B infection

 ANSWERS

34-1. E. The postcoital form of contraception, named the Yuzpe method after its founder, consists most commonly of two Ovral pills given in two doses, 12 hours apart. Ovral is composed of 50 μg ethinyl estradiol and 0.5 mg norgestrel. Lo/Ovral consists of 30 μg ethinyl estradiol and 1.0 mg norgestrel. Alesse consists of 20 μg ethinyl estradiol and 1.0 mg levonorgestrel. The goal is to give two doses, 12 hours apart, with each dose consisting of at least 100 μg ethinyl estradiol. In this question, the Alesse dosing achieves this concentration, whereas the Lo-Ovral does not. An IUD placed just after coitus will work as contraception; however, in this setting of possible exposure to STIs, an IUD is not the optimal management plan, given the potentially increased risk for PID. Vaginal misoprostol can be used as an abortifacient early in pregnancy but not periconceptually. Depo-Provera has not been studied as a form of postcoital contraception.

34-2. C. The two organisms to be covered here are primarily *N. gonorrhoeae* and *C. trachomatis*. Given the 15% cross-reactivity between cephalosporins and penicillin, it is not a good idea to give a cephalosporin to this patient who has a penicillin allergy when alternative treatments exist. In this case, the ceftriaxone would normally be given to cover *N. gonorrhoeae*, which also can be covered with one-time doses of ofloxacin, ciprofloxacin, and the 2-g dose of azithromycin. If ofloxacin or ciprofloxacin is used, the patient also needs coverage for *C. trachomatis* with either a one-time dose of azithromycin or a 1-week course of doxycycline.

34-3. D. This patient appears normally responsive to questions and is without a specific indication for a psychiatry consultation. Alternatively, a social services consultation to arrange follow-up care, possible counseling, and support groups is useful. Face x-ray films should be obtained to rule out an orbital fracture and a chest x-ray film to rule out a rib fracture. HIV prophylaxis should be offered, although patients often decline.

34-4. D. HPV is the cause of condyloma as well as cervical cancer. Unfortunately, there is no particular way to prevent its transmission other than barrier methods such as condoms. Chlamydia, gonorrhea, and HIV can all be prevented with prophylactic antibiotics, and hepatitis B can be prevented by administration of HB IgG.

 ## SUGGESTED ADDITIONAL READING

Gibb AM, McManus T, Forster GE. Should we offer antibiotic prophylaxis post sexual assault? *Int J STD AIDS.* 2003;14:99–102.
Amaral E. Current approach to STD management in women. *Int J Gynaecol Obstet.* 1998;63(suppl 1):S183–S189.

Vulvar Lump

ID/CC: A 25-year-old G_0 woman presents with a mass on her perineum.

HPI: B.C. reports that she had a very tender mass in the same region 6 weeks ago that was treated with drainage and a course of antibiotics. The mass initially rose over 2 to 3 days, causing significant discomfort when sitting and walking. The pain resolved quickly with treatment at that time, but she still feels a mass in the area, which is noticeably uncomfortable when she is physically and sexually active. Now she feels that over the past 2 days it has become larger and more painful.

PMHx: None

PSHx: Appendectomy at age 7

Meds: None

All: None

POb/GynHx: Sexually active and usually uses condoms. Genital HSV, last outbreak 1 year ago.

SHx: Single, graduate student in psychology. Occasional tobacco and ethanol use.

VS: Temp 97.2°F, BP 120/70, HR 85, RR 14

PE: *Abdomen:* soft, nontender, no distension, no palpable masses. *Pelvic:* normal except for a 5 × 4 cm cystic mass in the inferior aspect of the right. Labium majora, moderately tender, with minimal surrounding erythema (Figure 35-1).

Labs: GC and *Chlamydia* negative by DNA probe 6 weeks ago

THOUGHT QUESTIONS

- What is the differential diagnosis for vulvar masses?
- What kinds of cysts arise on the vulva?
- When do you treat them?

A differential diagnosis for benign growths on the vulva includes Bartholin gland cyst, epidermal inclusion cyst, lipoma, fibroma, hidradenoma, hydrocele, leiomyoma, nevus, and supernumerary mammary tissue. Malignant growths include squamous cell carcinoma, melanoma, adenocarcinoma, and sarcoma. The majority of vulvar masses are benign. Generally, three types of cysts arise in the vulva: Bartholin gland cysts, epidermal inclusion cysts, and hydroceles. Treatment is rendered for pain, infection, or recurrent cyst formation and usually involves a simple surgical procedure for release of the accumulated secretions.

CASE CONTINUED

The patient notices the mass when sitting down and is unable to engage in sexual intercourse secondary to the pain. As the pain has increased over the past couple of days, walking has become more uncomfortable. She denies a history of other STIs such as gonorrhea or chlamydia. She is worried about a persistent infection.

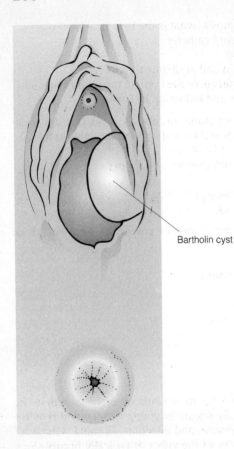

FIGURE 35-1.
Bartholin gland cyst. These cysts can become enlarged or infected. *(From Champion RH. Textbook of Dermatology. 6th ed. Oxford: Blackwell Publishing; 1999, with permission.)*

Bartholin cyst

QUESTIONS

35-1. What is the most common cystic mass in the vulvovaginal region?

A. Fibroma
B. Epidermal inclusion cyst
C. Hidradenoma
D. Nevus
E. Bartholin cyst

35-2. Given your diagnosis, what is the best treatment plan?
   A. Insertion of a Word catheter
   B. Marsupialization
   C. Needle aspiration and antibiotic treatment
   D. Incision and drainage of the cyst via the labium majora
   E. Warm sitz baths and follow-up in 1 week

35-3. This same presentation occurs in a 56-year-old postmenopausal woman. What is the most appropriate management?
   A. Insertion of a Word catheter
   B. Insertion of a Word catheter and biopsy of the cyst wall
   C. Marsupialization
   D. Incision and drainage of the cyst
   E. Excision of the cyst

35-4. What is the most common cause of Bartholin gland enlargement?
   A. Trauma
   B. Physiologic secretions
   C. Infection
   D. Unknown
   E. *Neisseria gonorrhoeae*

ANSWERS

35-1. E. Bartholin cyst is the most common cystic growth in the vulvovaginal area. It usually occurs in young women and requires treatment for pain, enlargement, and infection. Fibroma is the most common benign solid tumor of the vulva. It typically occurs along the insertion of the round ligament into the labium majora. Epidermal inclusion cysts usually are asymptomatic and present as a small hard lump containing sebaceous material. Hidradenomas are benign growths from apocrine glands. Nevi are common in the vulva and can be highly varied in appearance. They must be followed closely and biopsied or excised for acute changes in size, color, or shape.

35-2. A. This patient had a Bartholin gland abscess, which initially was treated by drainage and antibiotics. She now presents with a likely reinfection of the cyst, secondary to inadequate treatment at the initial presentation. Insertion of a Word catheter into this cystic cavity to form a fistulous tract will allow the gland to drain appropriately. A biopsy and/or excision procedure would be justified if there is a concern about an underlying malignant process. Marsupialization is indicated in recurrent Bartholin gland enlargement. This is a procedure where a portion of tissue is removed in an elliptical fashion, and the edges of the skin and cyst wall are approximated to form a pouch. This procedure allows for continued drainage and reepithelialization of the involved area.

35-3. B. In postmenopausal women with unilateral Bartholin gland enlargement, the possibility of an underlying malignancy must be considered. The possible types of malignancies include adenocarcinoma, adenoid cystic carcinoma, and squamous cell carcinoma of the vulvar. A biopsy of the cyst wall is warranted in this patient, as is placement of a Word catheter.

35-4. C. The most common cause of Bartholin gland enlargement is an infection. These infections are generally polymicrobial with anaerobic and aerobic organisms. Cultures of cyst contents are positive for *N. gonorrhoeae* in approximately 10% of cases. Nevertheless, all patients should be screened for STIs at the time of presentation with a Bartholin gland abscess. Fibrosis after an infection can lead to cyst formation from accumulation of the gland's mucinous secretions.

SUGGESTED ADDITIONAL READING

Hopkins MP, Snyder MK. Benign disorders of vulva and vagina. In Curtis MC, Hopkins MP, eds. *Glass's office gynecology.* 5th ed. Philadelphia, Pa: Lippincott Williams & Wilkins; 1999:417–426.

Droegemueller W. Benign gynecologic lesions: vulva, vagina, cervix, uterus, oviduct, ovary. In: Stenchever MA, Droegemueller W, Herbst AL, et al., eds. *Comprehensive gynecology.* 4th ed. St. Louis, Mo: Mosby, 2001:279–530.

Sweet RL, Biggs RS. *Infectious diseases of the female genital tract.* 4th ed. Philadelphia, Pa: Lippincott, Williams & Wilkins; 2002:562–566.

CASE **36**

Acute Vulvodynia

ID/CC: A 38-year-old G_2P_2 woman complains of persistent vulvar burning and pain.

HPI: V.M. reports acute onset of vulvar discomfort 9 months ago. She initially noticed the pain with penetration during intercourse but now the discomfort is constant. She describes the pain as a "burning" sensation. She has also had increased vaginal discharge. Use of over-the-counter antifungal creams worsened the pain. A doctor had examined her and prescribed oral fluconazole. She saw this physician several times with the same complaints, and he continued prescribing antifungals, which offered no relief. At this time she is concerned that the pain is a sign of some underlying disease that has not been diagnosed. She notes no pruritus and no vaginal irritation or discharge.

PMHx: Migraine headaches

PSHx: Umbilical hernia repair

Meds: Antifungals PRN, NSAIDs, sumatriptan

All: NKDA

POb/GynHx: Two forceps-assisted vaginal deliveries, 10 and 8 years ago. History of *Chlamydia* infection 12 years ago. Normal Pap smears, performed annually for past 3 years. Regular menses every 28 days. Uses condoms for birth control.

SHx: Married. Drinks two cups of coffee per day; social ethanol use; denies tobacco use.

VS: Temp 97.5°F, BP 102/60, HR 84, RR 14

PE: *Gen:* slightly anxious, thin woman. *Pelvic:* external genitalia—symmetric labia, no obvious lesions. *SSE:* vagina—physiologic discharge, mild erythema in the posterior vestibule, which is tender to touch; cervix—multiparous os, no lesions. *BME:* uterus—small, AV/AF, nontender. No palpable adnexal masses.

THOUGHT QUESTIONS

- What is vulvodynia?
- What are the causes of vulvodynia?
- What physical findings support this clinical diagnosis?

Vulvodynia is a complex clinical syndrome of unexplained vulvar pain—burning and/or stinging, often accompanied by sexual dysfunction, physical disability, and psychological distress. The pain usually has an acute onset, which can evolve into a chronic problem lasting months to years. Vulvodynia may have multiple causes, such as vulvar vestibulitis, cyclic vulvovaginitis, dysesthetic vulvodynia, and vulvar dermatoses. Given symptomatology overlap, the same differential diagnosis for vulvar pruritus must be considered in vulvodynia as well. Physical findings often are normal, limited to pain on palpation of the vestibule and/or present as inflammation in the vestibule or vagina. Because vulvodynia can be the initial presentation of both vulvar infections, such as candidiasis, and vulvar cancer, these conditions must be ruled out with culture, KOH prepared slides, colposcopy of the vulva, and biopsy.

CASE CONTINUED

V.M. does not recall any particular event preceding the onset of her symptoms. The patient denies history of physical or sexual abuse. You perform a thorough examination including a Pap smear, KOH/wet mount, and *Gonorrhea* and *Chlamydia* cultures. Upon colposcopic examination of the vulva, you note no particular acetowhite areas. You perform an unguided biopsy of the vulvar vestibule.

QUESTIONS

36-1. If on clinical examination you see multiple pits and scars on the vulva as well as areas with draining sinuses, what do you need to include in the differential diagnosis?

A. Psoriasis
B. Acanthosis nigricans
C. Behçet syndrome
D. Hidradenitis suppurativa
E. Squamous cell carcinoma

36-2. The Pap smear is normal. The KOH/wet mount preparation is normal. The biopsy returns as moderate to marked inflammation, with an abundance of plasma cells, most prominent in the stroma beneath the vestibular epithelium. What is her diagnosis?

A. Contact dermatitis
B. Cyclic vulvovaginitis
C. HPV infection
D. Lichen planus
E. Vestibulitis

36-3. What is your first-line therapy for this diagnosis?

A. Amitriptyline
B. Topical corticosteroid ointment
C. Oral fluconazole followed by topical antifungal medication
D. Topical estrogen
E. Sitz baths with Burow solution compresses

36-4. Eighteen months later despite topical steroid therapy she is distraught and complaining of intractable burning and pain in the vulvar region. What can you offer her?

A. Recombinant α-interferon injections into the vestibule
B. CO_2 laser ablation of the vestibular glands
C. Observation for spontaneous remission
D. Perineoplasty and gland excision
E. Empiric broad-spectrum antibiotics with concurrent topical steroid use

ANSWERS

36-1. D. Hidradenitis suppurativa is a chronic refractory infection arising from apocrine glands affecting the skin and subcutaneous tissue. Deep-seated, painful subcutaneous nodules are observed in the areas containing apocrine glands, such as the vulva and axilla. Occlusion of apocrine ducts from chronic infection results in progression of disease to multiple draining abscesses and sinuses. Dermatologic diseases that typically involve other areas of the body also can affect the vulva. Vulvar psoriasis generally appears in the intertriginous areas as red to reddish-yellow papules that bleed easily. Acanthosis nigricans is a raised, pigmented papillary lesion that can become quite extensive but rarely involves the vulva. Behçet syndrome is a triad of oral ulcers, genital ulcers, and ophthalmologic inflammatory changes, with possible involvement of the ocular mucosa. Squamous cell carcinoma is a slow-growing cancer that can present quite variably and frequently is painless. The basic tenet of vulvar lesions is to biopsy for diagnostic confirmation.

36-2. E. Vulvar vestibulitis is a syndrome consisting of pain on palpation of the vestibule or attempted vaginal entry. Physical findings consist of inflammation and erythema localized to the vestibule. It can be a chronic problem and often is multifactorial in origin. Typically, surgical specimens reveal areas of inflammatory changes, often characterized by an abundance of plasma cells and lack of polymorphonuclear leukocytes, with the vestibular stroma most prominently involved. There is no evidence of HPV changes on her Pap and biopsy. Similarly, she does not have yeast vulvovaginitis on the wet mount. Lichen planus lesions tend to be intensely pruritic and appear as chronic violaceous papules. In addition, some women with lichen planus develop a desquamative vaginitis, resulting in burning dysesthesia of the vulvovaginal area. Contact dermatitis usually presents with pruritus and, in severe cases, with evidence of excoriation, erythema, and edema.

36-3. B. First-line therapy for vulvar vestibulitis is topical steroid application. If an infectious cause is identified, concurrent treatment with antibiotics must be initiated. Amitriptyline, in addition to steroids, can be useful for patients in whom psychological factors appear to have a role in disease manifestation. Topical estrogen is used for management of atrophic vaginitis. Local care with sitz baths and compresses can confer significant relief from the "pain/itch" cycle of vulvar irritation caused by contact dermatitis and may be helpful for vulvar vestibulitis as well.

36-4. D. In the absence of a documented infection, addition of a broad-spectrum antibiotic is not recommended. In women with HPV disease, recombinant α-interferon injections into the vestibular glands have been effective in treating vulvar vestibulitis. CO_2 laser ablation of the vestibular glands has been shown to be ineffective and, conversely, can cause significant scarring and worsen the dyspareunia and pain. Spontaneous remission has been reported in up to 30% of women (within 6–12 months of the initial complaint) but seems unlikely to be the case here. In a small percentage of women, elimination of dietary oxalates (coffee, chocolate, tea, peanuts, spinach) can alleviate the pain. Gland excision and perineoplasty has produced relief in 75% to 90% of women who do not respond to medical management and should be discussed.

 SUGGESTED ADDITIONAL READING

Droegemueller W. Benign gynecologic lesions: vulva, vagina, cervix, uterus, oviduct, ovary. In: Stenchever MA, Droegemueller W, Herbst AL, et al., eds. *Comprehensive gynecology.* 4th ed. St. Louis, Mo: Mosby; 2001:279–530.

Wilkinson EJ, Stone IK. *Atlas of vulvar disease.* Baltimore, Md: Williams & Wilkins; 1995:149, 178–179.

McCormack WM, Spence MR. Evaluation of the surgical treatment of vulvar vestibulitis. *Eur J Obstet Gynecol Reprod Biol.* 1999; 86:135–138.

Mariani L. Vulvar vestibulitis syndrome: an overview of non-surgical treatment. *Eur J Obstet Gynecol Reprod Biol.* 2002;101: 109–112.

Acute Pelvic Pain II

ID/CC: A 20-year-old $G_2P_1T_1$ woman presents to your office complaining of worsening pelvic pain.

HPI: The pain started approximately 5 days ago and has gradually worsened. It is sharp, constant, and worse in the LLQ. She has had two episodes of diarrhea and mild nausea today. She denies fevers or chills. She also denies vaginal discharge or bleeding but has noted an abnormal vaginal odor.

SHx: None

Meds: None

PMHx: Hepatitis A, 3 years ago; Pneumonia, age 12

PSHx: None

PGynHx: LMP 10 days ago, regular cycles, no STDs, sexually active with new partner, uses OCPs

PObHx: Never pregnant

All: NKDA

THOUGHT QUESTION

■ What is included in the differential diagnosis at this point?

This patient's history is most consistent with PID. Because GI symptoms are common complaints, distinguishing PID from appendicitis sometimes is difficult. If the physical exam helps rule out appendicitis, an imaging study may be necessary. This patient may also have an ectopic pregnancy. You must rule out pregnancy with a negative pregnancy test. In fact, you must obtain a pregnancy test in any woman of reproductive age presenting with abdominal or pelvic pain because the diagnosis of pregnancy can significantly alter your management plan, regardless of the ultimate diagnosis.

CASE CONTINUED

VS: Temp 99.5°F, BP 107/68, HR 106, RR 16

PE: Uncomfortable appearing. *Abd:* soft, ND. Diffusely tender, worse in LLQ. Mild diffuse rebound. No guarding. Normal BS. *Pelvic:* Normal-appearing vagina and cervix. *BME:* cervical motion tenderness. Uterus normal size AV/AF, mildly tender to palpation. Tenderness in both adnexa (L > R), but no appreciable masses.

Labs: WBC: 8.9, Hct: 38.6, urine pregnancy test: negative, *Gonorrhea/Chlamydia* cultures pending

THOUGHT QUESTIONS

- What is your diagnosis now?
- How would the culture results influence treatment for this patient?
- How would the finding of an LLQ mass affect your treatment?

Major and minor criteria are used for the diagnosis of PID. The three major criteria are abdominal tenderness, adnexal tenderness, and cervical motion, all of which are shown by this patient. If a patient has all three major criteria in the absence of another etiology (e.g., appendicitis), she is diagnosed with PID. Minor criteria, such as fever or elevated WBC or ESR, are used to help establish the diagnosis of PID when all three major criteria are not met. PID is thought to be caused by an ascending cervical gonorrheal or chlamydial infection. However, once the infection is in the upper tract, it is polymicrobial. Treatment consists of a broad-spectrum cephalosporin and doxycycline (regardless of culture results). A stable patient who is able to tolerate oral medications and who can be compliant can be treated as an outpatient. Otherwise, admission for IV antibiotics is necessary.

Persistent PID can lead to tubo-ovarian abscesses (TOAs) or tubo-ovarian complexes (TOCs; pelvic adnexal infections that are not walled off and hence more responsive to antibiotic therapy). Finding an adnexal mass on exam should raise concern for a TOA or TOC. Pelvic ultrasound can confirm this diagnosis. Treatment is hospitalization for IV antibiotics. If antibiotic therapy fails, CT-guided drainage of the abscess or surgical removal of infected tissues is necessary.

QUESTIONS

37-1. A patient with a TOA does not respond to IV cefotetan and doxycycline treatment. The next step in management would be:
   A. Expand antibiotic coverage with ampicillin, gentamicin, and clindamycin.
   B. Laparoscopy for confirmation of the diagnosis.
   C. Laparotomy with unilateral salpingo-oophorectomy.
   D. Laparotomy with hysterectomy and bilateral salpingo-oophorectomy.

37-2. Of the following, the most common sequela of PID is:
   A. Fitz-Hugh-Curtis syndrome
   B. Infertility
   C. Toxic shock syndrome
   D. Bacterial vaginosis

37-3. A 17-year-old woman complains of an abnormal vaginal discharge. A mucopurulent discharge is seen, and a first-stream urine test is positive for *Gonorrhea*. Appropriate treatment for this patient is:
   A. A 10-day course of dicloxacillin
   B. A 7-day course of doxycycline
   C. An IM dose of ceftriaxone once
   D. Azithromycin 1 g once

37-4. Which of the following has been shown to be protective against PID?
   A. IUD use
   B. Oral contraceptive use
   C. Weekly douching with diluted vinegar solution
   D. Cigarette smoking

ANSWERS

37-1. A. If the first line of antibiotics fails, the appropriate treatment is to expand coverage to triple antibiotic therapy. Laparotomy and adnexal surgery are reserved for TOAs that are unresponsive to antibiotic therapy or those with gross rupture. Usually an unilateral salpingectomy is performed for unilateral TOAs. For bilateral TOAs, bilateral salpingectomy or a total abdominal hysterectomy is performed.

37-2. B. The two most common sequelae of PID are infertility, which is estimated to occur in 20% of all PID patients, and ectopic pregnancy, for which there is a 10-fold increased risk. Fitz-Hugh-Curtis syndrome, an ascending perihepatitis, is an occasional complication of PID. Toxic shock syndrome occurs rarely. It is caused by a *Staphylococcus aureus* toxin and has been associated with menstruation and tampon use and with postpartum and postabortal endometritis. Bacterial vaginosis is not a sequela of PID.

37-3. C. Both *Gonorrhea* and *Chlamydia* can cause a mucopurulent discharge. Both can be detected on a first-stream urine sample. The treatment for chlamydia cervicitis is a 7-day course of doxycycline 100 mg BID or a one-time 1-g dose of Azithromycin. Gonorrhea cervicitis can be treated with 250 mg ceftriaxone IM once.

37-4. B. Risk factors for PID include young age, multiple sexual partners, nonwhite and non-Asian ethnicity, being unmarried, recent history of douching, and cigarette smoking. IUDs are considered a risk factor for PID because they may increase the likelihood of ascending infection if cervicitis is present. OCPs have been found to be protective against PID. The mechanism is thought to involve alterations in cervical mucous. Barrier contraceptives provide the best protection against PID.

 ## SUGGESTED ADDITIONAL READING

Beigi RH, Wiesenfeld HC. Pelvic inflammatory disease: new diagnostic criteria and treatment. *Obstet Gynecol Clin North Am.* 2003;30:777–793.

Krivak TC, Cooksey C, Propst AM. Tubo-ovarian abscess: diagnosis, medical and surgical management. *Compr Ther.* 2004;30:93–100.

Menorrhagia

ID/CC: A 45-year-old G_3P_3 African-American woman presents complaining of heavy periods.

HPI: C.O. states that she currently is completing a menstrual period complicated by heavy bleeding requiring up to 30 pads per day for a 5-day period and is now down to five pads per day. In total, she has been bleeding for 12 days. In general she has had regular 28- to 30-day cycles, bleeding for 5 to 6 days and using five to six pads per day. During the past year, her periods have become less frequent but occasionally quite excessive. Ms. O. denies having spotting between menses. She has a history of significant cramping and breast tenderness with her menses but states that these complaints have improved over the past year. She denies having any weakness or dizziness but does complain of mild fatigue. She denies having any hot flashes, vaginal dryness, night sweats, or changes in weight over the past 6 months.

PMHx: Hypertension for 8 years, mild obesity

PSHx: Appendectomy as a child; one C/S with tubal ligation

Meds: Hydrochlorothiazide, 25 mg PO every day

All: NKDA

POb/GynHx: Two NSVDs, one C/S for breech presentation. Menarche age 11; menstrual cycle as above. Normal Pap smears, last performed 6 months ago. Distant history of chlamydial infection; denies PID. Sexually active with husband; tubal ligation.

SHx: Lives with husband, children grown; denies domestic violence. Quit smoking 5 years ago after 15-pack per year history; social ETOH use; denies other recreational drug use.

THOUGHT QUESTIONS

- What is the difference between menorrhagia, metrorrhagia, and menometrorrhagia?
- What is your differential diagnosis for this patient's complaint of menorrhagia?
- Should this patient be admitted to the hospital and/or receive a blood transfusion?

Menorrhagia is heavy or prolonged bleeding at the time of menses. Metrorrhagia is bleeding between menses. Menometrorrhagia is a combination of the two (i.e., menses that are heavy or prolonged with occasional intermenstrual bleeding).

In general the differential diagnoses for menorrhagia include the following: endometrial hyperplasia, endometrial cancer, anatomical sources including fibroids or polyps, adenomyosis, hormonal sources including anovulation, and bleeding disorders. The latter usually is a diagnosis made early in a patient's menstrual life and usually does not occur for the first time late in life unless the patient is acutely ill with a liver disorder and/or a coagulopathy. Polyps, cervical or endometrial, usually present as metrorrhagia but should remain part of a differential diagnosis.

Acute bleeding from menorrhagia requiring a blood transfusion or hospitalization for hemodynamic stabilization can occur. When evaluating a patient it is important that you first determine whether the patient is hemodynamically stable. A patient who is not stable may present quite obviously (e.g., brought in by ambulance with tachycardia, low blood pressure, and mental obtundation). However, most patients present with more subtle findings, such as dizziness and fatigue with tachycardia, orthostatic hypotension, and a low hematocrit.

CASE CONTINUED

VS: Lying BP 135/88, HR 76; sitting BP 138/88, HR 80; standing BP 140/90, HR 84. Weight 160 lb, Height 5 feet 5 inches

PE: *Gen:* NAD. *Lungs:* CTA. *Cor:* RR&R, no murmurs. *Abd:* obese, soft, nontender, no HSM. *Extremities:* no clubbing, cyanosis, or edema. *Pelvic:* no vulvar lesions; pink, moist mucous membranes. *SSE:* thin, white vaginal discharge, scant blood in vault; cervix within normal limits. *BME:* small anteverted nontender uterus, no adnexal masses noted.

Labs: Urine hCG negative, WBC 6.0, Hb 11.4, Hct 35.0, Plts 300,000. Endometrial biopsy sent.

Ten days later you receive the biopsy result, which shows no evidence of hyperplasia or carcinoma. You have Ms. O undergo a blood draw 21 days after completion of her menses to determine whether or not she ovulated. The findings above suggest that she did not ovulate during this cycle. You counsel her that her heavy menses likely is secondary to anovulation and you discuss therapies.

QUESTIONS

38-1. What hormone did you measure and what was the result that suggested anovulation?
    A. Progesterone—high
    B. Progesterone—low
    C. Estrogen—high
    D. Estrogen—low
    E. FSH—low

38-2. What treatment options are available for this patient?
    A. Low-dose oral contraceptive pills
    B. Hormone replacement therapy
    C. Cyclical progesterone
    D. All of the above
    E. B and C only

38-3. If this patient had presented with a long history of heavy menses and an enlarged uterus, what would her most likely diagnosis be?
    A. Adenomyosis
    B. Fibroids
    C. Endometrial polyps
    D. Endometrial cancer
    E. None of the above

38-4. Which of the following patients should undergo an endometrial biopsy to rule out endometrial cancer?
- A. A 40-year-old female with a history of breast cancer on tamoxifen with vaginal bleeding
- B. A 40-year-old female with bleeding between menses for the last 6 months
- C. A 32-year-old female with 4 months of abnormal bleeding after starting OCPs
- D. All of the above
- E. A and B only

ANSWERS

38-1. B. A review of the menstrual cycle demonstrates that, after ovulation, progesterone rises dramatically as it is secreted by the corpus luteum. This rise helps the endometrium to become more glandular and secretory in preparation for a possible fertilized ovum to implant. If ovulation does not occur, then you do not see this rise in progesterone. Measuring estrogen is not a useful test in this situation because it is difficult to interpret and to specify which result signifies anovulation.

38-2. D. The nonspecific diagnosis for this patient is dysfunctional uterine bleeding (DUB). This diagnosis of DUB is made when other conditions, anatomical lesions, and cancerous states have been excluded. The treatment for DUB secondary to anovulation involves many options. No treatment is an option for anovulation if the condition occurs infrequently. However, a more chronic anovulatory state (which is an estrogen-dominant state) can put a patient at risk for developing hyperplasia or carcinoma, so therapy with progesterone is recommended. In addition, a patient can become quite anemic from this chronic blood loss. All of the treatments listed will likely help to control the patient's cycles, limit bleeding, and add back some progesterone to protect against hyperplasia or carcinoma.

38-3. B. Uterine fibroids, also called leiomyomas or myomas, are a local proliferation of uterine smooth muscle cells and are very common. They can grow slowly or quickly over time, causing increasing symptoms. However, most women remain asymptomatic even with large fibroids. Symptoms include menorrhagia, pelvic pain, pelvic pressure, or pelvic fullness. The patient described could have any of the other diagnoses listed as well, but all would be much less common for this presentation.

38-4. E. Approximately 25% of endometrial cancer cases occur before menopause. Abnormal bleeding in a woman older than 38 to 40 years of age, especially if they have risk factors, mandates an endometrial biopsy. Known risk factors for endometrial hyperplasia and carcinoma include exposure to estrogen therapy without progesterone; tamoxifen therapy; diabetes mellitus; nulliparity; a family history of endometrial, colon, or breast cancer; early menarche (before age 12) and late menopause; obesity; and hypertension. In much younger women, abnormal bleeding is generally not related to cancer, although hyperplasia can occur. In addition, breakthrough bleeding while taking oral contraceptives during the first 3 to 6 months is quite common.

SUGGESTED ADDITIONAL READING

Marjoribank J, Lethaby A, Farquhar C. Surgery versus medical therapy for heavy menstrual bleeding. *Cochrane Database Syst Rev.* 2003;CD003855.

Lethaby AE, Cooke I, Rees M. Progesterone/progestogen releasing intrauterine system versus either placebo or any other medication for heavy menstrual bleeding. *Cochrane Database Syst Rev.* 2000;CD002126.

Lethaby AE, Irvine G, Cameron I. Cyclical progestogens for heavy menstrual bleeding. *Cochrane Database Syst Rev.* 2000; CD001016.

Metrorrhagia

ID/CC: A 46-year-old G_3P_3 Caucasian woman presents with complaints of vaginal spotting.

HPI: J.P. states that over the past 6 to 8 months she has noticed occasional vaginal spotting between menses. The bleeding lasts for 2 to 10 days and is quite light, not requiring a pad. Her periods remain regular, every 30 to 32 days, and she bleeds for 5 to 6 days using approximately four tampons each day. She is sexually active but is uncertain whether the spotting is related to sex. She denies having any pelvic pain. Her vaginal discharge is thick and white with some mild pruritus. She had a yeast infection about 3 months before, which she treated with an over-the-counter yeast medication. Ms. P. denies having any fever or chills, night sweats, or recent changes in weight. She is quite certain this is vaginal bleeding and denies having any rectal bleeding or changes in bowel movements.

PMHx: Type 2 diabetes mellitus for 5 years; moderate obesity

PSHx: None

Meds: Glyburide, occasional acetaminophen (Tylenol)

All: Penicillin, causing rash

POb/GynHx: Three NSVDs, uncomplicated. LMP 3 weeks prior. Menarche age 12; cycles as above. Distant history of chlamydial infection with PID. Sexually active, two partners in past 6 months, uses condoms. Last Pap 5 years ago was normal. She had an abnormal Pap many years ago, but on repeat "it was better" and she required no treatment.

SHx: Lives alone. Smokes half-pack per day for 20 years; occasional ETOH use; denies recreational drug use.

FHx: Type 2 diabetes mellitus in multiple family members, heart disease in an aunt and uncle.

THOUGHT QUESTIONS

- What is this patient's differential diagnosis?
- What tests would you like to perform on this patient and why?

The differential diagnosis for metrorrhagia includes cervical and endometrial polyps, cervical dysplasia and carcinoma, endometrial hyperplasia and carcinoma, cervicitis, and vaginal and vulvar lesions.

A KOH test should be performed because severe vaginal candidiasis when associated with excoriated areas can bleed. In addition, this patient is overdue for a Pap smear, and her vague history of an abnormal Pap in the past is worrisome. Cervicitis can cause spotting, so gonorrhea and chlamydia tests should be done. In addition, an endometrial biopsy is warranted, given the patient's age and her risk factors for endometrial hyperplasia and carcinoma (i.e., diabetes mellitus, obesity).

CASE CONTINUED

VS: Temp 98.4°F, BP 138/86, HR 88, RR 16, weight 174 lb, height 5 feet 4 inches

PE: *Gen:* obese female, NAD. *Lungs:* CTAB. *Neck:* normal-size thyroid without nodules. *Cor:* RR&R, no murmurs. *Abd:* obese, soft, nontender. *EGBUS:* mild erythema of labia minora and majora, no lesions noted. *SSE:* thick white vaginal discharge; no cervical lesions or polyps noted. *BME:* limited secondary to habitus; midposition uterus noted, approximately 5 to 6 week size, nontender; no adnexal masses appreciated. *Rectal:* guaiac negative, no hemorrhoids noted. *Extremities:* no clubbing, cyanosis, or edema.

Labs: Urine pregnancy test: negative; wet prep: normal, few WBCs; KOH: pseudohyphae noted (Figure 39-1); FSBG, 188; Pap smear, endometrial biopsy, cultures for *Gonorrhea* and *Chlamydia* sent.

The patient is told that she has a vaginal yeast infection. You prescribe fluconazole (Diflucan) 150 mg PO, one dose, and you refer her to her

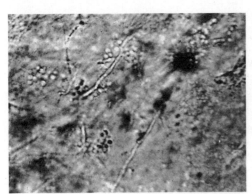

FIGURE 39-1.
Candida albicans.
Note the budding and
pseudohyphae. *(From
Crissey JT. Manual of
Medical Mycology.
Malden, Mass: Black-
well Science, 1995,
with permission.)*

primary doctor for re-evaluation of her current oral hypoglycemic regimen. The *Gonorrhea* and *Chlamydia* cultures return as negative 5 days later. Ten days later, the endometrial biopsy result returns without evidence of hyperplasia or carcinoma. However, gland proliferation suggestive of an endometrial polyp is noted. The Pap smear is normal. You schedule the patient for a pelvic ultrasound, which reveals a thickened endometrial stripe, possibly secondary to a polyp, without other pathologic evidence.

QUESTIONS

39-1. In the face of this possible diagnosis, what is a potential next step?
   A. Operative hysteroscopy with possible polypectomy
   B. Balloon ablation
   C. Laparoscopy
   D. No treatment needed
   E. Hysterectomy

39-2. Approximately what percentage of endometrial polyps are associated with cancer?
   A. Less than 1%
   B. 1% to 5%
   C. 6% to 10%
   D. 11% to 20%
   E. 21% to 30%

39-3. Which hysteroscopic distension medium is incorrectly matched to its possible complication?
  A. Glycine—anaphylactic shock
  B. Sorbitol—hyponatremia
  C. Dextran—pulmonary edema
  D. Hyskon—bleeding diathesis
  E. None of the above

39-4. Assume that during your office examination you visualized a cervical polyp measuring 1.0×0.5 cm. What is the next step?
  A. Biopsy a piece of the polyp and send it to pathology.
  B. Remove the polyp with polyp forceps and send it to pathology.
  C. Remove the polyp with cryosurgery.
  D. Remove the polyp in the operating room in case of bleeding.
  E. None of the above.

ANSWERS

39-1. A.; **39-2.** A. Endometrial polyps are an overgrowth of endometrial glands and stroma. Less than 1% are associated with adenocarcinoma. Removal is recommended, both to establish that no cancer is present as well as to eliminate the symptomatic bleeding. Removal can be accomplished in several ways. Hysteroscopy can be done in the office or the operating room, allowing the gynecologist to visualize the endometrium and to remove polyps or lesions if needed. A hysteroscope is a metal instrument and camera that is inserted into the vagina and cervix to allow visualization of the uterine cavity. Fluid is instilled into the uterus through a separate port to dilate the uterus and act as a medium for the operative procedure. The operative hysteroscope often is followed with curettage (scraping) of the endometrium so that the entire endometrium is sampled and can be evaluated by pathology.

39-3. A. In performing diagnostic and operative hysteroscopy, several distension media are available. It is important that the operator knows and understands the complications of each medium so as to prevent such complications or recognize them immediately should they occur. High-viscosity fluids such as Hyskon and dextran have been associated with anaphylactic shock, bleeding diathesis (through interference with platelet function and factor VII), and pulmonary edema. Low-viscosity and hyperosmolar fluids such as glycine and sorbitol are associated with hyponatremia, which can lead to cerebral edema and death.

39-4. B. Cervical polyps are generally benign focal overgrowths of cervical tissue. Their removal usually is quite easy and can be done in the office. Polyp forceps are used to grasp the polyp in its entirety, and then the polyp is twisted until it is removed. Bleeding is generally minimal and can be resolved with pressure. The specimen is sent to pathology to confirm that the polyp is benign.

 SUGGESTED ADDITIONAL READING

Gebauer G, Hatner A, Siebzehnrubl E, et al. Role of hysteroscopy in detection and extraction of endometrial polyps: study results of a prospective trial. *Am J Obstet Gynecol.* 2001;184:59–63.

Intermenstrual Vaginal Bleeding

CC/ID: A 40-year-old G$_3$P$_1$ woman presents to the office complaining of vaginal bleeding between menses.

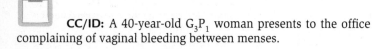

THOUGHT QUESTIONS

- What is in the differential diagnosis at this time?
- How would you focus your history to further refine the diagnostic possibilities?

There are many causes of intermenstrual bleeding in young women. Table 40-1 lists the more common causes.

Questions to elucidate the following would help narrow the list of possible causes, including

- Method of contraception, if any
- Menstrual cycle interval
- Timing of bleeding during the intermenstrual period
- Precipitating factors such as intercourse, trauma, or exercise
- Associated symptoms, such as pain, fever, vaginal discharge, nipple discharge, or hot flashes
- Medications that can decrease the efficacy of oral contraceptive pills (OCPs)

TABLE 40-1 Causes of Intermenstrual Bleeding in Young Women

Pregnancy	Threatened abortion or ectopic pregnancy
Ectropion	Normal exuberant growth of the transformation zone of the cervix that can bleed spontaneously or after intercourse
Mittelschmerz	Midcycle unilateral pelvic pain and vaginal spotting that occur at the time of ovulation
Hormonal imbalance	Irregular use or too low a dose of the contraceptive pill causing breakthrough bleeding Concurrent use of antiepileptic medications and oral contraceptives Endocrine dysfunction (thyroid, pituitary) Progesterone-only contraception: "mini" pill disturbs hormone levels in some patients Anovulatory cycles: cause erratic bleeding when the interval between cycles becomes too long
Infection	Endometritis: due to postpartum, postabortal, or postsurgical infection Cervicitis: likely due to gonorrheal or chlamydial infection Vaginal: trichomonal, monilial, or bacterial infection
Structural lesions	Injury due to intercourse or insertion of foreign objects Vaginal ulceration from use of diaphragms or pessaries Intrauterine device: can cause occasional spotting Postprocedural cervical abnormalities: cervical conization/ LEEP, cryotherapy Endometrial or cervical polyps Leiomyomas
Neoplasm/malignancy	Vaginal or vulvar condyloma Endometrial hyperplasia or cancer Cervical dysplasia or cancer Vaginal or vulvar dysplasia or cancer
Nongynecologic	Hemorrhoids, acute cystitis

CASE CONTINUED

HPI: The intermenstrual bleeding started approximately 4 months ago and became progressively more frequent. Her menses have occurred every 28 days since she started taking birth control pills 3 years ago. Prior to that time her menses were regular and occurred approximately every 28 to 30 days. She states that she takes the pill every day as directed. The abnormal bleeding occurs randomly during the intermenstrual period and usually constitutes light spotting.

She is sexually active with one partner (her husband of the last 10 years) and denies postcoital bleeding or dyspareunia. Bowel movements and urination are normal. Her review of systems is otherwise negative. Denies tobacco use; occasionally drinks alcohol.

LMP: 3 weeks ago

Last Pap smear: 7 months ago and normal

PMHx: Mild asthma

PSHx: LEEP 12 years ago

Meds: 30 µg estradiol, combination OCPs, albuterol
(Ventolin)

PGynHx: No STDs, remote HGSIL, normal Paps since

PObHx: Cesarean

All: NKDA

PE: Afebrile, vital signs normal, BMI = 22, appears healthy. *Abd:* soft, without masses. *Pelvic:* normal external genitalia. *Vagina:* normal rugae, no excoriations, lacerations, or abnormal discharge. *Cervix:* appears consistent with prior LEEP procedure (transformation zone not visible), does not bleed with manipulation with swab, no cervical motion tenderness. *Uterus:* normal size, anteverted, no uterine tenderness. *Adnexa:* normal, without tenderness; urine pregnancy test performed in your office is negative.

THOUGHT QUESTIONS

- Now what is on your differential diagnoses?
- What test should you perform next?

Your investigation so far now makes polyps or a neoplastic process the most likely diagnostic category. Breakthrough bleeding due to too low a dose of her birth control pill still is possible; however, she has been on a medium-dose OCP for several years without a problem. You have not yet ruled out endocrine dysfunction, but her history and physical exam findings make this less likely.

An endometrial biopsy should be performed in all women older than 35 years with abnormal bleeding to rule out endometrial cancer or premalignant cells such as atypical hyperplasia. You also should consider an endometrial biopsy in women aged 18 to 35 years with abnormal bleeding who have risk factors for endometrial cancer, such as obesity, chronic anovulation, history of breast cancer, and tamoxifen use.

You perform an endometrial biopsy, which reveals normal endometrium with exogenous hormone effect. No evidence of hyperplasia or atypia. You then obtain a transvaginal ultrasound, which shows an endometrium that is relatively thick near the fundus and measures 2 cm.

THOUGHT QUESTION

- What further imaging would confirm your diagnosis?

A focal thickening of the endometrium is most consistent with an endometrial polyp. A saline infusion sonogram (sonohysterogram) is the best study to confirm the presence of and evaluate endometrial polyps.

Endometrial polyps are localized overgrowths of the endometrial lining that project into the uterine cavity. They may be sessile (broad based) or pedunculated (on a narrow stalk). Malignancies have been reported in only 0.6% of cases of endometrial polyps.

Endometrial polyps are most common among women of reproductive age older than 20 years. The incidence rises steadily with increasing age and then gradually declines after menopause. The most frequent symptom of women with endometrial polyps is metrorrhagia (irregular, acyclic uterine bleeding). Postmenstrual spotting also is common. Less frequent symptoms include hypermenorrhea (prolonged and/or profuse uterine bleeding, also called menorrhagia), postmenopausal bleeding, and breakthrough bleeding during hormonal therapy.

Endometrial polyps can be removed by dilation and thorough curettage. However, removal of polyps or other structural abnormalities may be missed by blind curettage; therefore, hysteroscopic-guided curettage is often used.

QUESTIONS

40-1. A 44-year-old G_0 woman has been referred to you for management of abnormal bleeding. She reports irregular cycles every 2 to 5 months that are very heavy. On exam, she has a BMI of 35. Her CBC, TSH, and prolactin levels were checked by her primary physician, and all were normal. The endometrial biopsy you perform reveals a secretory endometrium without hyperplasia or atypia. An appropriate next step for this patient is to:

    A. Do nothing because her biopsy is benign and wait to see if normal menses resumes

    B. Insert a copper IUD

    C. Prescribe ethinyl estradiol daily for 21 days per month

    D. Prescribe combination OCPs

40-2. A 22-year-old G_1A_1 woman presents with a 3-month history of postcoital bleeding. She denies any abnormal discharge or pelvic pain. She and her partner use condoms regularly. Her cycles are regular, and her LMP was 1 week ago. A pelvic exam is unremarkable. Your initial laboratory evaluation of this patient should include:

    A. Endometrial biopsy

    B. Cervical biopsy

    C. Colposcopy

    D. Wet smear

40-3. A 16-year-old G_1A_1 girl presents to your office complaining of irregular spotting between menses. Menarche occurred at age 12. She underwent an uncomplicated first-trimester pregnancy termination 5 months ago and started combination OCPs immediately after the procedure. She states she takes her pills every day as directed. Her Pap smear performed just prior to starting OCPs was normal. Her review of systems is otherwise negative. The most likely cause of her abnormal bleeding is:

    A. Von Willebrand disease

    B. Cervical intraepithelial neoplasia

    C. Breakthrough bleeding

    D. Endometritis

40-4. A 19-year-old G₀ woman presents with irregular vaginal bleeding for at least 6 months. She is not sure how often her menses are. She has never been sexually active. She notes a watery vaginal discharge and vaginal burning for the last few months. On exam, she is thin and has moderately discolored teeth. Her pelvic exam is notable only for thin vaginal mucosa and moderate white blood cells but no clue cells on a wet smear. The most likely diagnosis is:

A. Bacterial vaginosis
B. Bulimia
C. Polycystic ovarian syndrome
D. Premature ovarian failure

ANSWERS

40-1. D. This patient's history and biopsy results are consistent with anovulatory bleeding. Anovulatory uterine bleeding is commonly caused by chronic unopposed estrogen. Unopposed estrogen can cause endometrial hyperplasia, a precursor to endometrial cancer. Anovulatory bleeding should be treated medically by either establishing regular withdrawal bleeding or providing progesterone to oppose estrogen-induced proliferation of the endometrium. A levonorgestrel IUD provides a small daily dose of progesterone to the uterine lining. Both combined OCPs and a 10-day course of progesterone such as norethindrone acetate will establish withdrawal bleeding.

40-2. D. Probable causes for postcoital bleeding in this patient include undiagnosed pregnancy, cervical dysplasia, cervicitis, vaginitis, trauma, an endometrial polyp, and ectropion. Pregnancy should be ruled out in all women of reproductive age who have abnormal bleeding. If this patient has not had a recent normal Pap smear, one should be performed to rule out cervical dysplasia. A wet smear is used to look for evidence of vaginal infection. An endometrial biopsy evaluates the endometrial lining for evidence of malignancy or premalignancy (i.e., atypical hyperplasia). At age 22, this patient is at low risk for these disorders unless she has a history consistent with chronic anovulation. Although an endometrial biopsy sometimes can show evidence of an endometrial polyp, an ultrasound or a sonohysterogram is a better test if you suspect a polyp. Cervical biopsy would only be done if a cervical lesion was suspected. Colposcopy is used to evaluate suspected cervical dysplasia.

40-3. C. Breakthrough bleeding (irregular spotting between menses) is the most common side effect of birth control pills. Low-dose birth control pills are more likely to cause breakthrough bleeding because the endometrium become relatively thinner (atrophic) and more fragile in a low-estrogen environment. Switching to a higher-estrogen OCP can help stabilize the endometrium. Von Willebrand disease is not likely in this patient because she has a several-year history of normal menses and her elective abortion was uncomplicated. Her recent Pap smear was normal, so dysplasia is unlikely. Although endometritis is a possible complication of a procedure such as a D&C, her history is not consistent with a chronic low-grade infection.

40-4. B. The absence of clue cells on the wet smear makes bacterial vaginosis unlikely. White blood cells on the slide and the finding of a thin vaginal epithelium are consistent with atrophic vaginitis. Atrophic vaginitis occurs in a low-estrogen environment, which could occur with either premature ovarian failure (high FSH) or hypogonadotrophic hypogonadism (low FSH). Either type of hypogonadism presents with oligomenorrhea or amenorrhea. Common causes of hypogonadotrophic hypogonadism in young women include anorexia/bulimia, strenuous exercise, and stress. This patient's presentation (thin and stained teeth) is very consistent with bulimia.

SUGGESTED ADDITIONAL READING

APGO Educational Series on Women's Health Issues. Clinical Management of Abnormal Uterine Bleeding. Crofton, Md: Association of Professors of Gynecology and Obstetrics; May 2002.

Maitra N, Kulier R, Bloemenkamp KW, et al. Progestogens in combined oral contraceptives for contraception. *Cochrane Database Syst Rev.* 2004;CD004861.

Painful Periods

ID/CC: A 32-year-old G_0 woman with severe, progressive dysmenorrhea.

HPI: P.D. notes that her periods have become increasingly worse over the past 4 years. She often has to miss work during the first and second days of her menses. The pain typically resolves 2 to 5 days after the end of her period. She receives only partial relief with ibuprofen. In addition, during the last 4 months she has experienced deep, sharp pain with intercourse. She has been in a monogamous relationship for the past 2 years.

PMHx: None

PSHx: None

POb/GynHx: Menarche age 14, LMP 3 weeks ago. Regular menses every 27 to 30 days, lasting 4 to 5 days, with moderate flow. No history of STI. Uses diaphragm.

Meds: Ibuprofen 200–400 mg PRN

All: NKDA

SHx: No tobacco use, occasional ethanol use.

FHx: 35-year-old sister who has been unable to conceive for 5 years; otherwise noncontributory.

VS: Afebrile, stable.

PE: *Abdomen:* soft, nontender. No guarding. No palpable masses. Normal external genitalia, normal vagina and cervix. No discharge. *Pelvic:* small uterus, retroverted, slightly tender to palpation and mild CMT tenderness. No obvious adnexal masses or tenderness.

Labs: WBC 6.4, Hb 11.2, UA negative, negative urine hCG

THOUGHT QUESTIONS

- What is your differential diagnosis?
- What additional studies would you recommend to make a diagnosis?
- What first-line treatment option would you recommend?

This patient has progressive, severe dysmenorrhea. The differential diagnosis includes primary and secondary dysmenorrhea. Primary dysmenorrhea is a diagnosis of exclusion when no organic cause can be identified. The age at presentation, the progressive nature of her complaint, the new-onset dyspareunia, and the physical findings all suggest an organic lesion. Endometriosis, adenomyosis, uterine fibroids, pelvic infection, uterine polyps, intrauterine contraceptive device, cervical stenosis or obstruction in menstrual flow at any point in the genital tract, and pelvic adhesions can cause secondary dysmenorrhea. This patient's clinical presentation is suggestive of endometriosis, the classic symptoms of which are dysmenorrhea, dyspareunia, and infertility. This patient has at least the first two symptoms. A positive family history is present in approximately 20% of endometriosis patients, and this patient reports that her sister has infertility (but we do not know the cause). Endometriosis is formally diagnosed by direct visualization and tissue diagnosis, usually via laparoscopy.

Cultures (or a DNA-based test) for *Neisseria gonorrhoeae* and *Chlamydia trachomatis* should be sent to rule out acute or chronic PID. Pelvic ultrasound is helpful in evaluating for the presence of uterine fibroids, polyps or IUD, and ovarian cysts, the latter of which may be seen in the context of endometriosis (endometriomas). Occasionally adenomyosis can be diagnosed with ultrasound, but this diagnosis often requires a pelvic MRI. Sonohysterogram and/or hysterosalpingogram to evaluate the uterine cavity and tubes are useful if submucosal fibroids or polyps are suspected or if uterine synechiae is a possibility.

A trial of oral contraceptives for at least 3 months and/or NSAIDs at adequate dosing and schedule would be reasonable options as initial therapy, assuming the ultrasound was negative.

CASE CONTINUED

Chlamydia and gonococci cervical studies by ligase chain reaction (LCR) are negative. Pelvic ultrasound is normal. You start her on birth control pills (combined, monophasic OCP) and recommend that she keep a menstrual pain calendar. She is to return for a follow-up visit in 3 months.

QUESTIONS

41-1. On her next visit she reports that her menstrual pain has decreased significantly in the last menses. Which of the following would you recommend?

    A. Continue OCP use until conception is desired.

    B. Discontinue OCP now and restart only if symptoms reappear.

    C. Discontinue OCP at age 35 because of increased risk for thromboembolic events.

    D. Long-term OCP use is not a good choice because it increases the risk for ovarian cancer.

    E. Recommend diagnostic laparoscopy to confirm the diagnosis

41-2. Six months later, she notes no improvement in her menstrual pain during the last five of six periods. The next best step in management is:

    A. Begin antidepressant treatment with selective serotonin reuptake inhibitors (SSRIs)

    B. Total abdominal hysterectomy, bilateral salpingo-oophorectomy, and appendectomy

    C. Laparoscopy

    D. GnRH agonist (Lupron)

    E. Vaginal hysterectomy

41-3. In relation to primary dysmenorrhea, which of the following is the *best* answer?

    A. It is more common among women with irregular cycles and dysfunctional uterine bleeding.

    B. Response rates to NSAIDs and OCPs as first-line therapy are similar.

    C. Pelvic exam usually is abnormal.

D. For best results, NSAIDs should be started after the onset of menses.

E. Typically symptoms develop after age 20 years.

41-4. Which of the following conditions usually is associated with the sign or symptom provided?

A. Cervical stenosis—menorrhagia

B. Endometriosis—uterosacral nodularities

C. Adenomyosis—irregularly enlarged uterus

D. IUD—fixed, retroverted uterus

E. Primary dysmenorrhea—infertility

ANSWERS

41-1. A. Continuing with OCPs until conception is desired is the best option. You have not ruled out endometriosis, which is a real consideration in this patient, for whom OCPs may have some additional value aside from pain control. In addition, if she only has pain with menses, she may use OCPs continuously, stopping only several times per year to induce withdrawal bleeds. Prolonged discontinuation of OCPs likely will result in recurrence of symptoms. There are no contraindications for use of oral contraceptives after age 35 unless there are concomitant risk factors that increase the risk for thromboembolic events, such as cigarette smoking. OCPs actually reduce the risk of ovarian cancer by twofold to threefold.

41-2. C. For patients with progressive dysmenorrhea who have not responded to primary therapy with NSAIDs and OCPs, the next step in management is laparoscopy for diagnosis and treatment. Antidepressants such as SSRIs may be efficacious in premenstrual dysphoric disorder (PMDD) or chronic pelvic pain. Therefore, making a formal diagnosis will help guide therapy. Total abdominal hysterectomy, with removal of tubes, ovaries, and appendix, may be considered in patients with severe endometriosis who have completed childbearing and for whom medical as well as less invasive surgical approaches have failed. Endometriosis can be treated with a GnRH agonist; however, confirmation by direct visualization is often recommended prior to initiation of treatment.

41-3. B. Primary dysmenorrhea is unusual in women with irregular cycles. In fact, it usually begins within 6 to 12 months after the onset of ovulatory (regular) cycles in young women. Treatment of primary dysmenorrhea can be accomplished with either NSAIDs or OCPs, with similar response rates. NSAIDs are more effective if therapy is initiated prior to the onset of menses and continued for 3 to 5 days. Before the diagnosis of primary dysmenorrhea is made, secondary dysmenorrhea should be ruled out, which generally can be accomplished with a careful history and physical.

41-4. B. Cervical stenosis usually is seen in patients with a history of prior surgical procedure to the cervix (e.g., cone biopsy, LEEP). It manifests with colicky lower abdominal pain and scant or light menstrual flow. A fixed, retroverted uterus and nodularities on the uterosacral ligaments are characteristic, albeit not exclusive, of endometriosis. Diffuse enlargement and tenderness of the uterus are typical findings of adenomyosis that can be best appreciated at the time of menstruation. Dysmenorrhea is a common complaint among IUD users, but no characteristic size, shape, or flexion of the uterus is associated with IUD dysmenorrhea. NSAIDs usually are effective in managing IUD-related dysmenorrhea. In addition to colicky lower abdominal pain, primary dysmenorrhea often is accompanied by nausea, vomiting, headaches, diarrhea, anxiety, syncope, and abdominal bloating. Reproductive fitness is not impaired in women with primary dysmenorrhea.

 SUGGESTED ADDITIONAL READING

French L. Dysmenorrhea. *Am Fam Physician.* 2005;15;71:285–291.

Marjoribanks J, Proctor ML, Farquhar C. Nonsteroidal anti-inflammatory drugs for primary dysmenorrhoea. *Cochrane Database Syst Rev.* 2003;CD001751.

Proctor ML, Roberts H, Farquhar CM. Combined oral contraceptive pill (OCP) as treatment for primary dysmenorrhoea. *Cochrane Database Syst Rev.* 2001;CD002120.

Abdominal Pain and Fullness Associated with Amenorrhea

ID/CC: A 14-year-old girl presents with complaints of lower abdominal pain and fullness.

HPI: I.H. has had no prior medical complaints. She presents to the emergency room with her mother now complaining of low, midline abdominal pain. She notes that this pain began approximately 48 hours ago. It had increased slowly at first but over the last 4 to 6 hours has dramatically worsened in severity. She reports prior episodes of this pain, although not as bad, for almost 1 year. The last episode of pain was approximately 1 month ago. She is slightly nauseous but has not had any emesis. She also notes that she has not had any fever or chills. She denies anorexia but reports feeling a fullness in her abdomen for several months. She has no changes in bowel habits but has noticed an increase in urinary frequency.

PMHx: Childhood illnesses

PSHx: None

Meds: Acetaminophen (Tylenol) for pain

All: NKDA

POb/GynHx: Has not reached menarche yet.

SHx: On isolated history, no self-report of tobacco, ethanol, or recreational drug use. Has never been sexually active.

VS: Temp 98.4°F, BP 118/76, HR 92, RR 16

PE: *Gen:* appears uncomfortable but in minimal distress. *Abdomen:* soft, no rebound or guarding, fullness consistent with mass in lower abdomen, slightly tender. *Pelvic:* normal external genitalia. Patient and parents refuse internal exam.

THOUGHT QUESTIONS

■ What is in the differential diagnosis?
■ What laboratory tests or studies would you order next?

Because of the question of an abdominal mass, the differential should include soft-tissue tumors of the abdomen and pelvis. Benign adnexal tumors from the uterus and adnexa also should be considered. Two common ovarian tumors that present as enlarged masses are cystadenoma and benign teratoma. Either of these tumors can undergo torsion, which can lead to increasing pain, although usually with concomitant nausea, vomiting, and peritoneal signs.

At this time, the usual laboratory tests for abdominal pain are reasonable: CBC to look for signs of infection, LFTs, and bilirubins, although the latter two are likely to be low yield in this patient. The most important test to obtain next is an imaging study of the abdomen and pelvis. If this is truly a pelvic mass, a pelvic ultrasound is the imaging modality of choice. However, this patient may decline a transvaginal ultrasound because of her virginal history. In that setting, an abdominal/pelvic CT certainly is reasonable to begin characterizing the mass.

CASE CONTINUED

Labs: WBC 7.6, Hct 36.7, Plts 269,000

You discuss the possible imaging modalities with the patient and her mother, and they agree to try the ultrasound, although they would prefer that it be performed abdominally.

US: *Pelvic, transabdominal:* normal uterus, left ovary measures 3.2 × 3.4 × 3.1 cm, right ovary measures 2.6 × 3.2 × 3.6 cm. No evidence of adnexal mass. Moderate free fluid in the cul-de-sac, large amount of fluid below cervix in vagina, thickened endometrium in uterus along with heterogeneous material. Transvaginal approach failed secondary to patient discomfort.

THOUGHT QUESTION

■ What is your differential diagnosis now?

With the new information provided by the transabdominal ultrasound, it is clear that there is an obstruction to the menstrual flow from the uterus. The multiple potential causes include abnormal fusion of the lower and upper genital tracts, transverse vaginal septum, imperforate hymen, and a variant of vaginal agenesis where there is just absence of distal vagina. The obstruction to flow has allowed a large collection of blood and menstrual tissue to collect in the upper vagina, and it has flowed retrograde through the fallopian tubes into the pelvis. This has led to the patient's cyclic pelvic pain.

CASE CONTINUED

You explain this information to the patient and her mother and order an MRI to further detail the pelvic anatomy. You also perform a gentle speculum examination at this point to help with diagnosis and to plan treatment. There is approximately 1 cm of depth to the vagina beyond the external labia (Figure 42-1). There is no obvious evidence of a hymeneal ring, and the obstruction to the upper vagina appears thin and fluctuant.

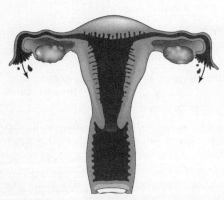

FIGURE 42-1.
The uterus and adnexa are normal but the outflow tract is occluded, leading to a collection of menses that has filled the vagina and backed up into the uterus and pelvis.

QUESTIONS

42-1. Based on the physical exam, what is the diagnosis?
A. Imperforate hymen
B. Transverse vaginal septum
C. Vaginal agenesis
D. Mayer-Rokitansky-Küster-Hauser syndrome
E. Not enough evidence to diagnose

42-2. On MRI, what other structures should be characterized in addition to the pelvic organs?
A. Adrenal glands
B. Appendix
C. Pancreas
D. Kidneys
E. Spine

42-3. Which treatment for recurrent miscarriages used from the 1950s to the 1970s was shown to be associated with müllerian abnormalities?
A. Ethinyl estradiol
B. Ethynodiol diacetate
C. Diethylstilbestrol (DES)
D. Desogestrel
E. Norethindrone acetate

42-4. This agent was also associated with which unusual disease of the genital tract?
A. Paget disease
B. Vaginal adenocarcinoma
C. Leiomyosarcoma
D. Ovarian adenocarcinoma
E. Squamous cell carcinoma of the cervix

 ANSWERS

42-1. A. The first three on the list are the most likely diagnoses prior to physical examination. Mayer-Rokitansky-Küster-Hauser syndrome is agenesis or dysgenesis of the müllerian system, whereas this patient has evidence of a normal uterus, cervix, and upper vagina. The fact that a hymeneal ring is not visualized makes transverse vaginal septum unlikely. Distal vaginal agenesis also is unlikely because the obstruction is relatively thin. Thus, the most likely diagnosis is imperforate hymen.

42-2. D. Patients with abnormalities of the genital tract and pelvic organs are at risk for renal anomalies as well. The most common are horseshoe kidney, unilateral renal agenesis, and ectopic or accessory ureters.

42-3. C.; **42-4.** B. DES is a progestogenic agent used in patients who had recurrent miscarriages from the 1950s up to the mid-1970s. There were case series of young patients with vaginal adenocarcinoma, also known as clear cell carcinoma, that eventually were associated with DES use by the mothers. As more evidence came in, associations with uterine anomalies, other genital tract anomalies, and cervical incompetence in pregnancy were discovered. The last patients were treated with DES about 25 years ago, so the legacy of this drug will dissipate over the next few decades.

 SUGGESTED ADDITIONAL READING

Reinhold C, Hricak H, Forstner R, et al. Primary amenorrhea: evaluation with MR imaging. *Radiology.* 1997;203:383–390.

Stelling JR, Gray MR, Davis AJ, et al. Dominant transmission of imperforate hymen. *Fertil Steril.* 2000;74:1241–1244.

Goldberg JM, Falcone T. Effect of diethylstilbestrol on reproductive function. *Fertil Steril.* 1999;72:1–7.

Wang J, Ezzat W, Davidson M. Transverse vaginal septum. A case report. *J Reprod Med.* 1995;40:163–167.

Chronic Pelvic Pain

ID/CC: A 25-year-old G_0 woman with an 8-month history of pelvic pain.

HPI: S.E. presents with moderate dysmenorrhea that has progressively worsened over time and become periodically incapacitating. At the onset of symptoms 3 years ago, her previous gynecologist placed her on oral contraceptive pills (OCPs). This therapy alleviated her symptoms for the subsequent year and a half, but the pain eventually returned and worsened. Over the last 8 months, S.E. describes the pain as constant, dull pelvic pain radiating to her lower back, with occasional sharp exacerbations. She has had pain during intercourse (dyspareunia) for the last 4 to 5 months. The chronicity of her pain has gradually increased to the point that it occurs almost daily. Ibuprofen, which initially provided adequate relief for the dysmenorrhea, is no longer effective. In addition, she has experienced decreased appetite, libido, and energy, as well as insomnia over the last 4 months. On review of systems, she notes increased urinary frequency and urgency. No hematuria. No GI symptoms.

PMHx: None

PSHx: Exploratory laparotomy at age 17 for suspected appendicitis, not confirmed. Diagnostic laparoscopy at age 22 for ruptured right ovarian cyst.

POb/GynHx: Menarche age 15, regular cycles every 27 to 30 days. LMP 3 weeks ago. No STDs.

Meds: Ibuprofen 600 mg PRN, with menses; OCPs

All: NKDA

SHx: Has lived with her boyfriend for more than 2 years. No tobacco use; occasional ethanol use.

VS: Afebrile, stable.

PE: *Abdomen:* soft, mild suprapubic tenderness. No guarding. Normal external genitalia, vagina, and cervix. *Pelvic:* smooth, regular 7- to 8-week size uterus, retroverted, fixed, mildly tender to palpation. No CMT. Fullness consistent with an adnexal mass on the left, and mild to moderate adnexal tenderness, right to left. Rectovaginal exam reveals some nodularity in the cul-de-sac.

THOUGHT QUESTIONS

- What is the differential diagnosis?
- What studies would you recommend to help you in the diagnosis?

This patient has chronic pelvic pain (CPP) given the duration (>6 months of pelvic pain) and the associated disturbances in both her mood and physical activity. The causes of CPP are multiple and may be gynecologic and nongynecologic. Although not exclusive, the initial catamenial relationship of her pain and the presence of dyspareunia are suggestive of a gynecologic source. Furthermore, the abnormal findings on pelvic exam are highly indicative of a gynecologic source for her pain. The history of dysmenorrhea gradually progressing to constant pain, dyspareunia, and a fixed retroverted uterus makes endometriosis highly likely in the differential diagnosis. Adenomyosis is also a common cause of secondary dysmenorrhea that can be progressive and associated with dyspareunia. Pelvic adhesions, in this patient likely due to the two prior pelvic surgeries, are another important consideration. Primary dysmenorrhea is unlikely because the pain is chronic, without pain-free intervals.

Laboratory studies have a limited role in the setting of CPP. Imaging studies such as pelvic ultrasonography have questionable value in the setting of a normal pelvic examination but may be helpful in this patient given her physical examination findings. Laboratory studies should be tailored to the patient's history. Urinalysis (UA) with micro and possible culture is indicated in this patient because of her history. Cervical cultures for *Gonorrhea* and *Chlamydia trachomatis* also should be obtained. CBC with a sedimentation rate may be helpful in detecting a chronic inflammatory response.

CASE CONTINUED

CBC, sedimentation rate, UA, and *Gonorrhea* and *Chlamydia* studies are all within normal limits. Her urine pregnancy test was negative. Pelvic ultrasound revealed a slightly enlarged, homogeneous uterus and a 4-cm left adnexal mass (Figure 43-1).

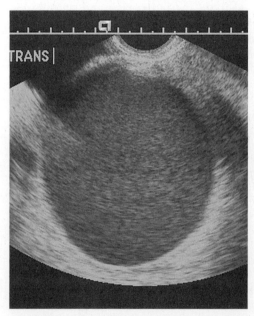

FIGURE 43-1.
Large endometrioma in the ovary. The mass is filled with heterogeneous material, mostly old blood. *(Image Provided by Departments of Radiology and Obstetrics and Gynecology, University of California, San Francisco).*

QUESTIONS

43-1. The next best step in management is:
A. Exploratory laparotomy
B. Repeat ultrasound in 6 to 8 weeks
C. Obtain cancer antigen 125 (CA-125) level
D. Laparoscopy
E. Increase ibuprofen dose

43-2. Appropriate surgical management in this patient would include which of the following?
- A. Copious irrigation and IV antibiotics
- B. Total abdominal hysterectomy and bilateral salpingo-oophorectomy
- C. Right salpingo-oophorectomy
- D. Ovarian cystectomy and fulguration or excision of peritoneal implants
- E. No intervention is necessary

43-3. After her surgery, the patient is started on which of the following to help keep her pain free?
- A. Cyclic oral contraceptives
- B. Continuous oral contraceptives
- C. GnRH analogue (Lupron)
- D. Fentanyl patches
- E. Narcotics PO

43-4. Which of the following is a common side effect(s) of GnRH analogues (Lupron)?
- A. Hot flashes and vaginal dryness
- B. Irreversible bone loss with 6 months of treatment
- C. Adverse impact on serum lipid levels
- D. Heavy menses
- E. None of the above

ANSWERS

43-1. D. The clinical picture is highly suggestive of endometriosis. A cystic adnexal mass with low-level echoes, although nonspecific, has a high likelihood of being an endometrioma. There is some controversy over the optimal treatment for mild endometriosis, but adhesive disease and endometriomas larger than 2 cm are best managed with surgery. In this symptomatic patient, diagnostic laparoscopy with subsequent laparoscopic surgery versus laparotomy (depending on the intraoperative findings) is the best next step.

43-2. D. The object of surgery in endometriosis is to ablate, electrocauterize, and/or excise all visible lesions and to restore anatomical relationships while preserving the reproductive organs to allow for future fertility. For all stages of endometriosis, laparoscopy offers similar results to laparotomy with less morbidity and lower cost. Radical or definitive surgery in endometriosis includes total abdominal hysterectomy, usually with bilateral salpingo-oophorectomy, and is reserved for patients who have not responded to conservative therapy and have completed childbearing.

43-3. B.; **43-4.** A. Medical therapy of endometriosis with hormones is generally performed in a stepwise fashion. The first step is cyclic oral contraceptives. If this fails, the next step is continuous oral contraceptives. If there is no pain relief from continuous oral contraceptives, a diagnostic and therapeutic laparoscopy should be performed in patients without a definitive diagnosis. In patients who have already been diagnosed, the next step is treatment with a GnRH agonist (Lupron), which sends the body into a premature menopausal state. In this patient who has been treated with cyclic OCPs but never a continuous regimen, the next step in her management after the surgery would be to attempt to control her pain in this way. Some patients will obtain relief from the surgery itself and, if they are interested in fertility, will decline any hormonal treatment whatsoever. For acute pain relief, NSAIDs are the first-line therapy. Opiates should be used only in the emergent setting where a patient requires pain relief for a defined period prior to surgery or in order for a particular hormonal treatment to work. If opiates are used chronically, the patient is likely to develop an addiction.

GnRH analogues produce a hypoestrogenic state similar to that seen in oophorectomized women. Side effects are related to the low-estrogen state and include hot flashes, vaginal dryness, mood swings, and sleep disorders. Long-term users (>6 months) of a GnRH analogue should be considered for "add-back" therapy, given concerns about its role in bone loss. Danazol, another agent used for treatment of endometriosis, has been shown to have a negative impact on serum lipid levels. However, this effect has not been demonstrated with GnRH analogues used for no more than 6 months.

 ## SUGGESTED ADDITIONAL READING

ACOG Committee on Practice Bulletins—Gynecology. ACOG Practice Bulletin No. 51. Chronic pelvic pain. *Obstet Gynecol.* 2004;103:589–605.

Marchino GL, Gennarelli G, Enria R, et al. Diagnosis of pelvic endometriosis with use of macroscopic versus histologic findings. *Fertil Steril.* 2005;84:12–15.

Hart R, Hickey M, Maouris P, et al. Excisional surgery versus ablative surgery for ovarian endometriomata. *Cochrane Database Syst Rev.* 2005;CD004992.

Abnormal Pap Smear

ID/CC: A 24-year-old $G_1P_0A_1$ woman presents to your office for a follow-up Pap smear.

HPI: She states that she had her last Pap smear at an annual gynecologic exam 9 months ago at a free clinic in another state. She does not have a copy of her results, but she reports that she was notified by phone that the results were abnormal and that she should have a repeat Pap in 4 to 6 months. Prior to this last test 9 months ago, her annual Pap smears had all been normal.

THOUGHT QUESTIONS

- What is the usual interval for Pap screening?
- What are the possible findings that are reported on a Pap smear?
- Which one is this patient likely to have?

The Pap smear is a screening test for premalignant or malignant lesions of the cervix. Normal intervals for screening depend on age and history (Table 44-1).

The Pap report consists of the following:
Specimen type: conventional slide versus liquid based, etc.
Specimen adequacy (reported as satisfactory or unsatisfactory): whether visualization is obscured by blood or inflammation
Result: negative or intraepithelial lesion or malignancy; if present, can also describe infection such as *Candida,* reactive cellular changes, atrophy, presence of endometrial cells

TABLE 44-1 Normal Intervals for Pap Screening

Initial screening	3 years after initiation of sexual intercourse or age 21
Interval	Annually until age 30
	Annually after age 30 if history of
	DES exposure
	Prior abnormal Pap
	Immune suppression (immunosuppressive illnesses or
	drugs, renal transplantation, HIV)
	History of high-risk HPV type
	Current smoking status
	Every 3 years for women after age 30 with three prior normal
	Pap smears or negative high-risk HPV type
Cease screening	For women after age 70 with three recent normal Pap smears
	in the past 10 years
	After total hysterectomy (hysterectomy not done for
	dysplasia or cancer)

Possible results on a Pap smear include the following:
  Squamous epithelial cell abnormalities
  Atypical squamous cells (ASC)
    Of undetermined significance (ASC-US)
    Cannot exclude high-grade (ASC-H)
  Low-grade intraepithelial lesion (LGSIL)
  High-grade intraepithelial lesion (HGSIL)
  Squamous cell carcinoma
  Glandular cell abnormalities
  Atypical glandular cells (AGC)
    Can identify source (i.e., endocervical vs. endometrial)
  Endocervical adenocarcinoma in situ
  Adenocarcinoma

This patient most likely had an ASC-US finding on her Pap smear, and a human papillomavirus (HPV) culture was not done at the time of her Pap smear (see management guidelines in Table 44-2).

TABLE 44-2 Abnormal Pap Test Management Guidelines

Result	Action
Satisfactory, negative	Routine follow-up
Unsatisfactory	Repeat smear
ASC-US	
Unknown HPV	Repeat in 4–6 months
Negative high-risk HPV	Repeat in 12 months
Positive HPV	Colposcopy
Immediately prior Pap also ASC-US	Colposcopy
ASC-H	Colposcopy
AGC	Colposcopy and endocervical sampling; endometrial biopsy should also be done in women over 35 or those with abnormal bleeding
LGSIL	Colposcopy
HGSIL	Colposcopy
Carcinome, Adenocarcinoma in-situ (AIS) or other malignant cells	Referral to gynecologic oncologist

CASE CONTINUED

Menses: LMP 3 weeks ago. Has regular cycles. Menarche at age 13.

PMHx: None

PSHx: D&C

Meds: None

PGynHx: *Chlamydia* infection 3 years ago; uses condoms and withdrawal

PObHx: First-trimester TAB

All: NKDA

SHx: Works as a waitress. Currently is sexually active with two partners. Has smoked one pack of cigarettes per day for the last 5 years. Occasional alcohol and marijuana use.

PE: Appears healthy. *Abd:* soft, without masses *Pelvic:* normal external genitalia without lesions. *Vagina:* normal rugae, no excoriations, lacerations, or abnormal discharge. *Cervix:* appears normal. Does not bleed with manipulation with swab, no cervical motion tenderness. *Uterus:* normal size, anteverted, no uterine tenderness. *Adnexa:* normal, without tenderness.

You perform a repeat Pap smear and HPV culture. The results are *Pap:* satisfactory, ASC-US; *HPV:* positive.

THOUGHT QUESTIONS

- What is the significance of a positive HPV test?
- What test should you do next?
- Describe this test. What information you can derive from it?

There are more than 100 serotypes of HPV. This virus is ubiquitous and is a common cause of condyloma, cervical dysplasia, and cancer. Some serotypes are considered high risk because they are more likely to cause dysplasia/cancer. HPV-16 confers the greatest risk. Others, such as types 6 and 11, are a very low risk for cancer and are more commonly associated with condyloma. A positive high-risk HPV increases the likelihood that the ASC-US finding on this patient's Pap smear is due to dysplasia.

You should perform a colposcopy on this patient. A colposcopy is an office procedure that involves inspecting the cervix carefully with a magnifying scope. The cervix is swabbed with a dilute vinegar solution in order to enhance visualization of dysplastic or neoplastic lesions. A green filter is used to further enhance visualization.

Colposcopy yields a visual diagnosis and allows for confirmatory biopsies of abnormal areas of the cervix. Dysplastic lesions tend to turn white when vinegar is applied. Architectural characteristics, such as mosaicism (a mosaic pattern caused by abnormal vasculature), are more common to high-grade lesions. Biopsies of any lesions of concern are sent for pathologic evaluation. Because most dysplasias occur at the transformation zone of the cervix, it is important that you can completely visualize this zone during colposcopy. If the transformation zone cannot be seen, the colposcopy is deemed "unsatisfactory," and endocervical curettage should be performed to rule out a lesion you cannot see.

The colposcopy is satisfactory, and you see an area that turns acetowhite at 10:00. Biopsy reveals LGSIL.

THOUGHT QUESTION

■ What are you management options now?

The management of women with LGSIL should be individualized based on the patient's immunocompetence, ability to follow up, and preference. Studies show that approximately 60% of biopsy-proven LGSIL regress spontaneously. Consequently, a patient who wishes to avoid ablative treatment and who can adhere to close observation can be followed with serial Pap smear surveillance. Once she has three normal Pap smears at 4- to 6-month intervals, she can return to annual screening. If the lesion progresses to HGSIL (20% of cases), the lesion does not regress in a reasonable amount of time, or the patient's preferences change, ablative treatment should be pursued. Ablation can be done with cryotherapy (freezing the surface of the cervix), excision (LEEP or cone biopsy), or laser.

QUESTIONS

44-1. After the above patient has consulted with you, she chooses surveillance rather than ablative treatment. She asks if there is anything she can do to minimize the chances that the dysplasia will become more severe. You inform here that the intervention that will most decrease her risk for progression to cervical cancer is to:

    A. Take oral contraceptive pills
    B. Use condoms exclusively
    C. Stop smoking
    D. Take daily folic acid supplements

44-2. A 44-year-old woman has a routine annual exam with you. Her Pap smears have always been normal, and her last one was 3 years ago. Her review of systems was negative. Her exam was unremarkable, and routine screening test were done. Her Pap smear shows atypical glandular cells. Further evaluation should be:

    A. Repeat the Pap smear in 4 months and proceed to colposcopy if glandular atypia persists
    B. Endometrial biopsy
    C. Colposcopy and endocervical curettage
    D. Colposcopy, endometrial biopsy, and endocervical curettage

44-3. An HIV-positive woman who is on antiretroviral therapy comes to see you for routine gynecologic exam. Her most recent CD4 count was 536, and her viral load was undetectable. The baseline HPV screening and Pap smear you perform are both negative. Appropriate follow-up cervical cancer screening for this patient should be:

A. Annual Pap smears

B. Repeat Pap smear in 6 months

C. Annual colposcopy with biopsy of suspicious lesions

D. Annual colposcopy with endocervical curettage and biopsy of suspicious lesions

44-4. You see a 28-year-old G_2P_1 woman for her first prenatal visit at 15 weeks gestation. The routine Pap smear that you send as part of her prenatal evaluation is reported as HGSIL. Your next step is to:

A. Increase her folic acid supplementation to 1 mg per day and repeat her Pap smear in 6 to 8 weeks.

B. Repeat her Pap smear 6 to 8 weeks postpartum.

C. Perform colposcopy with biopsy of lesions suspicious of HGSIL or worse.

D. Perform colposcopy with endocervical curettage and biopsy of all suspicious lesions.

 ANSWERS

44-1. C. Women who smoke have a nearly fourfold increased risk for cervical cancer. Cumulative exposure to cigarette smoking correlates with the risk for dysplasia. Some evidence indicates that folate deficiency enhances the progression to dysplasia. However, the effect of dietary supplementation with folic acid has not been proven. Conversely, taking oral contraceptive pills independently increases the risk for dysplasia by a factor of two. The exact causal relationship is unknown but is thought to be secondary to folic acid deficiency. Barrier methods have not been shown to affect the progression of dysplasia.

44-2. D. AGC is associated with premalignant or malignant lesions in approximately one third of cases. An AGC finding on Pap smear should prompt immediate referral for colposcopy and endocervical curettage. In women older than 35 years, an endometrial biopsy should also be done. This is also true for younger women with anovulatory bleeding or undiagnosed abnormal uterine bleeding. Performing just an endometrial biopsy would only be appropriate for a woman with atypical endometrial cells on cytology. Repeating cytology in 4 to 6 months can be done for ASC-US but not AGC.

44-3. B. HPV infection is considered a necessary condition for the development of cervical cancer. Immunocompromised women and particularly those who are HIV positive are at significantly higher risk for HPV infection and consequent cervical dysplasia. Moreover, these women have faster rates of progression to more severe disease. For HIV-seropositive women with CD4 counts >500/μL and normal cervical cytology and negative test for HPV at baseline, the current recommended interval between Pap smear is two Pap smears 6 months apart after the initial HIV diagnosis, then annually if results are normal. Some recent studies suggest screening can safely be extended to 3 years as long as CD4 counts remain high. Colposcopy is a diagnostic test. In this immunocompetent, HIV-positive patient, colposcopy should be used only if the patient's screening cytology is positive or if a prior history of dysplasia warrants colposcopic surveillance.

44-4. C. Any pregnant woman with LGSIL or greater on Pap smear should be evaluated with colposcopy. It is important to rule out invasive cancer because it may require treatment during the pregnancy. Any lesions that are suspicious for HGSIL or worse should be biopsied. Endocervical curettage should not be performed because of the risk for provoking miscarriage. If the colposcopy is unsatisfactory, repeating the colposcopy after 6 to 8 weeks may be useful because the progression of the pregnancy may make the transformation zone more visible. Repeating the Pap smear postpartum is appropriate only if the screening Pap reveals ASC-US. Although folic acid supplementation reduces the risk for neural tube defects, it has not yet been shown to make dysplasia regress.

 ## SUGGESTED ADDITIONAL READING

Wright TC Jr, Cox JT, Massad LS, et al. 2001 consensus guidelines for the management of women with cervical cytological abnormalities. *JAMA.* 2002;287:2120–2129.

Wright TC Jr, Cox JT, Massad LS, et al. 2001 consensus guidelines for the management of women with cervical intraepithelial neoplasia. *Am J Obstet Gynecol.* 2003;189:295–304.

VI

Reproductive Endocrinology

CASE **45**

Amenorrhea I

ID/CC: A 28-year-old G₂P₁ woman presents with an 8-month history of amenorrhea.

HPI: She had a normal vaginal delivery 2 years ago and breast-fed for 1 year. She was amenorrheic until approximately 9 months ago, when she had two menses spaced 6 weeks apart. Since then she has not menstruated. She had taken medroxyprogesterone acetate (DMPA [Depo-Provera]) for 6 months immediately after delivery but stopped because she felt she did not need it. On review of systems, she denies headache or visual changes but reports that she is still able to express milk from both breasts. Her depression was diagnosed a few months after delivery of her child. She reports her mood has improved since she started taking paroxetine (Paxil) 12 months ago.

PMHx: Depression

PSHx: D&C 8 years ago; cone bx 6 years ago

Meds: Paxil

PGynHx: h/o HGSIL; menarche at age 12; irregular cycles for last 4 years; denies STDs

All: NKDA

THOUGHT QUESTIONS

- What important test should you obtain before you proceed?
- How is amenorrhea considered in terms of etiology?
- Why are the possible anatomical causes for this patient's amenorrhea unlikely?

You should rule out pregnancy with a urine or serum β-hCG test. Although unlikely, she may have ovulated in the last few months and become pregnant at that time.

The two types of amenorrhea are defined by the patient's menstrual history. *Primary amenorrhea* is defined as the absence of menses in women who have not undergone menarche by age 16 (or age 14 with the concurrent absence of normal growth and development and secondary sexual characteristics). *Secondary amenorrhea* is the absence of menses for three cycles or a maximum of 6 months in women with a history of menstruation. Within these two types, possible causes for amenorrhea fall into three broad categories: anatomical/outflow abnormalities, end-organ (ovarian) disorders, and central disorders. Table 45-1 lists some causes of amenorrhea.

Possible anatomical causes for secondary amenorrhea in this patient include uterine adhesions or scarring (Asherman syndrome) caused by her prior D&C and cervical stenosis, a consequence of surgical or obstetric trauma. Neither is likely because she has menstruated after her surgical procedures and twice since her vaginal delivery.

TABLE 45-1 Causes of Amenorrhea

	Primary Amenorrhea	Secondary Amenorrhea
Anatomic/outflow abnormality	Imperforate hymen Transverse vaginal septum Vaginal atresia Müllerian agenesis Testicular feminization	Asherman syndrome Cervical stenosis
End-organ disorder	Primary ovarian failure (hypergonadotropic hypogonadism) Savage syndrome Turner syndrome (45, XO) Gonadal agenesis (46, XY) Swyer syndrome 17-α-hydroxylase deficiency	Premature ovarian failure Polycystic ovarian syndrome
Central disorder	Kallmann syndrome (absent GnRH) Pituitary stalk compression Pituitary tumors	Hypothyroidism Pituitary tumors Chest wall and nipple stimulation Drug induced CNS disease

CASE CONTINUED

PE: Overweight at 172 lb. Neck supple, without masses. *Breasts:* normal, able to express milky fluid from both. *Pelvic:* well-estrogenized pelvic tissues. Cervix consistent with previous cone biopsy. Uterus normal, anteverted and mobile. No adnexal masses.

THOUGHT QUESTION

- What initial labs would be useful?

Pertinent Labs and Studies:
Urine pregnancy test: negative
TSH: 9.7 mU/L (normal 0.5–4.5 mU/L)
PRL: 37 ng/mL (normal 2–15 ng/mL)

THOUGHT QUESTIONS

- What further tests, if any, are necessary?
- How would you treat this patient's amenorrhea?

Once you have ruled out pregnancy, you should check TSH and prolactin levels. If these levels are normal, then the next step is to check the FSH level to rule out premature ovarian failure. In this patient, both TSH and prolactin levels are elevated. Hypothyroidism leads to elevated TRH, which in turn stimulates pituitary cells to secrete prolactin. Hence, hyperprolactinemia is a direct consequence of this patient's hypothyroidism. An isolated elevation in prolactin level should trigger an evaluation for drug-induced hyperprolactinemia and an MRI to rule out a hypothalamic or pituitary lesion such as a pituitary macroadenoma.

You may wish to obtain a free T_4 level to confirm the diagnosis. In addition, an MRI of the head may reveal hypertrophy or hyperplasia of the pituitary. This, along with the patient's amenorrhea and galactorrhea, should resolve quickly with treatment of her hypothyroidism.

In addition, you should consider discontinuing her Paxil once her TSH level normalizes because her depression may have been induced by her hypothyroidism.

QUESTIONS

45-1. You are evaluating a patient who has a 3-year history of secondary amenorrhea. Her TSH level is normal, but her prolactin level is elevated. You review her medications. Which of the following could be the cause of the hyperprolactinemia?

    A. The large doses of ibuprofen she takes for chronic pain
    B. The fluoxetine she takes for depression
    C. The clozapine she takes for agitation
    D. The famotidine she takes for GERD

45-2. If the patient you have just seen in the case above had complained of visual changes, the most likely visual or ocular defect found on physical exam would be:

    A. Bitemporal hemianopsia
    B. Retinal hemorrhages
    C. Lateral nystagmus
    D. Amaurosis fugax

45-3. A 34-year-old G_2P_1 woman has not had a menstrual cycle for 9 months. Prior to this time her cycles were irregular. Her TSH and PRL levels are normal. The next step in management is:

    A. Measure serum FSH.
    B. Perform a progestin challenge test.
    C. Begin treatment with oral contraceptives.
    D. Perform pelvic ultrasound to evaluate for ovarian neoplasm.

45-4. A 22-year-old professional dancer (G_0) presents with absence of menses for 6 months. Prior to this time, her cycles had been irregular and became less frequent. On exam, she is 5 feet 6 inches, weighs 98 lb, and appears healthy. Her pelvic exam is notable only for thin vaginal mucosa. The cause of her amenorrhea is most likely:

    A. Premature ovarian failure
    B. Hypogonadotrophic hypogonadism
    C. Sheehan syndrome
    D. Pregnancy

ANSWERS

45-1. C. Medications that antagonize dopamine cause elevated prolactin because dopamine suppresses prolactin secretion by the pituitary. Clozapine is the only dopamine antagonist in this list. Medications that antagonize dopamine include antipsychotics (phenothiazines, etc.), tricyclic antidepressants, estrogen, monoamine oxidase inhibitors, and opiates.

45-2. A. In the setting of hyperprolactinemia with visual disturbances, a pituitary lesion is likely. A pituitary mass or an enlarging pituitary can compress the optic chiasm and lead to bitemporal hemianopsia. Retinal hemorrhages are due to severe hypertension or, in infants, rotational acceleration ("shaken baby syndrome"). Lateral nystagmus typically is due to vestibular pathology. Amaurosis fugax is transient monocular blindness due to occlusion of the retinal artery by emboli arising from the carotid arteries.

45-3. B. The next diagnostic step is to perform a progestin challenge test. This is performed by giving oral progesterone for 10 days and then observing for a withdrawal bleed. Absence of a withdrawal bleed indicates hypoestrogenism (hence no endometrial lining). The serum FSH level would then help determine if the hypoestrogenism is hypergonadotrophic or hypogonadotrophic.

45-4. B. Atrophy of the vaginal mucosa suggests a low-estrogen state. Pregnancy is extremely unlikely in this setting. Sheehan syndrome is hypopituitarism due to ischemic injury to the pituitary gland. This condition is rare and, in women, usually follows severe obstetric hemorrhage. In addition to hypoestrogenism, patients have hypothyroidism and corticosteroid deficiencies. Premature ovarian failure is possible but unlikely in a 22-year-old woman. Mild to moderate hypothalamic dysfunction causes hypogonadotropic hypogonadism and is being increasingly recognized as a common cause of menstrual cycles irregularities among female athletes and dancers.

SUGGESTED ADDITIONAL READING

Schletche JA. Clinical practice. Prolactinoma. *N Engl J Med.* 2003;349:2035–2041.

Reindollar RH, Novak M, Tho SP, et al. Adult-onset amenorrhea: A study of 262 patients. *Am J Obstet Gynecol.* 1986;155:531–543.

CASE **46**

Infertility I

ID/CC: A 32-year-old G_0 woman presents to your clinic complaining of inability to conceive.

HPI: She reports regular menstrual cycles every 28 days since stopping birth control pills 3.5 years ago. For the last 2.5 years, she and her husband have had regular unprotected intercourse. She reports mild cramping with her cycles, which is relieved with ibuprofen (Motrin). She denies prior pelvic surgery or IUD use. She was diagnosed with PID 9 years ago and was treated with antibiotics. Her husband is 38 years old and has not fathered children before. He is not with her today.

PMHx: Unremarkable

PSHx: Knee surgery

Meds: None

PGynHx: LMP 2 weeks ago, normal Pap smears, menarche at age 13

All: NKDA

THOUGHT QUESTIONS

- Based on the history, what are the likely causes for this couple's infertility?
- What lab test for her would be most helpful?
- Which single lab test for him would be most helpful?

Infertility is the inability to conceive after 1 year of unprotected intercourse. The causes are grouped into three categories:

male factor (accounts for 40%), female factor (40%), and unknown etiology (20%). Causes of male factor infertility include endocrine disorders, abnormal spermatogenesis, abnormal sperm motility, and sexual dysfunction. Causes of female factor infertility include endocrine abnormalities (anywhere along the hypothalamic-pituitary-ovarian axis) that result in anovulation or oligo-ovulation and anatomical abnormalities that result in barriers to conception. Because this patient menstruates regularly, she is having ovulatory cycles. She may have peritoneal factors such as endometriosis or pelvic adhesions or tubal factors affecting fertility. Her history of PID puts her at risk for tubal occlusion. A hysterosalpingogram, which is a radiologic dye study of the uterine cavity and tubes, would help establish tubal patency. Because her husband has not fathered children before, male factor may be the cause here. A semen analysis would identify any abnormalities in sperm count, volume, morphology, and motility.

 CASE CONTINUED

PE: Normal-appearing, Tanner V. *Breasts:* normal without nipple discharge. *Pelvic:* well-estrogenized pelvic tissues. Normal cervix. Uterus normal, anteverted and mobile. No adnexal masses.

You give her lab slips for tests she and her husband should complete.

Labs and Studies:
Semen Analysis
    Volume: 3 cc   Normal: 2–5 cc
    Count: 15 million/cc   Normal: 20–250 million/cc
    Motility: 20%   Normal: >50%
    Morphology: 10%   Normal: >60%
Hysterosalpingogram: Bilateral patent fallopian tubes

 THOUGHT QUESTIONS

- What further evaluation of either partner is necessary?
- What initial fertility treatment would be appropriate for this couple?

The semen analysis reveals markedly abnormal sperm motility and morphology. A first step is to repeat the semen analysis to rule out a transient abnormality. If the abnormality is confirmed, a physical exam and endocrine evaluation are warranted. The endocrine evaluation should include thyroid function tests and serum testosterone, prolactin, and FSH levels. In addition, a post-ejaculatory urine analysis may identify retrograde ejaculation.

Treatment is directed toward overcoming the particular cause of the couple's infertility. For example, oligo-ovulation can be treated with gonadotropic medications that stimulate the ovaries. In this case, a low sperm volume is the only abnormality. Intrauterine insemination (IUI), a procedure in which washed sperm are directly placed in the uterus (bypassing the cervical mucus barrier), can be attempted.

QUESTIONS

46-1. If intrauterine insemination is unsuccessful, the next best treatment for this couple would be:
A. Ovulation induction with clomiphene citrate
B. Ovulation induction with gonadotropin treatment
C. In vitro fertilization (IVF)
D. Donor ovum IVF

46-2. The semen analysis of the male partner of an infertile couple reveals normal morphology and motility but a low sperm volume and count. The likely cause for this is:
A. Mumps orchitis
B. Radiation exposure
C. Varicocele
D. Retrograde ejaculation

46-3. A young couple both aged <30 comes to your office concerned that they have not conceived after attempting for the last 6 months. Her cycles are regular (every 27–30 days), but she notes that they are very light. She occasionally has painful menses for which she takes 3 to 4 doses of ibuprofen over 2 days of her cycle. She also reports midcycle pain. Your next step in management is:
A. Reassure them that they do not have a diagnosis of infertility.
B. Complete history and physical for both partners.
C. Semen analysis and hysterosalpingogram.
D. Perform a postcoital test.

46-4. Clomiphene citrate acts by:
   A. Binding to the FSH receptor on the ovary and stimulating follicle development.
   B. Binding to the estrogen receptor in the hypothalamus and stimulating pulsatile GnRH.
   C. Binding to the progesterone receptor in the uterus and providing luteal phase support.
   D. Blocking the GnRH receptor in the pituitary.

ANSWERS

46-1. C. The goal of intrauterine insemination is to overcome low sperm counts by decreasing the barriers (cervix, cervical mucous) sperm must cross to reach the ovum. If this fails, the next treatment is to directly place sperm in even closer proximity to an egg. This can only be done with IVF. In some cases, a single sperm is injected directly into an egg (intracytoplasmic sperm injection). This couple would not benefit from either form of ovulation induction because she is ovulating normally.

46-2. D. Retrograde ejaculation occurs when sperm are propelled into the bladder rather than the urethra. This diagnosis can be confirmed with evaluation of postejaculatory urine. A varicocele is the abnormal dilation of veins in the spermatic cord. The associated rise in testicular temperature is thought to impair semen quality but not quantity. Mumps orchitis and radiation exposure both result in abnormal sperm morphology.

46-3. A. The per cycle fecundity rate for couples attempting to conceive in any given month is 20%. Over the course of 12 months, 80% to 85% of couples will achieve spontaneous pregnancy, and 90% will do so within 18 months. Couples who have unsuccessfully attempted pregnancy with appropriately timed, unprotected intercourse for 1 year warrant an infertility evaluation.

46-4. B. Clomiphene citrate acts an antiestrogen by competitively binding to the estrogen receptor in the hypothalamus. This leads to increased pulsatile GnRH, which causes increased FSH and LH release from the pituitary and subsequent ovarian follicle growth and ovulation.

SUGGESTED ADDITIONAL READING

Male Infertility Best Practice Policy Committee of the American Urological Association; Practice Committee of the American Society for Reproductive Medicine. Report on varicocele and infertility. *Fertil Steril.* 2004;82(suppl 1):S142–S145.

Male Infertility Best Practice Policy Committee of the American Urological Association; Practice Committee of the American Society for Reproductive Medicine. Report on evaluation of the azoospermic male. *Fertil Steril.* 2004;82(suppl 1):S131–S136.

Brugh VM 3rd, Lipshutz LI. Male factor infertility: evaluation and management. *Med Clin North Am.* 2004;88:367–385.

Hirsutism

ID/CC: A 21-year-old G_1P_0 woman complains of increasing hair on her face, upper back, and abdomen.

HPI: A.H. has noticed an increase in the amount of hair on her face over the last 6 months. During that time, she has developed acne and has noticed some hair on her upper back as well as hair that extends above her underwear and bathing suit on her abdomen. This has led her to shave and use depilatory creams, but she has only mild success with these strategies and is quite upset. On review of systems, she denies changes in energy level, bowel or bladder habits, appetite, or diet. However, she has gained 10 lb over the past year, and her menses have become increasingly irregular.

PMHx: Asthma, no hospitalizations

PSHx: None

POb/GynHx: Menarche at age 12 with regular cycles until 2 years ago, at which time her menses became less frequent, ranging from 35 to 60 days (oligomenorrhea); first-trimester pregnancy termination (3 years ago), which she associates with the change in her cycles; no STIs; not currently sexually active.

Meds: Albuterol (Ventolin) inhaler

All: NKDA

SHx: Junior in college majoring in economics; social ethanol and tobacco use; no recreational drug use.

VS: Temp 98.0°F, BP 132/84, HR 88, RR 16, weight 144 lb, height 5 feet 4 inches

PE: *Gen:* healthy young woman, NAD, appears stated age. *HEENT:* no obvious moon facies. *Neck:* no LAD, no thyromegaly, acanthosis nigricans. *Back:* normal spine, no hump. *Chest:* RR&R/CTA. *Abdomen:* soft, nontender, no masses. *SSE:* normal vaginal mucosa, cervix normal without lesions, Pap smear performed. *BME:* uterus AV/AF, adnexa not palpated secondary to habitus.

THOUGHT QUESTIONS

- What additional history and physical information would you like?
- What laboratory tests should be performed?

This patient, who has concerns about her hirsutism, should be questioned regarding the timing of symptoms (chronic vs. acute), whether she has any signs of virilism (presence or development of male secondary sexual characteristics in a woman, including deepening of voice, male-pattern baldness, clitoral enlargement, irregular menses, and increased facial and body hair), and whether there is any evidence of virilism in her family history. If the patient had signs/symptoms of virilism, the differential diagnosis would include testosterone-secreting tumors, adrenal tumors, and congenital adrenal hyperplasia (CAH).

To help sort out the differential, the following laboratory tests should be performed: DHEAS, testosterone, and 17-hydroxyprogesterone (17-OHP). If the DHEAS level is elevated, an adrenal source of androgens would be likely. Elevation of testosterone level is suggestive of germ cell tumors of the ovary. CAH, a deficiency in the 21-hydroxylase enzyme, leads to an elevated 17-OHP level because of accumulation of cortisol precursors. In addition, the mineralocorticoids cannot be processed without the deficient enzyme (Figure 47-1). Without any lab abnormalities, a diagnosis of polycystic ovary syndrome (PCOS) should be considered. In addition to her presenting complaint of hirsutism, she has experienced recent weight gain and irregular menses. Standard workup for these conditions include a pregnancy test, prolactin and TSH levels, and a test for ovulation.

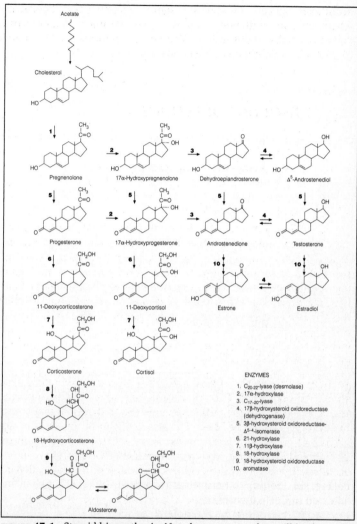

FIGURE 47-1. Steroid biosynthesis. Note key enzymes that will lead to a precursor accumulation. *(From Mishell DR, Davajan V, Lobo RA. Infertility, Contraception, and Reproductive Endocrinology. 3rd ed. Cambridge, Mass: Blackwell Science, 1991, with permission.)*

CASE CONTINUED

Labs: LH, FSH, TSH, DHEAS, prolactin, and testosterone levels
are all within normal limits. Her 17-OHP level is mildly elevated at
350 ng/dL.

QUESTIONS

47-1. The next step in her diagnosis should be:
   A. ACTH stimulation test
   B. Check cortisol level
   C. Check GnRH level
   D. No further tests necessary; she has Cushing disease
   E. No further tests necessary; she has CAH

47-2. If her only test abnormalities were an elevated LH/FSH
ratio, her diagnosis would be:
   A. PCOS
   B. CAH
   C. Gonadoblastoma of the ovary
   D. Adrenal tumor
   E. Idiopathic hirsutism

47-3. In addition to managing her primary diagnosis, which of the
following could be used to treat both her hirsutism and oligomenorrhea?
   A. Spironolactone
   B. Dexamethasone
   C. Finasteride
   D. Bromocriptine
   E. Oral contraceptive pills

47-4. In addition to her primary diagnosis, what other tests are
indicated in this patient?
   A. 24-hour urinary catecholamines
   B. Head MRI
   C. CT of the adrenal glands
   D. Glucose loading test
   E. Creatinine clearance

ANSWERS

47-1. A. patients with adult-onset CAH may or may not have elevated DHEAS and testosterone levels. The initial screening test for adult-onset CAH is the 17-OHP level. A level that is extremely elevated (>800 ng/dL) is diagnostic for 21-hydroxylase deficiency. If the 17-OHP level is mildly elevated (between 200 and 800 ng/dL), the next step is an ACTH stimulation test. Markedly elevated levels after the ACTH stimulation test also are diagnostic.

47-2. A. An elevated LH/FSH ratio is a classic indicator for diagnosing PCOS. Many clinicians still use it. However, if her other laboratory test results are normal and she has irregular menses and hirsutism, a clinical diagnosis of PCOS could be made.

47-3. E. The treatment of hirsutism is multifaceted. Spironolactone acts to inhibit androgen production and as a direct inhibitor of 5a-reductase, the enzyme that facilitates the peripheral conversion of circulating testosterone to the much more potent androgen dihydrotestosterone (DHT). Finasteride also inhibits 5a-reductase. Dexamethasone acts to suppress ACTH secretion and, in turn, adrenal androgens. Oral contraceptives are important in these patients both to regulate menstruation as well as to suppress the generation of hormones that lead to hirsutism; they possibly include ACTH, DHEAS, ovarian androgens, and the gonadotropins LH and FSH. Bromocriptine is not used in patients with hirsutism but rather in cases of hyperprolactinemia, particularly in association with pituitary microadenomas, to suppress prolactin production.

47-4. D. Patients with hyperandrogenism have a high association with insulin resistance and type 2 diabetes. One classic physical finding in these patients is acanthosis nigricans, a velvety thickening on the back of the neck. Thus, it is important to screen these patients with a fasting glucose and a 75-g glucose loading test. If the patient had an elevated DHEAS level suggestive of an adrenal tumor, a CT followed by a check for urinary catecholamines would be indicated. An MRI to rule out a pituitary tumor is warranted in a patient with elevated fasting prolactin level of unknown cause.

SUGGESTED ADDITIONAL READING

Trakakis E, Laggas D, Salamalekis E, et al. 21-Hydroxylase deficiency: from molecular genetics to clinical presentation. *J Endocrinol Invest.* 2005;28:187–192.

New MI. An update of congenital adrenal hyperplasia. *Ann N Y Acad Sci.* 2004;1038:14–43.

Tekin O, Avci Z, Isik B, et al. Hirsutism: common clinical problem or index of serious disease? *Med Gen Med.* 2004;6:56.

Amenorrhea II

ID/CC: A 17-year-old girl comes to your office with her mother. They are concerned because she has not yet begun to menstruate.

HPI: She and her mother feel her development has been normal to date. She has no medical illnesses. She denies cyclic abdominal pain. She has not yet engaged in sexual intercourse. She is the youngest of three children. Her older sister had menarche at age 13. Her review of symptoms is negative.

PMHx: None

PSHx: None

Meds: None

PGynHx: No prior gynecologic exam, no gynecologic infections

All: Penicillin (PCN) allergy resulting in rash

THOUGHT QUESTIONS

- How would a history of cyclic abdominal pain narrow your differential diagnosis?
- In addition to the pelvic exam, what aspects of the physical exam will help with the differential diagnosis?

Cyclic abdominal pain suggests that this patient is having menstrual cycles but that there is an obstruction to flow leading to retrograde menstrual flow into the abdomen causing peritoneal irritation. A vaginal septum, imperforate hymen, cervical atresia, or isolated rudimentary uterine horn can cause primary amenorrhea in this manner.

An important component of the physical exam for primary amenorrhea is evaluation of secondary sex characteristics. Absence of breasts (due to absent estrogen) suggest gonadal agenesis or failure, deficiencies in steroid synthesis, or disruptions in the hypothalamic-pituitary axis. Lagging breast development may be due to varying degrees of gonadal dysgenesis.

CASE CONTINUED

PE: Normal-appearing. *Breasts:* appear normal, Tanner V. *Pelvis:* normal external genitalia. Short vagina ends blindly at 3 cm. Uterus not palpable.

THOUGHT QUESTION

■ What would be the most useful test to obtain at this point?

This patient is phenotypically female but with absent uterus and cervix. Breast development indicates the presence of estrogen. The differential diagnosis includes müllerian agenesis (normal ovaries, hence estrogen present) and testicular feminization (defect in the testosterone receptor, hence testosterone peripherally converted to estrogen). You can distinguish the two by obtaining a karyotype.

CASE CONTINUED

Labs and Studies:
An ultrasound confirms an absent uterus and cervix. No pelvic masses are seen. Karyotype analysis reveals 46, XY.

THOUGHT QUESTION

■ What treatments should you pursue?

Individuals with testicular feminization have functioning testes that usually are not completely descended. They have an almost 50% risk for developing testicular cancer, so the testes should be removed surgically. After the procedure, estrogen replacement should be given to maintain secondary sex characteristics and prevent osteoporosis. Historically, these patients also undergo surgical reconstruction to enhance their vagina, which is a foreshortened blind pouch. However, this also can be accomplished with serial dilation using vaginal dilators over a period of 6 to 9 months, which allows them to forego the risks of surgery.

QUESTIONS

48-1. You see an 18-year-old woman with primary amenorrhea. On exam she has a uterus but no breast development. A karyotype reveals 46,XY. Her amenorrhea and exam are consistent with:

A. Gonadal agenesis
B. Müllerian agenesis
C. Absent GnRH secretion
D. 17-*a*-hydroxylase deficiency

48-2. A 16-year-old girl with primary amenorrhea has a normally developed vagina and uterus but no breast development. Karyotype is 46, XX. The next step in diagnosis is to obtain:

A. Urine pregnancy test
B. Serum FSH
C. Serum free testosterone
D. 24-hour urine cortisol collection

48-3. A 15-year-old girl presents to your office because she has not started menstruating. She underwent thelarche 3 years ago. She denies sexual activity and is otherwise healthy. Her physical exam is normal. Your next step is to:

    A. Advise her that some females do not start menstruating until age 16. She should come back if she has not started menstruating by then.

    B. Obtain a pregnancy test because she should have started menstruating by age 14.

    C. Obtain a karyotype analysis.

    D. Check a serum FSH.

48-4. An individual with Kallmann syndrome will have which of the following characteristics?

    A. Phenotypic female without uterus but normal breast development, 46, XX

    B. Phenotypic female with uterus but no breast development, 46, XY

    C. Phenotypic female without uterus or breast development, 46, XY

    D. Phenotypic female with uterus but no breast development, 46, XX

ANSWERS

48-1. A. Absence of testes (gonadal agenesis in XY individual) means that neither müllerian-inhibiting factor (MIF) nor testosterone is produced. Hence the uterus and cervix form from the müllerian ducts, but breasts do not develop because there is no peripheral conversion of testosterone to estrogen. 46,XY individuals with absent GnRH secretion or 17-*a*-hydroxylase deficiency produce MIF but not sex hormones, hence the uterus and upper vagina would be absent. In müllerian agenesis, ovarian estrogen secretion is normal, and the patient should have breast development.

48-2. B. This patient is hypoestrogenic. A serum FSH would reveal whether this is due to a hypothalamic or pituitary defect (low FSH) or to gonadal failure (high FSH). A 24-hour cortisol collection is used to diagnose Cushing syndrome. A serum testosterone can be helpful in diagnosing the cause of hirsutism in females. Levels above 200 ng/dL suggest an adrenal mass.

48-3. A. Primary amenorrhea is defined as the absence of menses in women who (1) have not undergone menarche by age 16 or (2) have not had a period by age 14 in the absence of normal growth and development and appearance of secondary sex characteristics. Although 15 years is relatively late for menarche, it is not outside the realm of normal. A normal physical exam excludes an anatomical or outflow tract abnormality.

48-4. D. Kallmann syndrome is the congenital absence of pulsatile GnRH. As a result, the pituitary does not release FSH or LH, nor do the ovaries produce estrogen. The resulting phenotype is a uterus that is present (no MIF) but absent breast development (no estrogen).

 SUGGESTED ADDITIONAL READING

Folch M, Pigem I, Konje JC. Mullerian agenesis: etiology, diagnosis, and management. *Obstet Gynecol Surv.* 2000;55:644–649.
Pletcher JR, Slap GB. Menstrual disorders. amenorrhea. *Pediatr Clin North Am.* 1999;46:505–518.

Infertility II

ID/CC: A 27-year-old G_1P_0 woman presents to your clinic complaining of inability to conceive.

HPI: She reports irregular menstrual cycles for the last 6 years. Her cycles come every 28 to 50 days and are at times heavy. For the last 1.5 years, she and her husband have had regular unprotected intercourse. She has never used contraception. She denies prior PID or pelvic surgery. Her husband also is 27 years old and has not fathered children before. On review of systems, she denies galactorrhea and has noted a 20-lb weight gain and a slight increase in facial hair over the last 3 years.

PMHx: Unremarkable

PSHx: Appendectomy

Meds: None

PGynHx: LMP 3 weeks ago. Normal pap smears. Menarche at age 12.

PObHx: First-trimester termination at age 19

All: NKDA

THOUGHT QUESTIONS

- Based on the history, what are the likely causes for this couple's infertility?
- What lab tests for her would be most helpful?
- Which lab test for him would be most helpful?

Given this patient's irregular menses, anovulation is the likely cause of infertility. Common causes for anovulation include polycystic ovary syndrome (PCOS), premature ovarian failure, thyroid disorders, hyperprolactinemia, and medications. A semen analysis is useful to exclude male factors as causes for infertility. An endocrine evaluation of this patient will help identify causes of anovulation. At minimum this should include thyroid studies and FSH and prolactin levels.

CASE CONTINUED

PE: Moderate central obesity, moderate facial hair on upper lip and chin, Tanner V. Normal breasts without nipple discharge. Abdomen with diamond escutcheon. Well-estrogenized pelvic tissues. Normal cervix. Uterus normal, anteverted and mobile. No adnexal masses.

Labs and Studies: FSH 8 mIU/mL, LH 19 mIU/mL, testosterone 18 nmol/L, 17-OH Progesterone 14 nmol/L, PRL 14 ng/mL, TSH 2.9 μU/mL; HSG: bilateral patent fallopian tubes; semen analysis: normal.

THOUGHT QUESTIONS

- What is your most likely diagnosis now?
- What is the best first treatment for this couple?
- What additional test may be useful at this juncture?

PCOS is a constellation of symptoms that usually include infertility, menstrual disturbances, hirsutism, and obesity. In PCOS, excess LH stimulates cystic changes in the ovary, which in turn causes increased androgen secretion from the ovarian stroma. An LH/FSH ratio >2:1 suggests PCOS, but because the ratio is not particularly sensitive, the diagnosis is increasingly made by excluding other causes of anovulation. Her elevated free testosterone levels are also consistent w/PCOS, but they are not high enough to suggest an androgen-secreting tumor. Because this patient has a functioning hypothalamic-pituitary-ovarian axis, she may ovulate with clomiphene citrate treatment. Clomiphene citrate acts as an antiestrogen at the estrogen receptor in the hypothalamus. This leads to increased GnRH, then FSH and LH and subsequent follicle growth and ovulation.

A subset of women with PCOS also have insulin resistance. An elevated fasting insulin to glucose ratio would diagnose insulin-resistant PCOS and indicate that this patient may be able to ovulate if treated with metformin. In some cases, metformin treatment suffices; otherwise, it is used in conjunction with clomiphene citrate.

QUESTIONS

49-1. The most common complication of clomiphene citrate is:
A. Ovarian torsion
B. Multiple gestations
C. Ovarian hyperstimulation
D. Premature ovarian failure

49-2. This patient should be screened with increased frequency for:
A. Insulin resistant (type 2) diabetes
B. Ovarian cancer
C. Ovarian cysts
D. Endometrial cancer

49-3. Which of the following is associated with the lowest risk of ectopic pregnancy?
A. Pelvic surgery
B. In vitro fertilization (IVF)
C. Gonadotropin ovulation induction
D. Salpingitis

49-4. An appropriate candidate for clomiphene citrate treatment is:
A. A 41-year-old woman who failed gonadotropin ovulation induction
B. A 27-year-old woman with Asherman syndrome
C. A 28-year-old woman with mild hypothalamic amenorrhea
D. A 29-year-old woman with DES syndrome

ANSWERS

49-1. B. There is an 8% risk for multiple gestations with clomiphene citrate. Ovarian hyperstimulation and possible subsequent torsion are complications of ovulation induction using gonadotropins such as menotropins (Pergonal). Premature ovarian failure is not a complication of clomiphene citrate use.

49-2. A. PCOS is a constellation of symptoms that usually include infertility, menstrual disturbances, hirsutism, and obesity. Patients with PCOS are at risk for hyperinsulinemia and insulin resistance. They also manifest abnormal lipid profiles, which place them at risk for hypertension and coronary artery disease. Because chronic anovulation causes elevated estrogen levels, these patients are at risk for endometrial and breast cancer, not ovarian cancer. Endometrial hyperplasia/cancer can be prevented by provoking regular withdrawal bleeding, hence specific screening for this is not necessary.

49-3. C. Pelvic surgery and salpingitis can cause tubal occlusion and hence are risk factors for ectopic pregnancy. IVF can result in ectopic pregnancy if fertilized embryos are pushed up into the tube when they are placed in the uterus. Gonadotropin ovulation induction is associated with multiple gestations but not ectopic pregnancy.

49-4. C. Clomiphene citrate is the first-line treatment for mild hypothalamic amenorrhea. A patient who has failed gonadotropin induction needs IVF. Asherman syndrome is the presence of adhesions in the endometrial cavity and is a rare complication of endometrial surgery. Diethylstilbestrol (DES) is a medication that was commonly given to pregnant women in the 1950s and 1960s. In utero exposure results in characteristic changes to the cervix, vagina, and uterus (T-shaped uterus), which increase the risk of infertility, spontaneous abortion, and premature labor. There is no treatment for DES exposure.

SUGGESTED ADDITIONAL READING

Lakhani K, Prelevic GM, Seifalian AM, et al. Polycystic ovary syndrome, diabetes and cardiovascular disease: risks and risk factors. *J Obstet Gynaecol.* 2004;24:613–621.

Ehrmann DA. Polycystic ovary syndrome. *N Engl J Med*. 2005;352: 1223–1236.

Duckitt K. Infertility and subfertility. *Clin Evid*. 2004;11:2427–2458.

American College of Obstetrics and Gynecology Practice Bulletin. Management of infertility caused by ovulatory dysfunction. *Obst Gynecol*. 2002;99:347–358.

CASE **50**

Irregular Menses and Mood Swings

ID/CC: A 48-year-old G_2P_2 woman complains of frequent hot flashes and irregular menstrual cycles.

HPI: M.A. reports an 8-month history of hot flashes and irregular menstrual cycles varying from 25 to 45 days. Previously she had had regular 30-day cycles without any intermenstrual bleeding. She sheepishly adds that her family has noted that her moods have been quite labile, which she has noticed as well.

PMHx/PSHx: None

Meds: Vitamins

All: NKDA

POb/GynHx: No STIs. Two NSVDs. No contraception.

FHx: Cardiac disease and hypertension in parents, no cancers.

SHx: No tobacco use. Occasional ethanol use.

VS: Temp 96.8°F, BP 142/82, HR 80, RR 14, weight 160 lb

PE: *Breasts:* symmetrical, no masses, no nipple discharge. *Abd:* soft, nontender, no distension, no palpable masses. *Pelvic:* external genitalia within normal limits; vagina—with rugae and physiologic discharge; cervix—multiparous os, no lesions. *BME:* uterus—small, AV/AF, nontender. No palpable adnexal masses.

Labs: Hb 11.2

THOUGHT QUESTIONS

- What physiologic state classically encompasses her complaints?
- What diagnostic tests would you be interested in obtaining?
- How would you manage her symptoms?

This patient's complaints of irregular menstrual cycles, vasomotor instability, and mood changes are characteristic of the perimenopausal period (transition period to the menopause). The average age of menopause in the United States is 50 to 51 years, with menopausal symptoms beginning typically any time after age 40. The decreasing estrogen production and response to stimulatory hormones of the ovaries lead to a breakdown in the feedback cycle of the hypothalamic-pituitary-ovarian axis and ultimately to an increase in circulating FSH levels. Thus the diagnosis of menopause usually is made clinically with symptoms of diminished estrogen and confirmed by an elevated FSH level.

In this patient, an endometrial biopsy is warranted given the history of new-onset metrorrhagia in an older woman. Results of the biopsy will evaluate the endometrium for endometrial polyps, hyperplasia, or cancer and will help confirm her perimenopausal status. In the absence of other pathologic abnormalities and medical contraindications, it would be appropriate to consider hormone therapy (HT) for relief of moderate to severe vasomotor symptoms. However, in light of the associated higher incidence of cardiovascular and thromboembolic events, and breast cancer in women on HT, alternative therapies should be explored.

CASE CONTINUED

She denies passage of heavy clots, postcoital bleeding, dyspareunia, or dysuria. In fact, her bleeding has been light to normal. Nevertheless, you recommend an endometrial biopsy. The results reveal disordered proliferation of the endometrium without evidence of hyperplasia or cancer. FSH level was 35.

QUESTIONS

50-1. Which of the following treatment regimens is most appropriate for her at this point?
- A. Combination oral contraceptives
- B. Continuous combined conjugated estrogens (Premarin, 0.625 mg) and medroxyprogesterone acetate (Provera, 2.5 mg) every day
- C. Unopposed continuous low-dose estrogen therapy
- D. Placement of progestin-releasing IUD
- E. Transdermal estrogen therapy

50-2. At age 50, she discontinued taking the oral contraceptive pills (OCPs) without further vasomotor sequelae. She had no bleeding for the next 12 months but now complains of irregular vaginal bleeding over the last 6 months. What do you now do in light of these complaints?
- A. Perform a Pap smear
- B. Observation only
- C. Perform an endometrial biopsy
- D. Order a pelvic ultrasound
- E. Do a hysteroscopy, and dilation and curettage

50-3. What if you performed an endometrial biopsy and the results return as atrophic endometrium? What would you recommend?
- A. Estrogen plus progestin therapy
- B. Endometrial ablation
- C. Observation and rebiopsy in 6 months
- D. Dilation and curettage
- E. Progestin alone therapy

50-4. She returns to the clinic the following year with a history of a lower-extremity deep venous thrombosis and a dual x-ray absorptiometry (DEXA) scan with a T-score of 2.5 standard deviations below the mean. She wishes to discuss her treatment options. What do you recommend?
- A. Combination HT
- B. Raloxifene
- C. Alendronate
- D. Isoflavones
- E. Ginseng

ANSWERS

50-1. A. OCPs are widely accepted in the management of the transition to menopause and are the best choice for this patient. OCPs will relieve her menopausal symptoms, suppress irregular bleeding, and provide her with a predictable bleeding pattern. Many peri-menopausal women are ovulatory despite irregular cycles, and OCPs will provide effective contraception. At age 50, these women can be switched to the combined HT regimens. However, although a continuous combined HT regimen will provide vasomotor symptom relief, it will not manage the irregular bleeding and could actually worsen erratic bleeding. Additionally, recent findings from the Women's Health Initiative study raise concerns about increased risk for cardio-vascular, thromboembolic, and breast cancer events in women on prolonged HT. Unopposed estrogen therapy and transdermal estrogen therapy without progestins is not recommended because it increases the risk for endometrial hyperplasia/cancer. Progestin therapy can relieve menopausal symptoms, particularly hot flashes, and can be used for patients who have contraindications to estrogen use. However, there is a high incidence of unpredictable bleeding. Alternative therapies for vasomotor symptoms include phytoestrogens, acupuncture, clonidine, and amitriptyline.

50-2. C. An evaluation of this postmenopausal woman is warranted. A Pap smear alone is not sufficient to evaluate post-menopausal bleeding. Observation is contraindicated for the same reason. An endometrial biopsy is necessary to evaluate for possible endometrial abnormalities such as atrophy, polyps, hyperplasia, or cancer. Although ultra-sonography has 90% sensitivity for identifying endometrial abnormalities in women with postmenopausal bleeding using an endometrial thickness cutoff of 5 mm, ultrasonography cannot define the pathology. Nevertheless, it is a helpful test, particularly when an endometrial biopsy is not possible, or before deciding to proceed with a hysteroscopy and dilation and curettage.

50-3. C. The importance of working up abnormal uterine bleeding during the menopausal transition with an endometrial biopsy cannot be overemphasized. Follow-up of atrophic endometrium involves a re-evaluation at 6 months. A cyclic sequential HT regimen can provide the patient with predictable withdrawal bleeding periods and a lower incidence of breakthrough bleeding; however, the recently published findings of the Women's Health Initiative study with regard to risk for breast cancer and cardiovascular and thromboembolic events for women on continuous combined HT must be considered. Endometrial ablation selectively destroys the endometrium and is a relatively new approach in managing dysfunctional uterine bleeding during the menopausal transition. When polyps are determined to be the cause of dysfunctional uterine bleeding, curettage can be therapeutic. There is no real indication for a hysterectomy. It may be difficult to control abnormal uterine bleeding during the menopausal transition with cyclic progestin therapy because the ovaries may cycle intermittently.

50-4. C. Pharmacologic treatment should be offered to women with osteoporosis as defined by a T-score <2.5, women with existing osteoporotic fracture, and women without osteoporotic fracture and T-score <2.0. Pharmacologic treatments approved by the U.S. Food and Drug Administration (FDA) include alendronate, risedronate, raloxifene, and calcitonin. Addition of alendronate to a diet supplemented with calcium and vitamin D and a regular exercise routine can be instrumental for managing bone density loss. However, the major concern with bisphosphonates is the propensity for gastric irritation. Raloxifene is not recommended for this patient because raloxifene, like estrogen, increases the risk for thromboembolic events threefold. Combination HT is associated with a reduced risk for fractures but is not advised in this scenario. Clinical efficacy and safety of isoflavones have not been fully characterized. Ginseng is thought to have estrogenic properties, but to date no studies have demonstrated its effects on bone remodeling.

 SUGGESTED ADDITIONAL READING

McKinlay SM, Brambilla DJ, Posner JG. The normal menopause transition. *Maturitas*. 1992;14:103–115.

Writing Group for the Women's Health Initiative Investigators. Risks and benefits of estrogen plus progestin in healthy postmenopausal women: principal results from the Women's Health Initiative Randomized Controlled Trial. *JAMA*. 2002;288:321–333.

Writing Group for the Women's Health Initiative Investigators. Effects of conjugate equine estrogen in postmenopausal women with hysterectomy: the Women's Health Initiative Randomized Controlled Trial. *JAMA*. 2004;291:1701–1712.

Bone health and osteoporosis: a report of the Surgeon General. Rockville, Md: U.S. Department of Health and Human Services; 2004.

VII

Pelvic
Relaxation

Incontinence

ID/CC: A 62-year-old G_2P_1 woman presents with complaints of incontinence.

THOUGHT QUESTION

- What are the types of incontinence, and how can they be differentiated by history?

Continence involves several factors: (1) structural integrity of the bladder and urethra (no holes), (2) ability of the urethral sphincters to withstand increases in intra-abdominal and intravesicular pressure, and (3) the ability to inhibit bladder contractions. There are four types of incontinence:

Stress incontinence: Urine loss with exertion or straining, associated with pelvic relaxation and displacement of the urethrovesical junction. Patients describe leaking small quantities of urine when coughing or exercising.

Urge incontinence: Urine leakage due to involuntary and uninhibited contraction of the detrusor muscle. Patients cannot suppress the urge to void, and often large quantities of urine are lost.

Overflow incontinence: Loss of urine due to poor or absent bladder contractions that lead to urinary retention, increasing distension and eventual overflow of the urine out the urethra. Patient's present with frequent or constant dribbling and symptoms of either stress or urge incontinence.

Total incontinence: Typically the result of a urinary fistula formed between the bladder and vagina. Patients present with a painless continuous loss of urine. In the United States, the most common risk factors for such a fistula are pelvic surgery and pelvic radiation.

The type of incontinence usually can be diagnosed using the history and physical exam. Sometimes, the patient's history is consistent with a mixed type of incontinence (both stress and urge components). In this case, urodynamic testing, which measures bladder and urethral pressures as the bladder is filled, can be helpful to determine the cause(s) of incontinence.

CASE CONTINUED

HPI: She reports that she leaks large amounts of urine one to three times per day. It occurs when she has the urge to void but she cannot make it to the bathroom in time. Sometimes, when she is almost home and thinks about voiding, it suddenly happens. She denies leakage when she coughs, laughs, or exercises. She has taken to wearing adult diapers because she cannot predict when the leakage will happen.

PMHx: Diabetes (type 2)

PSHx: Appendectomy, C-section

Meds: None

PGynHx: No STDs, normal Pap smears, menopause at age 51

PObHx: SAB, C-section 30 years ago

All: NKDA

THOUGHT QUESTION

■ Based on the history, what type of incontinence do you think this patient has?

This patient's history is consistent with urge incontinence. It usually is caused by involuntary detrusor contractions during the filling phase of bladder function. The urge to urinate or the thought of urination can prompt the detrusor to contract. Because of this the quantity leaked can be large.

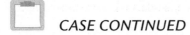

     CASE CONTINUED

PE: Healthy-appearing woman. *Pelvic:* normal external genitalia and vaginal mucosa. Cervix normal, no descent with strain. Uterus small. No apparent rectocele or cystocele.

     THOUGHT QUESTION

■ What diagnostic tests would be helpful at this point?

Urinalysis and urine cultures should always be obtained to rule out infection as a cause of incontinence. A cystometrogram uses pressure sensors to measure bladder and sphincter tone as the bladder is filled. An early detrusor reflex and the patient's inability to inhibit the desire to void suggest detrusor instability.

     CASE CONTINUED

Labs and Studies:
Urinalysis and urine cultures are both normal. The cystometrogram reveals involuntary detrusor contractions starting at 150 cc of bladder filling.

THOUGHT QUESTION

■ How would you treat this patient?

The usual treatment for urge incontinence involves the use of medications to inhibit or relax the detrusor muscle. Anticholinergics inhibit the cholinergic enervation of the detrusor muscle. β-Adrenergic agonist and smooth muscle relaxants both relax the detrusor muscle. There is no effective surgical treatment for urge incontinence.

QUESTIONS

51-1. You are seeing a patient with detrusor instability. The most appropriate treatment is:
A. Tolterodine (Detrol)
B. Surgical correction of bladder neck hypermobility
C. Daily oral nitrofurantoin treatment
D. Prazosin

51-2. A 68-year-old woman complains of frequent urinary dribbling. A measured void is 150 cc, and the postvoid residual is 400 cc. A possible cause of her symptoms is:
A. Diabetes mellitus
B. Daily use of prazosin
C. Bladder neck hypermobility
D. Cervical dysplasia

51-3. Which of the following physical exam findings is correctly paired with the associated type of incontinence?
A. Positive cotton-tipped swab (Q-tip) test—Urge incontinence
B. Absent bulbocavernous reflex—Overflow incontinence
C. Elevated postvoid residual—Stress incontinence
D. Cystocele—Urge incontinence

51-4. Which of the following statements regarding the events leading to micturition is true?
A. Stretch receptors in the bladder wall send a signal to the CNS to relax the detrusor muscle.
B. Activation of the sympathetic nerves via the hypogastric nerve allows for micturition by relaxing the bladder neck and internal sphincter.
C. Sympathetic control of the bladder is derived from S2–4 of the spinal cord.
D. Activation of the parasympathetic pelvic nerves results in contraction of the detrusor muscle and micturition begins.

ANSWERS

51-1. A. α-Adrenergic antagonists such as prazosin reduce urethral closing pressure and exacerbate urge incontinence. Anticholinergics inhibit detrusor muscle contraction. β-adrenergics and muscle relaxants relax the detrusor. There is no surgical treatment for detrusor instability. Nitrofurantoin prophylaxis is used for patients with frequent recurrent urinary tract infections.

51-2. A. This patient's symptoms are consistent with overflow incontinence. Neurologic deficits such as lower motor neuron disease, autonomic neuropathy, spinal cord injuries, and multiple sclerosis can cause detrusor insufficiency, which leads to bladder overflow. Bladder neck hypermobility is associated with stress urinary incontinence. α-Adrenergic antagonists such as prazosin reduce urethral closing pressure and can cause symptoms of urge incontinence. Outflow tract obstruction (i.e., advanced cervical cancer) can cause bladder overdistension. However, cervical dysplasia is unlikely to cause any mass effect.

51-3. B. The bulbocavernosus reflex provides evidence of the integrity of the S2-4 sacral reflexes. The detrusor muscle, which is enervated by S2-4, contracts reflexively after voluntary relaxation of the pelvic floor and urethral muscle. Urge incontinence is due to detrusor overactivity. An absent reflex indicates decreased/absent detrusor activity and would likely be associated with overflow incontinence.

The Q-tip test involves inserting a Q-tip coated with an anesthetic gel into the urethra and measuring the angle of displacement when the patient strains. Hypermobility of the urethra is consistent with stress incontinence. A cystocele (bladder prolapsed into the vagina) is due to laxity of the pelvic floor ligaments and musculature. Cystoceles can be associated with stress incontinence and overflow incontinence.

51-4. D. Micturition involves (1) stretch receptors in the bladder wall sending a signal to the CNS to begin voiding. This triggers (2) inhibition of the sympathetic fibers from T10-L2 (hypogastric nerve), causing relaxation of the urethra and external sphincter and then (3) activation of the parasympathetic pelvic splanchnic nerves to contract the detrusor muscle.

 ## SUGGESTED ADDITIONAL READING

Drutz HP, Alnaif B. Surgical management of pelvic organ prolapse and stress urinary incontinence. *Clin Obstet Gynecol.* 1998;41: 786–793.

Nygaard IE, Heit N. Stress urinary incontinence. *Obstet Gynecol.* 2004;104:607–620.

Heesakkers JP, Vriesema JL. The role of urodynamics in the treatment of lower urinary tract symptoms in women. *Curr Opin Urol.* 2005;15:215–221.

CASE **52**

Vaginal Mass

   ID/CC: A 64-year-old G₃P₃ woman complains of pressure in her vagina and occasionally feeling "something down there" when she strains.

HPI: She denies pain or vaginal bleeding. Review of systems reveals that she often has dysuria and that she occasionally leaks small amounts of urine when she coughs, laughs, or exercises. She tries to limit her physical activity so as to minimize urine leakage.

PMHx: Hypothyroidism, chronic bronchitis

PSHx: None

Meds: Levothyroxine (Synthroid), albuterol (Ventolin)

PGynHx: No STDs, normal Pap smears, menopause at age 48, no hormone replacement therapy (HRT)

PObHx: Forceps delivery for first child, then two NSVDs

All: NKDA

SHx: Denies EtOH or recreational drug use; 30 pack per year history of tobacco use but quit 5 years ago.

THOUGHT QUESTIONS

- What diagnoses could lead to this patient's symptoms?
- What risk factors does this patient have for each of the possible diagnoses?

The sensation of a mass in the vagina can be due to the following:

Pelvic organ prolapse (POP). Occurs when the pelvic ligaments weaken to the point where the pelvic organs sag into the vagina. This includes bladder prolapse (cystocele), uterine prolapse, and rectal prolapse (rectocele). Risk factors for POP include factors that chronically increase intra-abdominal pressure (chronic cough, ascites, pelvic tumors, straining due to chronic constipation) and those that weaken the pelvic supporting ligaments (history of traumatic vaginal delivery, age).

Neoplasm. Both benign and malignant neoplasms can cause the sensation of a vaginal mass. Malignant neoplasms include vaginal and cervical cancer, although these patients more commonly present with bleeding, pain, and pruritus. Possible benign neoplasms include cervical polyps or prolapsing uterine fibroids.

Hemorrhoids. These are dilations of hemorrhoidal veins in the anus. External hemorrhoids can protrude (or protrude further than baseline) upon straining, giving the sensation of a mass. Hemorrhoids are due to frequent straining with defecation, which in turn is due to chronic constipation.

This patient has multiple risk factors for pelvic relaxation, including chronic cough (chronically increased intra-abdominal pressure), history of obstructed labor or traumatic delivery (forceps delivery), aging, and menopause.

CASE CONTINUED

PE: Appears older than stated age. *Pelvic:* External genitalia and vaginal mucosa moderately atrophied, moderate bulge in the anterior vaginal wall (Figure 52-1). Cervix appears normal, descends to way down vagina with straining. Uterus small. Cervix descends to almost the level of the introitus on standing and straining.

THOUGHT QUESTIONS

- What could account for the bulge at the anterior vaginal wall on this patient's exam?
- How does this relate to her incontinence?
- What initial therapies can you try in this patient?

The vaginal bulge most likely is a cystocele. Cystoceles occur when the bladder herniates into the vaginal vault. Other possibilities include a urethral diverticulum or a Skene gland abscess, but these are rare. The prolapsing bladder probably is accompanied by bladder neck relaxation. This leads to stress urinary incontinence. Kegel exercise (tightening and relaxing of the pubococcygeus muscle throughout the day) can strengthen the pelvic musculature and thereby reduce pelvic organ prolapse. It also works to increase the external urethral sphincter tone and reduce stress incontinence. Estrogen replacement also can help by reversing atrophy of the vaginal mucosa and improving tissue tone.

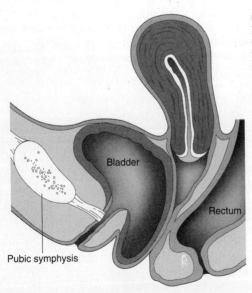

FIGURE 52-1.
Defect in the anterior vaginal wall leads to herniation of the bladder into the vagina down to the introitus and beyond.

Cystocele

QUESTIONS

52-1. If Kegel exercise and estrogen replacement fail in this patient, what other therapy can you try?
A. Treatment with prazosin
B. Placing a vaginal pessary
C. Placing a cervical cap
D. Improving management of her chronic bronchitis

52-2. Surgical treatment of stress urinary incontinence includes:
A. Urethral dilation procedure
B. Urethral sling procedure
C. Hysteroscopic myomectomy procedure
D. There are no effective surgical procedures to treat stress urinary incontinence

52-3. A 36-year-old G_3P_3 woman comes to your office reporting loss of urine when she coughs or jogs. This started shortly after her third vaginal delivery 2 years ago. You diagnose mild stress urinary incontinence. The first best step in treatment for this patient is:
A. Begin Kegel exercises
B. Begin HRT
C. Begin a course of oxybutynin chloride (Ditropan)
D. Fit the patient for a pessary

52-4. A 78-year-old woman presents to your office for an annual exam. On exam you find uterine prolapse to 2 cm before the introitus and a moderate cystocele. She denies any symptoms consistent with pelvic organ prolapse or urinary incontinence. The best management for this patient is to:
A. Do nothing now and monitor for symptoms
B. Fit a pessary
C. Start her on HRT
D. Perform a vaginal vault suspension procedure in the operating room

ANSWERS

52-1. B. Vaginal pessaries provide mechanical support of the pelvic organs. They are placed in the vagina and hold the pelvic organs in their normal positions. Using a pessary requires a very motivated patient as it requires routine removal and replacement for cleansing. A cervical cap is a contraceptive. It does not provide pelvic organ support. Prazosin (α-antagonist) would relax sphincter tone, worsening incontinence. Improved management of chronic bronchitis will not reverse pelvic organ prolapse.

52-2. B. Common surgical procedures for stress incontinence fall into three main categories: (1) *anterior colporrhaphy,* which is designed to close an open bladder neck, (2) *bladder neck suspension procedures* to correct hypermobility, and (3) *sling procedures* to correct intrinsic sphincteric weakness. Although this is quite technical, you should be aware that surgery is commonly used to treat stress incontinence, that urethral dilation would only make matters worse, and that a hysteroscopic myomectomy involves the removal of fibroids from the uterus and is a different procedure altogether.

52-3. A. Kegel exercises result in increased resting and active pelvic muscle tone and have been shown to be effective in treating mild stress incontinence. Medical treatment for stress incontinence involve α-adrenergics, which increase sphincter tone, not anticholinergics such as Ditropan. This patient does not need hormone replacement because she is not menopausal.

52-4. A. A woman who has pelvic organ prolapse but is asymptomatic does not need treatment. However, she is at high risk for developing symptoms and may require treatment at that time. Depending on her desires and surgical risk factors, appropriate treatments would include the use of a pessary or surgical procedures to reduce prolapse. Hormone replacement will not treat pelvic organ prolapse.

 ## SUGGESTED ADDITIONAL READING

Swift S. Current opinion on the classification and definition of genital tract prolapse. *Curr Opin Obstet Gynecol.* 2002;14: 503–507.

Shull BL. Pelvic organ prolapse: anterior, superior, and posterior vaginal segment defects. *Am J Obstet Gynecol.* 1999;181:6–11.

VIII

Gynecologic Oncology and Breast Disease

Vulvar Pruritus

ID/CC: A 57-year-old G_3P_3 postmenopausal woman complains of vaginal and vulvar itching.

HPI: D.L. reports that she has been in good health except for worsening vulvovaginal pruritus over the last few years. She noticed the onset of itching soon after menopause. She had some relief initially with estrogen cream prescribed by her doctor. Then she tried over-the-counter antifungal creams but to no avail. Her symptoms are particularly bad in the nighttime. Ms. D. denies any postmenopausal vaginal bleeding but notes that sexual intercourse is painful.

PMHx: Basal cell carcinoma (BCC)

PSHx: Excision procedures for BCC

Meds: Vitamins, calcium

All: NKDA

POb/GynHx: Three vaginal deliveries. Menarche at age 15, menopause at 55. No HRT. No history of STIs or abnormal Pap smears.

SHx: Lives with husband. Remote history of tobacco use.

VS: Temp 97.6°F, BP 135/80, HR 76, RR 18

PE: *Gen:* well-developed, well-nourished slightly overweight woman. *External genitalia:* fused labia minora and majora with focal areas of raised, shiny white plaques around the posterior fourchette and at the 4 o'clock position. *Pelvic:* cervix flush with vagina—no lesions; atrophic vagina; uterus—small; no palpable adnexal masses.

Labs: Pap smear (1 year ago): atrophy; mammogram (last year): negative.

THOUGHT QUESTIONS

- What have her symptoms been attributed to?
- What other possible causes of vulvar pruritus and vulvodynia need to be investigated?
- How would you manage her?

Her report of symptomatic relief with local estrogen cream suggests an atrophic component to her symptoms. Overgrowth of organisms such as *Candida, Trichomonas,* and *Gardnerella* are common causes of vulvar pruritus. Yeast dermatitis usually is diagnosed by a KOH preparation, although the sensitivity of the test is variable (25%– 80%). One also could perform a Gram-stain examination, which is almost 100% sensitive for a yeast infection. Besides infection, dysplasia, cancer, and vulvar dystrophy are other causes of chronic vulvar pruritus. This patient needs a complete workup with a KOH/wet mount and Gram stain to evaluate for infection. Colposcopic-directed biopsies to evaluate for disease processes such as vulvar dysplasia, vulvar cancer, or vulvar dystrophy also are warranted.

CASE CONTINUED

The KOH/wet mount was normal, and Gram stain revealed no evidence of a yeast infection. You perform a colposcopic examination using topical acetic acid to isolate suspicious areas of the vulva. You identify several areas of acetowhite epithelium and take biopsies of these areas of the vulva. Ms. D. is very anxious for some alleviation of her itching.

QUESTIONS

53-1. What is the most common cause of vulvar pruritus?
A. Estrogen deficiency
B. Yeast dermatitis
C. Contact dermatitis
D. Bacterial vaginosis
E. Trichomoniasis

53-2. What would you recommend the patient do for symptomatic relief while awaiting the biopsy results?
  A. Testosterone gel
  B. Nothing
  C. Topical clotrimazole cream
  D. Hydrocortisone cream
  E. 5% imiquimod topical cream

53-3. The colposcopic examination revealed areas of acetowhite epithelium at the posterior fourchette and at the 4 o'clock position. Punch biopsies were performed without difficulty. What would you expect the final pathologic report to show?
  A. Chronic inflammation
  B. Vulvar intraepithelial neoplasia (VIN) II–III
  C. Condyloma
  D. Superficial spreading melanoma
  E. Lichen sclerosus et atrophicus

53-4. What is the best management for a patient with VIN III?
  A. Topical steroid cream application
  B. Wide local excision
  C. Trichloroacetic acid (TCA) application
  D. Skinning vulvectomy
  E. Combination topical steroid and testosterone creams

ANSWERS

53-1. B. The most common reason for vulvar pruritus is yeast dermatitis secondary to candidal species. Vaginal discharge from bacterial vaginosis and trichomoniasis, common vaginal infections, can cause vulvar irritation, dyspareunia, and pruritus. Estrogen deficiency is a common etiology of vulvar pruritus in postmenopausal women. Finally, acute contact dermatitis caused by perfumed soaps, laundry detergents, tight-fitting or synthetic undergarments, or vaginal hygienic products can cause intense vulvar pruritus.

53-2. D. Symptomatic relief while awaiting biopsy results can be achieved with a topical steroid cream. Local measures to diminish irritation, such as cotton underclothing, avoidance of strong detergents/soaps, and use of bath salts, also can help control the itching. Testosterone gel or cream in combination with a topical steroid would be appropriate treatment for lichen sclerosus et atrophicus. Imiquimod is indicated only for treatment of condyloma.

53-3. B. The colposcopic findings are consistent with the diagnosis of VIN. Vulvar dysplasia appears as multifocal discrete whitish, thickened lesions. Vulvar dystrophies such as lichen sclerosus et atrophicus typically appear thin, with areas of scarring or contractures. Skin fissures may be present because of excoriation. Condyloma appears as solitary or clustered, pedunculated, papillary lesions. Melanoma is the most frequent nonsquamous cell carcinoma of the vulva and presents as irregularly pigmented, variegated lesions that can be flat, ulcerated, or nodular.

53-4. B. Various modalities exist for treatment of premalignant changes in the vulva. Circumscribed VIN II–III lesions, like those described in this patient, can be treated with a wide local excision procedure. Skinning vulvectomy or CO_2 laser therapy are forms of therapy for superficial multifocal disease. Topical steroid or testosterone creams are not treatment options for vulvar dysplasia. TCA is effective treatment for small condyloma acuminata lesions.

 SUGGESTED ADDITIONAL READING

Disaia PJ, Creasman WT. *Clinical gynecologic oncology.* 6th ed. St. Louis, Mo: Mosby; 2002;47–50.

Herbst AL. Neoplastic diseases of the vulva. In: Stenchever MA, Droegemueller W, Herbst AL, et al., eds. *Comprehensive gynecology.* 4th ed. St. Louis, Mo: Mosby; 2001:999–1022.

Apgar BB, Cox JT. Differentiating normal and abnormal findings of the vulva. *Am Fam Physician.* 1996;53:1171–1180.

Hart WR. Vulvar intraepithelial neoplasia: historical aspects and current status. *Int J Gynecol Pathol.* 2001;20:16–30.

Vaginal Spotting/Routine Gynecologic Exam

ID/CC: A 26-year-old G$_0$ woman presents for an annual gynecologic exam.

HPI: A.D. states that overall she is doing well. Her last exam and Pap smear, she believes, were 3 years ago, and the results were normal. She currently is sexually active with one male partner for the past 5 months and uses oral contraceptive pills (OCPs). She has been taking OCPs for 3 months and has had some episodes of spotting, which are bothersome to her. She notes no change in her vaginal discharge, which she says is generally white and thin. Her last clinical breast exam was 3 years ago. She examines her own breasts at home every couple of months.

PMHx: Asthma, well-controlled by medication. No hospitalizations.

PSHx: Tonsillectomy as a child. Appendectomy at age 18.

Meds: Albuterol metered-dose inhaler (MDI) PRN; norethindrone acetate/ethinyl estradiol (Loestrin)

All: NKDA

POb/GynHx: Menarche age 13, 28- to 30-day cycles, 5 days of moderate bleeding. Last Pap smear 3 years ago. No history of abnormal Pap smears. History of chlamydia in college. Denies history of PID.

SHx: Works as a paralegal. Lives with a roommate. Has smoked one pack of tobacco per day for 8 years; social ETOH use; denies recreational drug use.

FHx: Significant for heart disease in her father at age 60, history of ovarian cancer in a maternal aunt at age 64.

THOUGHT QUESTIONS

- What is part of a routine gynecologic exam in this patient? How about a patient at age 40? 50?
- What high-risk behaviors and risk factors does this patient have and how do they relate to a routine gynecologic exam?
- Why might this patient have episodes of spotting or "breakthrough bleeding"?

A routine gynecologic examination can differ, depending on the individual needs and risk factors. In general, all patients should receive a thorough discussion of their gynecologic history with a focus on current issues: menstrual history, sexual history, obstetric history, a discussion of birth control if pertinent, infection history, and general gynecologic history (i.e., ovarian cysts, fibroids). A full examination concentrates on the breasts, abdomen, external genitalia, and pelvic organs. Thus, speculum, bimanual, and rectal examinations are required for all patients. Any sexually active patient should be offered a screen for STIs. Pap smears are performed every 1 to 3 years depending on the age of the patient and the medical history. The additional use of human papilloma virus (HPV) DNA screening may be appropriate in some women but is controversial. Mammograms are currently recommended every 2 years in patients older than 40 and annually in patients older than 50.

Most notably, Ms. D.'s smoking history is worrisome not only because of her asthma but also as a significant risk factor for cervical cancer. Her family history of ovarian cancer should be further explored. Patients with a family history of ovarian cancer may benefit from the use of OCPs. Thus, discussing this with her may encourage her to continue their use despite the episodes of bleeding.

Breakthrough bleeding while taking OCPs in young women is very common during the first 3 to 6 months of use. If the breakthrough bleeding continues, she may benefit from using a different OCP. A change from a monophasic to a multiphasic with an increased amount of estrogen may help to prevent breakthrough bleeding. Other diagnoses associated with spotting in a patient taking OCPs include cervicitis (especially with a chlamydial infection), cervical polyp, endometrial polyp, and cervical cancer. In older patients, spotting can be associated with endometrial hyperplasia, endometrial cancer, polyps, anovulation, or atrophy.

CASE CONTINUED

VS: Temp 98.3°F, BP 104/68, HR 74, RR 14, weight 140 lb, height 5 feet 5 inches

PE: *Gen:* NAD. *HEENT:* unremarkable. *Neck:* no thyroid nodules or enlargement. *Breasts:* no masses or axillary LAD. *Lungs:* CTAB. *Cor:* RR&R without murmurs. *Abd:* soft, nontender, no distension. *Extremities:* no clubbing, cyanosis, or edema. *Pelvic:* normal female genitalia, otherwise unremarkable. *SSE:* thin white discharge; no cervical lesions. *BME:* small anteverted uterus, no adnexal masses.

Labs: Wet prep: no clue cells or trichomonads, few WBCs. KOH: no pseudohyphae

As part of the routine exam you collect a sample for a Pap smear. You discuss with Ms. D. that the episodes of vaginal bleeding may be related to her OCP use. She decides to continue the current OCP but will return in 3 months if she continues to have spotting. You discuss with her the need to quit smoking, and she agrees to try with the assistance of the nicotine patch.

Two weeks later, the patient's Pap smear returns with the following result: "low-grade squamous intraepithelial lesion (LGSIL), endocervical cells present."

QUESTIONS

54-1. Given the Pap result of LGSIL, what is your recommendation to this patient?
   A. Repeat the Pap smear immediately
   B. Repeat the Pap smear in 6 to 8 months
   C. Colposcopic exam of the cervix with directed biopsies
   D. Loop electrosurgical excision procedure (LEEP)
   E. Cone biopsy

54-2. If instead the Pap smear result was "atypical squamous cells of unknown significance (ASCUS)," what might be your recommendation?

A. Repeat the Pap smear immediately
B. Repeat the Pap smear in 3 to 6 months or colposcopic exam now
C. Colposcopic exam now
D. LEEP
E. Cone biopsy

54-3. If instead the Pap smear result was "atypical glandular cells of undetermined significance (AGUS)," what would be your recommendation?

A. Repeat the Pap smear immediately
B. Repeat the Pap smear in 3 to 6 months
C. Colposcopic exam now
D. LEEP
E. Cone biopsy

54-4. Which serotypes of HPV are associated with cervical cancer?

A. 6, 11
B. 16, 18, 31
C. 42, 48, 52
D. All of the above
E. None of the above

ANSWERS

54-1. C. Pap smears are a screening tool for cervical cancer. The procedure involves scraping cells from the transformation zone of the cervix, but the test is not a biopsy. Thus, the results received can be open to interpretation and how one manages a patient with dysplasia can be controversial. In general it is agreed that all patients with a Pap smear suggesting high-grade squamous intraepithelial lesion (HGSIL) proceed directly to colposcopic exam with directed biopsies. Also, most practitioners agree that patients with LGSIL proceed directly to colposcopic exam with directed biopsies. This certainly would be the case in this patient who is a smoker. The follow-up for a patient with a first-time result of ASCUS is more controversial.

54-2. B. A good rule of thumb is to proceed directly to colposcopic exam in a patient with risk factors for cervical cancer or at risk for noncompliance with close follow-up. In a patient with a history of normal Pap smears with one risk factor, repeating the Pap in 4 to 6 months also is reasonable.

54-3. C. AGUS is a very different entity from ASCUS. First, there are two types of cervical cancer: squamous and adenocarcinoma (glandular). The spectrum of dysplasia associated with squamous cell cancer includes ASCUS, LGSIL, and HGSIL. AGUS is considered a dysplastic entity associated with adenocarcinoma of the cervix and endometrium. The percentage of AGUS patients with a significant lesion is much higher than those with ASCUS. Thus, colposcopic exam, endocervical curettage, and endometrial biopsy (in older patients) is required.

54-4. B. The serotypes 16, 18, and 31 are correlated with cervical cancer. The serotypes 6 and 11 are associated with condyloma only.

 SUGGESTED ADDITIONAL READING

Saint M, Gildengorin G, Sawaya GF. Current cervical neoplasia screening practices of obstetrician/gynecologists in the United States. *Am J Obstet Gynecol.* 2005;192:414–421.

Sherman ME, Lorincz AT, Scott DR, et al. Baseline cytology, human papillomavirus testing, and risk for cervical neoplasia: a 10-year cohort analysis. *J Natl Cancer Inst.* 2003;95:46–52.

Sawaya GF, McConnell KJ, Kulasingam SL, et al. Risk of cervical cancer associated with extending the interval between cervical-cancer screenings. *N Engl J Med.* 2003;349:1501–1509.

Wright TC Jr, Cox JT, Massad LS, et al. 2001 Consensus Guidelines for the management of women with cervical cytological abnormalities. *JAMA.* 2002;287:2120–2129.

Postmenopausal Vaginal Bleeding

ID/CC: A 65-year-old G_0 woman presents with irregular vaginal bleeding over the last 6 months.

HPI: S.H. notes that she has not had any vaginal bleeding or abnormal discharge since menopause at age 53. She first noticed a watery discharge and scant irregular vaginal bleeding 6 months ago. Her gynecologic exam last year was normal. Occasionally S.H. has had mild abdominal cramps but denies any weight loss or anorexia.

PMHx: Type 2 diabetes, hypertension

Meds: Glyburide, hydrochlorothiazide, ACE inhibitor lisinopril (Prinivil)

All: NKDA

PSHx: Breast biopsy for benign cyst

POb/GynHx: G_0. Polycystic ovary syndrome (PCOS). No STIs, no abnormal Pap smears.

SHx: Unmarried, lives with sister. No ethanol or tobacco use.

VS: Temp 97.8°F, standing BP 150/80, HR 80; sitting BP 140/72, HR 78; RR 14, weight 143 lb, height 5 feet 1.5 inches

PE: *Oral:* mucosa moist and pink. *Abd:* soft, nontender, no distension, no palpable masses. *Pelvic:* atrophic external genitalia and vagina; cervix—nulliparous os, no lesions. *BME:* uterus—approx 8-week size, AV/AF, nontender. No palpable adnexal masses.

THOUGHT QUESTIONS

- What is in the differential diagnosis for this patient?
- What is the most common finding in women with postmenopausal bleeding?
- What is the diagnosis of most concern and how would you work it up?

　　　　The differential diagnosis for postmenopausal uterine bleeding includes bleeding from adjustment to hormone replacement therapy, endometrial atrophy, atrophic vaginitis, endometrial or cervical polyps, endometrial hyperplasia, fibroids, and endometrial carcinoma. The most common cause of postmenopausal bleeding is endometrial atrophy (Table 55-1). Only 10% of patients with postmenopausal bleeding have endometrial cancer, but >90% of women with endometrial carcinoma complain only of abnormal uterine bleeding. A thorough physical examination including a Pap smear, endometrial biopsy, and CBC must be performed. You could consider transvaginal ultrasonography as an adjunctive study to the endometrial biopsy.

CASE CONTINUED

You send off samples for a Pap smear, endometrial biopsy, and CBC. The Pap smear shows atypical glandular cells of undetermined significance (AGUS). The pathology report from the endometrial biopsy reveals a focus of well-differentiated adenocarcinoma in the background of complex atypical hyperplasia. The CBC is normal with Hb 12 and Hct 37.

TABLE 55-1 Common Causes of Postmenopausal Bleeding

Cause	Percentage
Atrophic endometrium	65–75
Hormone replacement therapy	15–25
Cancer of the endometrium	9–12
Endometrial hyperplasia	5–10
Endometrial or cervical polyps	2–12

S.H. returns to your clinic for a discussion of the diagnosis and potential management options. You explain to her that her risk factors for endometrial cancer include diabetes, hypertension, and nulliparity. In addition, you discuss that the overall 5-year survival rate for all-comers with endometrial cancer is approximately 65% and is ≥75% for those with stage I disease (Figure 55-1).

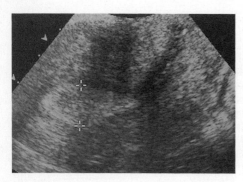

FIGURE 55-1.
The 12-mm thickness of the endometrium here is worrisome for hyperplasia or polyp. A typical post-menopausal endometrium should be <5 mm in thickness. *(Image provided by Departments of Radiology and Obstetrics and Gynecology, University of California, San Francisco).*

QUESTIONS

55-1. Upon initial presentation to the office, the diagnostic test with the best sensitivity and specificity for endometrial cancer is:
 A. Endometrial biopsy
 B. Ultrasonography
 C. Abdominal and pelvic CT
 D. Wet mount
 E. Pap smear

55-2. What percentage of complex atypical hyperplasia progresses to carcinoma?
 A. 1%
 B. 3%
 C. 8%
 D. 15%
 E. 29%

55-3. Given the finding of well-differentiated adenocarcinoma, the most appropriate management is:
   A. Observation and rebiopsy in 3 months
   B. Treatment with progestins and careful follow-up
   C. Dilation and curettage (D&C)
   D. Hysterectomy and bilateral salpingo-oophorectomy (BSO)
   E. Pelvic irradiation

55-4. The surgical pathology report notes the presence of a well-differentiated endometrioid adenocarcinoma with 30% invasion of the myometrium. What is her FIGO stage?
   A. Stage IA, grade 1
   B. Stage IB, grade 1
   C. Stage IB, grade 3
   D. Stage IC, grade 1
   E. Stage IIA, grade 3

ANSWERS

55-1. A. The diagnostic test of most value is an endometrial biopsy, which has a diagnostic accuracy of 90% to 98%. A physical examination rarely reveals evidence of endometrial carcinoma or hyperplasia. A Pap smear is not reliable, as <50% of women with endometrial carcinoma have an abnormal Pap result. Currently, more data are needed before transvaginal ultrasonography can substitute for tissue diagnosis in the workup of postmenopausal bleeding, although an endometrial thickness <5 mm in a postmenopausal woman is consistent with atrophy. A wet mount would only evaluate for bacterial vaginosis, yeast, or *Trichomonas*. CT would be useful if the clinical examination was limited secondary to habitus or discomfort.

55-2. E. Endometrial hyperplasia classification is based on the findings that only cytologically atypical lesions progress to cancer. Hyperplasias are classified as simple or complex based on architecture, and are designated as atypical hyperplasia based on cytology. Progression from hyperplasia to cancer occurs in 1% of women with simple hyperplasia and in 3% of women with complex hyperplasia. Whereas 8% of women with simple atypical hyperplasia progress to carcinoma, 29% of those with complex atypical hyperplasia develop carcinoma.

55-3. D. Treatment of endometrial cancer typically involves surgical staging, hysterectomy with BSO. Postoperative radiation is considered for advanced and/or poorly differentiated endometrial carcinoma. Progestins may be used to treat hyperplasia in select

TABLE 55-2   Staging of Endometrial Cancer

Stage	Characteristics
IA G123	Tumor limited to endometrium
IB G123	Invasion to <½ myometrium
IC G123	Invasion to >½ myometrium
IIA G123	Endocervical gland involvement
IIB G123	Cervical stromal invasion
IIIA G123	Invasion of serosa or adnexa or positive peritoneal cytology
IIIB G123	Vaginal metastases
IIIC G123	Metastases to pelvic or para-aortic lymph nodes
IVA G123	Invasion of bladder and/or bowel mucosa
IVB	Distant metastases including intra-abdominal and/or inguinal lymph node

Histopathology	Grouped by differentiation of adenocarcinoma
Grade 1	<5% nonsquamous or nonmorular solid growth pattern
Grade 2	6% to 50% nonsquamous or nonmorular solid growth pattern
Grade 3	>50% nonsquamous or nonmorular solid growth pattern

patients who are poor candidates for surgery or in those who desire future childbearing. Close follow-up study with endometrial biopsies is indicated in these patients. A D&C is of no diagnostic or therapeutic value in this patient with endometrial cancer. Observation and rebiopsy are inappropriate here.

55-4. B. In endometrial cancer, both grade and depth of invasion discriminate the risk of nodal disease. As grade becomes less differentiated, there is a greater probability of deep myometrial invasion and, subsequently, pelvic and para-aortic lymph node involvement. Greater depth of invasion (>50% myometrial involvement) is associated with a higher probability of extrauterine tumor spread, treatment failure, and recurrence. Nevertheless, regardless of grade, 1% of women with endometrial involvement have pelvic or para-aortic lymph node metastases (Table 55-2).

 ## SUGGESTED ADDITIONAL READING

Trope CG, Alektiar KM, Sabbatini PJ, et al. Corpus epithelial tumors. In: Hoskins WJ, Perez CA, Young RC, eds. *Principles and practice of gynecologic oncology.* 4th ed. Philadelphia, Pa: Lippincott Williams & Wilkins; 2005:823–872.

Brinton LA, Berman ML, Mortel R, et al. Reproductive, menstrual, and medical risk factors for endometrial cancer: results from a case-control study. *Am J Obstet Gynecol.* 1992;167:1317–1325.

Dijkhuizen FP, Mol BW, Brolmann HA, et al. The accuracy of
  endometrial sampling in the diagnosis of patients with
  endometrial carcinoma and hyperplasia: a meta-analysis.
  Cancer. 2000;89:1765–1772.
Creasman WT, Morrow CP, Bundy BN, et al. Surgical pathologic
  spread patterns of endometrial cancer. A Gynecologic Oncology
  Group Study. *Cancer.* 1987;60:2035–2041.

Abdominal Distension

ID/CC: A 72-year-old G_3P_2 woman complains of abdominal distension and anorexia.

HPI: A.D. had been in her usual state of good health until approximately 4 months ago, when she noticed increasing abdominal girth and worsening abdominal discomfort. She also reports anorexia and mild fatigue. She denies any alteration in her bowel movements but has had a few episodes of urinary incontinence. She also denies any postmenopausal uterine bleeding.

PMHx: Ductal carcinoma-in-situ (CIS) of breast, age 53

PSHx: Wide local excision on right breast

Meds: Calcium, multivitamin, vitamin D, alendronate

All: NKDA

POb/GynHx: Two NSVDs, one SAB. Menarche at age 13, menopause at age 51. No history of abnormal Pap smears. No STIs.

SHx: Lives alone, widowed. Has one ethanol drink per night; no tobacco use.

VS: Temp 97.2°F, BP 130/74, HR 90, RR 20, O_2 saturation 93%

PE: *Chest:* CTAB except decreased breath sounds at the bases. *Breasts:* well-healed scar on right breast, no masses, no discharge, symmetrical. *Abd:* moderate distension with fluid wave, mild tenderness, firm 12-cm abdominal mass arising from the pelvis. *Pelvic:* atrophic genitalia and vaginal mucosa; cervix within normal limits, stenotic os. *BME:* cervix immobile, large pelvic mass.

THOUGHT QUESTIONS

- What is the differential diagnosis?
- Will tumor markers such as cancer antigen 125 (CA-125) be helpful?
- How would you manage this patient's care at this point?

The differential diagnosis for abdominal distension in this patient includes ovarian carcinomatosis, ascites from hepatic disease, pancreatic cancer, and metastatic carcinoma. CA-125 levels can be elevated in nongynecologic and gynecologic conditions such as epithelial ovarian cancer, endometrial cancer, endometriosis, adenomyosis, uterine leiomyomata, cirrhosis, peritonitis, pancreatitis, pancreatic cancer, and colon cancer (Table 56-1).

Studies to assess the ascites and rule out metastatic disease are necessary. Imaging studies of the abdomen/pelvis, a mammogram, and a chest x-ray film are in order. These studies will assist in evaluating the site of origin of the mass (e.g., pancreas vs. ovary) and help define the extent of disease. An ultrasound would be most helpful in assessing for adnexal masses; a CT scan of the abdomen and pelvis would yield more information about the involvement of the disease process in the abdominal organs, intestines, and lymph nodes.

TABLE 56-1 Gynecologic and Nongynecologic Conditions Associated with Elevated CA-125 Levels

Gynecologic Cancers	Nongynecologic Cancers	Benign Gynecologic Conditions	Benign Nongynecologic Conditions
Epithelial ovarian cancer	Pancreatic cancer	Normal and ectopic pregnancy	Pancreatitis
Fallopian tube cancer	Lung cancer	Endometriosis	Cirrhosis
Endometrial cancer	Breast cancer	Fibroids	Peritonitis
Endocervical cancer	Colon cancer	Pelvic inflammatory disease	Recent laparotomy

From Callahan T, Caughey A, Heffner L. *Blueprints obstetrics and gynecology.* 4th ed. Baltimore, Md: Lippincott Williams & Wilkins; 2006.

CASE CONTINUED

In taking her family history, you learn that her mother died of ovarian cancer when she was in her 60s, and a maternal aunt developed ovarian cancer and died at age 50. You perform a Pap smear and order an abdominal/pelvic ultrasound and CT, a screening mammogram, and a chest x-ray film. The ultrasound findings of significant ascites and bilateral solid, cystic adnexal masses with septations and nodularity (Figure 56-1) are confirmed on CT. The Pap smear and mammogram are normal. Her chest x-ray film is normal.

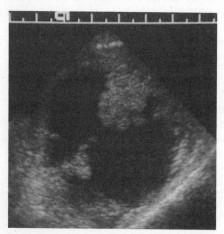

FIGURE 56-1.
Large complex mass in the ovary. The excrescences in the interior of the cyst are particularly worrisome. *(Image provided by Departments of Radiology and Obstetrics and Gynecology, University of California, San Francisco).*

QUESTIONS

56-1. You explain to her that she probably has ovarian cancer. She asks you how the disease spreads, and you inform her that the cancer *most* commonly spreads by:
    A. Direct exfoliation from the ovaries
    B. Hematogenous spread
    C. Lymph node metastases
    D. Transperitoneal dissemination
    E. Parenchymal involvement of the brain and lung

56-2. The next step in her management is:
A. Diagnostic laparoscopy
B. Chemotherapy with a platinum-based regimen
C. Total abdominal hysterectomy, bilateral salpingo-oophorectomy, lymph node dissection, omentectomy, tumor debulking
D. Laparoscopically assisted vaginal hysterectomy, bilateral salpingo-oophorectomy, lymph node sampling
E. Bilateral salpingo-oophorectomy, lymph node dissection, omentectomy

56-3. Findings at the time of surgery included 6 L of ascites, few <1.0-cm implants on the surface of the liver, enlarged para-aortic lymph nodes, and bilateral, solid cystic ovarian masses. All the sites were histologically confirmed to contain adenocarcinoma. What stage of ovarian cancer did she present with?
A. Stage IIIA
B. Stage IIIB
C. Stage IIIC
D. Stage IV
E. Stage IIC

56-4. Given this patient's family history, you should inform the patient's two daughters that:
A. They are not at increased risk for ovarian or breast cancer.
B. They should be screened with annual pelvic examinations only.
C. They should be screened with CA-125 levels to decrease mortality.
D. They should be screened with ultrasonography to decrease mortality.
E. Prophylactic oophorectomy decreases the risk of ovarian cancer.

ANSWERS

56-1. **A.** Ovarian cancer primarily spreads by direct exfoliation of malignant cells by either rupture or penetration of the ovarian capsule and implantation on other tissues. The disease then spreads along the circulatory path of peritoneal fluid flow and the lymphatic drainage system. Tumor involvement of the omentum, paracolic gutters, and cul-de-sac may be quite extensive. Hematogenous metastases are rare in ovarian cancer; therefore, parenchymal involvement of the lung, liver, and brain is rare.

56-2. C. Ovarian cancer staging is done clinically via exploratory laparotomy and evaluation of all areas at risk for metastatic disease. A rigorous staging procedure is necessary because postoperative therapy is based upon anatomic staging as well as other factors, such as histologic subtype of the tumor. The technique for surgical staging of ovarian cancer involves multiple cytologic washings or aspiration of ascites, removal of the adnexal mass/tumor, complete abdominal exploration, removal of the remaining ovary(s), uterus, and fallopian tubes, omentectomy, pelvic and para-aortic lymph node sampling, and biopsies of the peritoneum including the diaphragm.

56-3. C. She has stage IIIC ovarian cancer. Stage III disease is defined as tumor involving one or both ovaries with peritoneal implants outside of the pelvis and/or positive retroperitoneal or inguinal nodes, or tumor limited to the pelvis but with histologically verified malignant extension to the small bowel or omentum. The presence of superficial liver metastasis also indicates stage III. In stage IIIC the tumor implants are at least 2 cm in diameter, and the retroperitoneal/inguinal nodes are positive for cancer. The 5-year survival for stage IIIC epithelial ovarian cancer is 18%, with an overall 5-year survival rate of 31%. Survival rate has been shown to be influenced by the histologic grade of the tumor and the extent of residual disease after surgical debulking (Table 56-2).

TABLE 56-2 Ovarian Cancer Staging

Stage I	Confined to the ovaries IA. Limited to one ovary, no tumor on ovarian surface, capsule intact, negative cytology IB. Limited to both ovaries, no tumor on ovarian surface, capsule intact, negative cytology IC. Stage IA or IB but with tumor on ovarian surface, ruptured capsule, or positive cytology
Stage II	Involving one of both ovaries, with pelvic extension IIA. Extension and/or metastases to the uterus or fallopian tubes IIB. Extension to other pelvic tissues
Stage III	Involving one or both ovaries, with implants outside the pelvis and/or positive retroperitoneal or inguinal lymph nodes; superficial liver metastases IIIA. Grossly limited to pelvis, negative lymph nodes, microscopic disease on abdominal peritoneal surfaces IIIB. Implants outside the pelvis in the abdominal peritoneal surfaces <2 cm in diameter, negative lymph nodes IIIC. Abdominal implants >2 cm in diameter and/or positive lymph nodes
Stage IV	Distant metastases; positive pleural effusion, parenchymal liver metastases

56-4. E. Pedigree analysis can estimate a family member's risk of ovarian cancer. Patients with a family history suggestive of hereditary ovarian cancer syndrome (where more than two first-degree relatives have ovarian cancer or related cancer) have a 30% to 50% chance of developing ovarian cancer. A.D.'s daughters are at increased risk for developing ovarian cancer given their family history. Routine screening involves the combination of annual or biannual pelvic examinations, CA-125 levels, and transvaginal ultrasonography. However, no screening technique, even in high-risk patients, has significantly reduced mortality from ovarian cancer. Prophylactic oophorectomy can decrease the risk of ovarian and breast cancers, but it does not remove the risk for peritoneal carcinomatosis. BRCA1 screening can also be considered. Studies suggest that BRCA1 mutations occur in 5% of women diagnosed with ovarian cancer prior to age 70. BRCA mutations are being studied extensively to elucidate their roles in breast and ovarian cancers. BRCA1 is a tumor suppressor gene on chromosome 17q21, whereas the BRCA2 cancer susceptibility gene is located on chromosome 13q12–13. BRCA2 mutations also increase the risk for ovarian cancer but to a lesser extent than do BRCA1 mutations.

 SUGGESTED ADDITIONAL READING

Ozols RF, Rubin SC, Thomas GM, et al. Epithelial ovarian cancer. In: Hoskins WJ, Perez CA, Young RC, eds. *Principles and practice of gynecologic oncology.* 4th ed. Philadelphia, Pa: Lippincott Williams & Wilkins; 2005;823–872.

Bristow RE, Tomacruz RS, Armstrong DK, et al. Survival effect of maximal cytoreductive surgery for advanced ovarian carcinoma during the platinum era: a meta-analysis. *J Clin Oncol.* 2002;20: 248–259.

Welcsh PL, Owens KN, King MC. Insights into the functions of BRCA1 and BRCA2. *Trends Genet.* 2000;16:69–74.

Frank TS, Critchfield GC. Identifying and managing hereditary risk of breast and ovarian cancer. *Clin Perinatol.* 2001;2:395–406.

CASE 57

Painless Vaginal Bleeding

ID/CC: A 39-year-old G_4P_1 woman presents to the emergency department with complaints of vaginal bleeding and profuse vaginal discharge over the past 6 months.

HPI: P.C. denies any abdominal pain but reports a minimum 6-month period of irregular vaginal bleeding, periodically with large clots. She has noticed increased foul-smelling watery vaginal discharge. Ms. C. reports occasional chills. She denies any nausea or vomiting, changes in bowel and bladder habits, or recent change in weight.

PMHx/PSHx: Three D&Cs

Meds: None

All: NKDA

POb/GynHx: Three TABs, SVD 20 years ago. Last Pap smear 5 years ago, within normal limits. History of gonorrhea, chlamydia infection 2 to 3 years ago.

SHx: Homeless. Smokes 1.5 packs of cigarettes per day; history of EtOH, heroin, and cocaine use.

VS: Temp 96.7°F, BP 110/62, HR 76m, weight 95 lb, height 5 feet 3 inches

PE: *Gen:* cachectic-appearing woman in mild distress. *HEENT:* poor dentition, pale mucosa, neck without masses. *Abd:* soft, nontender, no distension, bilateral shoddy inguinal lymph nodes. *Pelvic:* cervix with a polypoid, friable, fungating mass protruding through the os. Vagina without lesions. *BME:* cervix is firm and nodular, enlarged to approximately 4 to 5 cm; parametria and pelvic sidewalls appear free; positive CMT. *Rectovaginal (RV):* confirms the above findings, thin rectovaginal septum.

Labs: Urine pregnancy test negative, WBC 1.1, Hb 9.0, Cr 1.2.

THOUGHT QUESTIONS

- What is the differential diagnosis for this woman with painless vaginal bleeding?
- Should the laboratory finding of leukopenia be of concern in her workup?
- What further diagnostic tests would help focus the differential diagnosis?

The differential diagnosis would have to include cervical carcinoma, prolapsing cervical polyp, condyloma, myoma, and infected degenerating/necrotic polyp or myoma. WBC of 1.1 is worrisome in this patient with cachexia, anemia, painless cervical mass, and history of polysubstance use, all of which suggest a possibly immunocompromised state. If she is clinically stable, a Pap examination, endocervical curettage, and biopsy of this mass must be performed.

CASE CONTINUED

You are concerned about an immunocompromised health status and obtain her consent for hepatitis, HIV, CD4, and viral load testing. You also perform biopsies of the cervical mass and obtain a social work consultation. The test results confirm your suspicions that she is HIV positive and has adenocarcinoma of the cervix.

THOUGHT QUESTIONS

- What is the staging workup for cervical cancer?
- What is the management of cervical cancer?

Cervical cancer is clinically staged via an examination under anesthesia, as well as cystoscopy and proctoscopy to assess for local spread of disease. CT scans of the abdomen, pelvis, and chest should be obtained. Although cervical cancer is clinically

TABLE 57-1 Staging Cervical Cancer

Stage I	Confined to the cervix IA. Microscopic disease IB. Clinically identifiable lesions
Stage II	Extracervical, but not to the pelvic walls or distal third of the vagina IIA. No parametrial involvement IIB. Parametrial involvement
Stage III	Extension to the pelvic wall or distal vagina IIIA. Not to the pelvic wall IIIB. To the pelvic wall
Stage IV	Beyond the true pelvis IVA. To the bladder or rectum IVB. Distant metastases

staged, these imaging studies help evaluate for metastatic disease (Table 57-1 and Figure 57-1). A radical hysterectomy would benefit a patient with invasive cervical cancer confined to the cervix, uterine corpus, and vagina (stage IIA or less). More advanced disease, stage IIB and beyond, is treated with combined radiation therapy and adjuvant cisplatin-based chemotherapy. In fact, radiation therapy and radical hysterectomy have been found to be equally effective in treating stage IB disease.

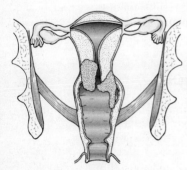

FIGURE 57-1.
The cervical cancer is bulky, larger than 4 cm, but is confined to the cervical corpus. *(From Callahan T, Caughey A, Heffner L. Blueprints Obstetrics and Gynecology. 4th ed. Baltimore, Md: Blackwell Publishing, 2006, with permission.)*

QUESTIONS

57-1. The hospital resident who consulted you about this patient wants to know the true relationship between cervical neoplasia and human papillomavirus (HPV). You explain that:

A. HPV serotype 16 is the most common HPV serotype in invasive cervical cancer and also is the most common HPV type in women with normal cytology.

B. Sexual/behavioral risk factors are not surrogates for cervical cancer.

C. HPV DNA is infrequently found to be integrated into the DNA of cervical cancer cells.

D. There is no relationship between cigarette smoking and HPV-associated dysplasia of the cervix.

E. HPV prevalence is lowest in a population of young sexually active individuals.

57-2. Her presentation is most concerning for an occult cervical carcinoma. The CT scan of her abdomen and pelvis does not show hydronephrosis or ureteral obstruction. What stage cervical carcinoma does this patient have?

A. Stage IA

B. Stage IB1

C. Stage IB2

D. Stage IIA

E. Stage III

57-3. Which of the following would be appropriate if she was hemodynamically unstable because of extensive bleeding from an erosive cervical tumor?

A. Transfuse with blood products and perform an emergent laparotomy, abdominal hysterectomy and bilateral salpingo-oophorectomy

B. Transfuse and perform a trachelectomy (amputation of the cervix)

C. Transfuse and treat with high-dose progestins

D. Transfuse and pack the vagina

E. Transfuse, pack the vagina, and consult interventional radiology for possible embolization of the hypogastric vessels

57-4. Which of the following is true?
A. The cervix is rarely involved in cancer of the endometrium
B. Invasive cervical cancer is an AIDS-defining disease
C. Adenocarcinoma is the most common variety of invasive cervical cancer
D. Primary vaginal cancer is a more common tumor than primary cervical cancer in postmenopausal women
E. Surgical therapy is recommended for treatment of all stages of cervical cancer

ANSWERS

57-1. A. HPV has been linked to the development of cervical dysplasia and squamous cell carcinoma of the cervix. Molecular analyses reveal that HPV DNA is integrated into the host cell's DNA in >90% of cervical cancer cells. HPV serotypes 6 and 11 are associated with condyloma, whereas serotypes 16, 18, and 31 are correlated with the development of preinvasive and invasive cervical squamous cell carcinomas. Sexual/behavioral risk factors, such as multiple sexual partners, early age at onset of sexual activity, and history of STIs, place women at increased risk for cervical dysplasia and cancer. Sexual partners of women with cervical cancer have been found to be at increased risk for HPV-associated diseases and penile cancer. Abnormal Pap test history, cigarette smoking, and infection with HIV are all risk factors for cervical dysplasia. HPV prevalence is variable depending on the population studied, but it is highly prevalent in a population of young sexually active individuals. HPV testing can be highly sensitive but lacks the specificity to be useful as a screening test for preinvasive and invasive cervical cancer.

57-2. C. Cervical carcinoma is a disease that is staged clinically and primarily by pelvic examination. It can be modified by findings on chest x-ray film, intravenous pyelogram, or CT that demonstrate ureteral obstruction or a nonfunctioning kidney, but not by operative findings. Clinical stage is the most important prognostic factor in cervical carcinoma. This patient has a 4- to 5-cm nodular lesion of the cervix that does not appear to involve the parametrial tissues, rectovaginal septum, or pelvic sidewalls. She has stage IB2 cancer of the cervix.

57-3. E. When a patient is clinically unstable, intravenous access needs to be obtained and aggressive resuscitation started with fluids and blood products. In this case, where the source of bleeding is diffuse from a tumor on the cervix, one can try to apply pressure to the cervix with a vaginal pack while resuscitation is ongoing. Consultation with interventional radiology for possible embolization of hypogastric vessels is appropriate. If the bleeding is not controlled with these less invasive measures, one will have to go toward an exploratory laparotomy and a modified radical hysterectomy, where paracervical and parametrial tissues are removed. A simple abdominal hysterectomy has little role in the therapy for invasive cervical cancer, although it may be performed for women with preinvasive or microinvasive disease. A radical trachelectomy is a conservative variant of a modified radical hysterectomy for young patients with early invasive cancer of the cervix who desire future childbearing. Progestins have no role in controlling bleeding from a cervical tumor.

57-4. B. In 1993, invasive cervical carcinoma was added to the CDC class C list of AIDS-defining illnesses. HIV-infected patients are at increased risk for cervical neoplasia and for disease progression and persistence. Screening of HIV-infected women for abnormal cervical cytology is controversial, but most practitioners would adopt a conservative approach with closer intervals of examinations. The cervix is commonly involved in cancer of the endometrium and vagina. In fact, endometrial cancer can extend into the cervix by direct or lymphovascular extension or multifocal disease. Primary vaginal cancer represents only 1% to 2% of malignancies of the female genital tract, and most lesions involving the cervix and vagina are designated cervical primaries. Squamous cell carcinoma is the most common invasive cervical cancer histology, followed by adenocarcinoma. Of the two modalities for primary treatment of invasive cervical cancer, surgery is limited to patients with early-stage disease, whereas radiation therapy can be used in all stages of disease.

SUGGESTED ADDITIONAL READING

Randall ME, Michael H, Vermorken J, et al. Uterine cervix. In: Hoskins WJ, Perez CA, Young RC, eds. *Principles and practice of gynecologic oncology.* 4th ed. Philadelphia, Pa: Lippincott Williams & Wilkins Philadelphia; 2005:743–822.

Franco EL, Duarte-Feranco E, Ferenczy A. Cervical cancer: epidemiology, prevention and the role of human papillomavirus infection. *CMAJ.* 2001;164:1017–1025.

Jay N, Moscicki AB. Human papillomavirus infections in women with HIV disease: prevalence, risk and management. *AIDS Read.* 2000;10:659–668.

Yalvac S, Kayikcioglu F, Boran N, et al. Embolization of uterine artery in terminal stage cervical cancers. *Cancer Invest.* 2002;20:754–758.

Family History of Breast and Ovarian Cancer

 ID/CC: A 48-year-old G_4P_2 woman presents with a family history significant for premenopausal breast cancer in two of her sisters and ovarian cancer in the third sibling at age 49.

HPI: C.S. is here to discuss cancer risk reduction strategies. She is otherwise healthy and without any significant complaints.

PMHx/PSHx: None

Meds: None

All: NKDA

POb/GynHx: Menarche at age 11, regular cycles every 28 days.

SHx: Married with two daughters and one son.

VS: Temp 97.8°F, BP 114/62, HR 80, RR 18

PE: *Chest:* CTAB. *Breasts:* no palpable masses or nodules. *Pelvic:* normal external genitalia, vaginal mucosa, and cervix. *BME:* small AV/AF uterus, no palpable adnexal masses.

THOUGHT QUESTIONS

- Given her family history, what cancer(s) is she most susceptible to?
- What other information in her family history would you like to know?
- How do you assess her risk for cancer?

A possible hereditary ovarian cancer (HOC) syndrome should be considered if a family includes two or more women with early-onset breast or ovarian cancer (usually at age <50 years). A woman diagnosed with breast cancer before age 50 or with ovarian cancer at any age should be asked about any first-, second-, or third-degree relatives on either side of the family, with either diagnosis. History of male breast cancer at any age and of breast and ovarian cancer in the same individual raise concern about the possibility of HOC in the family. A detailed family history is the cornerstone of effective genetic counseling and risk assessment. Counselors use various mathematical models and tools, such as BRCAPRO software, to help identify candidates for genetic testing. Empiric approaches based on epidemiologic data that indicate age-specific risks of breast or ovarian cancer or direct assessment of gene mutation status then are used to assess risk of disease and provide a rationale for recommended health behaviors.

     CASE CONTINUED

She recalls that her paternal grandfather died of colon cancer and several other members of the family had colorectal cancer (two paternal uncles), breast cancer (paternal aunt, maternal grandmother, maternal grandaunt, maternal aunt), and prostate cancer (father, maternal uncle).

![question mark icon]   QUESTIONS

58-1. Approximately 10% of epithelial ovarian cancer and 7% of breast cancer cases are associated with an autosomal dominant pattern of inheritance. Which gene mutation is responsible for the majority of HOCs?
   A. BRCA1
   B. BRCA2
   C. TP53
   D. PTEN
   E. her-2/neu

58-2. This patient's family history is of concern because of the second manifestation of HOC besides hereditary breast/ovarian cancer syndrome. In addition to testing for BRCA mutations, you would consider genetic testing for:

   A. Lynch syndrome I
   B. Lynch syndrome II
   C. Cowden syndrome
   D. Li-Fraumeni syndrome
   E. Gardner syndrome

58-3. You recommend that the patient undergo genetic evaluation. During this discussion you tell her that:

   A. Risk prediction models that predict the risk of breast cancer in the general population, such as the Gail model, are applicable to women with hereditary mutations.
   B. A personal history of early-onset cancer is the most powerful tool to determine the pretest probability of harboring a hereditary cancer mutation.
   C. A negative test result in the absence of a known mutation in the affected family member rules out the likelihood of hereditary risk of cancer.
   D. Mutations in BRCA1 and BRCA2 from either side of the family confer an increased risk for breast/ovarian cancer.

58-4. One of the patient's sisters tested positive for a BRCA1 mutation. How do you propose to best address your patient's increased risk for breast and ovarian cancers?

   A. Oral contraceptive pills
   B. Annual transvaginal sonography and cancer antigen 125 (CA-125) measurement
   C. Prophylactic bilateral salpingo-oophorectomy
   D. Prophylactic bilateral mastectomy
   E. Annual pelvic and mammographic examinations

 ANSWERS

58-1. A. BRCA1 and BRCA2 mutations are responsible for the majority of HOCs, with 70% of cases attributed to BRCA1 and 20% of the cases to BRCA2. Other mutations implicated in HOCs include mutations in the DNA mismatch repair genes MLH1 and MSH2, as well as other single genes. Mutation in TP53 appears to be an early event in a distinct subset of ovarian cancers. PTEN has been shown to be down-regulated in a proportion of ovarian cancers, whereas the proto-oncogene her-2/neu has not been clearly shown to be involved in ovarian cancer.

58-2. B. Epidemiologic studies point to the existence of two distinct manifestations of HOC. The first is the breast/ovarian cancer syndrome linked to BRCA1 and, to a lesser extent, BRCA2. The second manifestation is ovarian cancers associated with an excess of endometrial and colorectal cancers in a variant of hereditary nonpolyposis colorectal cancer (HNPCC) syndrome, also known as Lynch syndrome II. Lynch syndrome I is the other variant of HNPCC, which is defined by early-onset site-specific colorectal cancer and an excess of synchronous and metasynchronous colorectal cancer. Endometrial cancer represents a component tumor of Cowden syndrome, a disease characterized by benign hamartomas of multiple organs, including skin, intestines, breast, and thyroid. Patients with Li-Fraumeni syndrome have a very high risk of developing osteosarcoma, soft-tissue sarcoma, breast cancer, brain tumors, adrenocortical cancer, and leukemia. Mutations in TP53 are associated with Li-Fraumeni syndrome. Gardner syndrome is an autosomal dominant condition associated with familial adenomatous polyposis of the colon and mesodermal tumors such as dermoid tumors and osteomas of the skull.

58-3. D. Risk prediction models for the general population, such as the Gail and Claus models, are not applicable to women with BRCA mutations because these models underestimate the risk conferred by mutations inherited in an autosomal dominant fashion. The most powerful tool for determining the pretest probability of hereditary cancer is the family history of cancer. It is essential to consider history from both sides of the family for the possibility of hereditary cancers. In a family with a history suggestive of HOC, the most informative testing strategy focuses on identifying a specific BRCA mutation in an affected family member. A negative test result in the absence of a known mutation in the affected family member reduces the likelihood of hereditary cancer but does not eliminate it entirely.

58-4. C. Prophylactic bilateral salpingo-oophorectomy is believed to reduce the risk of ovarian cancer in women with BRCA1 and BRCA2 mutations by 95%. Evidence suggests that it also reduces the risk of breast cancer by nearly 50%. An NIH consensus panel on ovarian cancer has concluded that prophylactic oophorectomy should be considered in women with HOC syndromes who are 35 years of age "and older"or after completion of childbearing. Oral contraceptive pills have been demonstrated to reduce the risk of ovarian cancer in women with BRCA1 and BRCA2 mutations by approximately 60%. With regard to breast cancer, oral contraceptive use does not appear to increase its incidence in the general population or women with germline mutations. As screening tools for ovarian cancer, transvaginal sonography lacks specificity, whereas serum CA-125 measurements are quite unreliable. Nevertheless, these test should be performed at least annually in women with BRCA mutations who wish to retain their ovaries. Prospective cohort studies are being conducted to assess the risks and benefits of this screening approach in high-risk women. Prophylactic mastectomy significantly reduces the risk of breast cancer, but it is chosen by only a minority of women given the efficacy of early-stage breast cancer surveillance.

SUGGESTED ADDITIONAL READING

Boyd J, Berchuck A. Oncogenes and tumor-suppressor genes. In: Hoskins WJ, Perez CA, Young RC, eds. *Principles and practice of gynecologic oncology.* 4th ed. Philadelphia, Pa: Lippincott Williams & Wilkins; 2005:93–122.

Antoniou A, Pharoah PD, Narod S, et al. Average risks of breast and ovarian cancer associated with BRCA1 and BRCA2 mutations detected in case series unselected for family history: a combined analysis of 22 studies. *Am J Hum Genet.* 2003;72: 1117–1130.

Lynch HT, Casey MJ. Current status of prophylactic surgery for hereditary breast and gynecologic cancers. *Curr Opin Obstet Gynecol.* 2001;13:25–30.

Kauff ND, Satagopan JM, Robson ME, et al. Risk-reducing salpingo-oophorectomy in women with a BRCA1 or BRCA2 mutation. *N Engl J Med.* 2002;346:1609–1615.

Vaginal Bleeding and Family History of Colorectal and Endometrial Cancer

ID/CC: A 40-year-old G_1P_0 woman presents for a new patient consultation and reports a history of new-onset menorrhagia.

HPI: M.C. has no new complaints, although she has noticed increased menstrual flow over the last 4 months. A review of systems is otherwise negative. The patient's family history reveals that her father developed colon cancer at age 47; her older brother was diagnosed with colon cancer at age 45; and her paternal grandmother was treated for endometrial cancer when she was in her late 40s. In addition, her maternal grandmother developed ovarian cancer at age 67. You are concerned about her familial cancer risk.

PMHx/PSHx: None

Meds: None

All: NKDA

POb/GynHx: Menarche at age 12, regular menstrual cycles every 30 days.

SHx: Engaged.

VS: Temp 97.6°F, BP 130/76, HR 82, weight 132 lb, height 5 feet 2.5 inches

PE: *Chest:* CTAB. *Breasts:* no masses. *Abdomen:* soft, nontender. *Pelvic:* normal without adnexal masses or uterine enlargement.

THOUGHT QUESTIONS

- This patient's pedigree is of concern for a hereditary cancer syndrome. What genetic mutations would be most compatible with this history?
- Is the age of disease onset informative?
- Is flexible sigmoidoscopy an effective screening tool in a family with this cancer history?

Approximately 6% of cases of colorectal cancer in women are due to hereditary factors. Hereditary nonpolyposis colorectal cancer (HNPCC; Lynch I and II syndromes) is responsible for up to 5% of colorectal cancers in women, whereas familial adenomatous polyposis (FAP) accounts for ≤1% of colorectal cancer diagnoses. Lynch I syndrome is the site-specific familial cancer syndrome in which only colon cancer is inherited. Lynch II syndrome encompasses an increased incidence extracolonic adenocarcinomas at a variety of sites, including the endometrium, stomach, ovary, pancreas, biliary tract, small bowel, ureter, and renal pelvis. Additionally, of the so-called "sporadic" cases of colon cancer, 19% develop in women with at least one first-degree relative with colon cancer. A family history of a single first-degree relative with colorectal cancer places a patient at a twofold to threefold increased risk. Early age at onset is the one of the most striking characteristics of HNPCC-associated cancers (mean age 40 years vs. 70 years for the general population). Early-onset colorectal cancer is suggestive of HNPCC. Likewise, endometrial cancer that arises in association with HNPCC usually develops in the perimenopausal setting. Therefore, surveillance strategies must be initiated at a relatively early age and include a complete colonoscopy given the propensity for HNPCC-associated colon cancer proximal to the splenic flexure.

CASE CONTINUED

You believe that her family history is most compatible with HNPCC. You perform a pelvic examination, Pap smear, and endometrial biopsy. You recommend that she seek a consultation with a cancer geneticist and consider colorectal cancer screening. You discuss the different colorectal cancer screening strategies with her and strongly encourage her to research her family history for medical conditions affecting both sides of the family.

QUESTIONS

59-1. Which of the following statements regarding HNPCC is true?
- A. The majority of mutations responsible for HNPCC occur in two DNA mismatch repair genes, MSH6 and PMS1.
- B. The finding of microsatellite instability (MSI) in tumor tissue DNA in itself does not indicate the cancer was due to HNPCC mutation.
- C. HNPCC is clinically associated with a profusion of colonic polyps at an early age.
- D. HNPCC-associated colon cancer typically is located in the distal colon and amenable to screening by flexible sigmoidoscopy.
- E. Endometrial cancer is an uncommon extracolonic HNPCC tumor site.

59-2. The patient's Pap smear result was normal but the endometrial biopsy showed evidence of disordered proliferative endometrium. Her own genetic testing showed that she does not carry the HNPCC mutation found in her other family members. What course of action do you recommend?
- A. Routine pelvic examination
- B. Prophylactic subtotal colectomy
- C. Prophylactic hysterectomy—bilateral salpingo-oophorectomy
- D. Annual colonoscopy, transvaginal sonography, cancer antigen 125 (CA-125) level
- E. Annual colonoscopy, transvaginal sonography, CA-125 level

59-3. If the patient's genetic testing had shown a mutation in the MSH2 gene, what is her risk of colorectal and endometrial cancers by age 70?
- A. 2% and 1.5%, respectively
- B. 20% and 15%, respectively
- C. 30%–40% and 25%–30%, respectively
- D. 70%–82% and 42%–60%, respectively
- E. 95% and 80%, respectively

59-4. The patient's 22-year-old niece also underwent genetic testing, which revealed the presence of an HNPCC mutation. She wants to know when she should begin screening examinations and at what intervals.

    A. Colonoscopy beginning at age 20–25 at 5-year intervals
    B. Colonoscopy beginning at age 20–25 at 2-year intervals
    C. Gastroscopy beginning at age 30–35 at 1- to 2-year intervals
    D. Annual fecal occult blood testing beginning at age 20–25
    E. Annual urine cytology and endometrial biopsy beginning at age 30

ANSWERS

59-1. B. Most HNPCC is associated with mutations in the DNA mismatch repair genes MSH2 and MLH1. Mutations of MSH6, PMS1, and PMS2 have been implicated in a smaller number of HNPCC families. MSI is a phenomenon present in 90% of HNPCC-associated colorectal cancers, compared to 15% to 20% of sporadic tumors. The finding of MSI does not indicate that the tumor was due to HNPCC mutations, but it does lead one to perform further genetic testing. On the other hand, a negative result in the absence of compelling clinical criteria usually does exclude HNPCC. Diffuse polyposis is not a feature of HNPCC. However, precursor adenomas are found in HNPCC and evidence exists showing a reduction in HNPCC-associated colon cancer incidence and mortality with early colonoscopic evaluations. Early-onset endometrial cancer is the second most common manifestation of extracolonic HNPCC in women.

59-2. A. If an at-risk patient (based on family history) does not carry the mutation identified in her affected family members, her risk of cancer is no greater than that of the general population. Therefore, this patient can, forego the increased surveillance or other recommended health strategies for HNPCC. Prophylactic surgeries are considered only in patients with mutation-proven HNPCC. Prophylactic colectomy may be strongly considered in those with adenomas identified at an early age or with adenomas showing MSI. Prophylactic hysterectomy—bilateral salpingo-oophorectomy should be considered at the time of surgery for an HNPCC-associated colorectal cancer. Trials investigating the benefits of various gynecologic cancer screening and prevention strategies in women with HNPCC are underway.

59-3. D. Individuals with MSH2 or MLH1 mutations have a 70% to 82% risk of colorectal cancer and a 42% to 60% risk of endometrial cancer by age 70, compared to the general population risk of 2% and 1.5%, respectively. Of note, the increased risk for HNPCC-related cancers is seen at an early age and hence the recommendations for early age of screening. Patients with HNPCC who develop cancer are at a greatly increased risk for a second malignancy. They have a 30% risk for developing a second cancer within 10 years, as compared to the general population risk of 3%.

59-4. B. General population screening test for colon cancer, such as fecal occult blood testing and flexible sigmoidoscopy, are not sufficiently sensitive for patients with HNPCC. Recommended surveillance strategies by the International Collaborative Group on HNPCC are as follows:

- Colonoscopy beginning at age 20–25 at 2 year-intervals
- Gynecologic examination, transvaginal sonography, CA-125 beginning at age 30–35 at 1- to 2-year intervals
- Gastroscopy beginning at age 30–35 at 1- to 2-year intervals only if at least one family member is affected
- Urine cytology and ultrasonography beginning at age 30–35 at 1- to 2-year intervals only if at least one family member is affected

Studies of increased surveillance for endometrial and ovarian cancers in women with HNPCC mutations are ongoing. Endometrial biopsy is to be performed as symptoms arise. Routine surveillance for the other malignancies associated with HNPCC is not considered practical.

SUGGESTED ADDITIONAL READING

Wijnen JT, Vasen HF, Khan PM, et al. Clinical findings with implications for genetic testing in families with clustering of colorectal cancer. *N Engl J Med.* 1998;339:511–518.

Lu KH, Dinh M, Kohlmann W, et al. Gynecologic cancer as a "sentinel cancer" for women with hereditary nonpolyposis colorectal cancer syndrome. *Obstet Gynecol.* 2005;105:569–574.

Lynch TH, Kaul K. Microsatellite instability, clinical implications, and new methodologies. *J Natl Cancer Inst.* 2000;92:511–512.

Burke W, Petersen G, Lynch P, et al. Recommendations for follow-up of individuals with an inherited predisposition to cancer. I. Hereditary nonpolyposis colon cancer. *JAMA.* 1997;277:915–919.

Breast Lump

ID/CC: A 29-year-old G₀ woman presents with a painful lump in her right breast.

HPI: S.C. noticed the onset of breast pain approximately 4 weeks ago. She initially thought that the pain was due to a strained muscle, but then she felt a small tender area on the outer part of her right breast when she was in the shower. She denies any abnormal nipple discharge.

PMHx/PSHx: None

Meds: Medroxyprogesterone acetate (DMPA)

All: NKDA

POb/GynHx: Menarche at age 13, regular cycles until amenorrhea due to DMPA. No STIs.

SHx: Recently married. Two cups of coffee per day.

VS: Temp 97.6°F, BP 110/60, HR 76, RR 16

PE: *Chest:* CTAB. *Breasts:* symmetrical, nontender, no skin changes, no galactorrhea or other discharge; right breast—palpable 2.5-cm smooth, round, mobile mass, minimally tender, at 10 o'clock 3 cm from the nipple; left breast—within normal limits (Figure 60-1).

THOUGHT QUESTIONS

- What is the differential diagnosis for a painful lump in the breast of a premenopausal woman? Of an older woman?

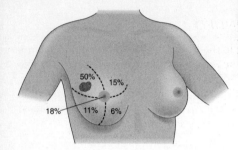

FIGURE 60-1.
Diagram of common locations for breast masses. In this case, the location is at 10 o'clock.

- What characteristics are associated with benign versus malignant masses?
- What other pertinent facts in her history would you like to know?

In a premenopausal woman, the differential diagnosis includes cysts, fibrocystic change, fat necrosis, or an abscess. Fat necrosis typically results from trauma to the breast. Although an abscess usually occurs in the postpartum period from progression of mastitis, subareolar abscesses have also been seen in older, nonlactating women. Sclerosing adenosis sometimes present as a hard, fixed, tender mass, as can cystosarcoma phyllodes, a rare, rapidly enlarging, but usually benign tumor that potentially can be a locally aggressive tumor. Malignancy should always be considered in an older woman, even though the majority of invasive tumors tend to be painless (unless it is an advanced stage invasive cancer).

When attempting to differentiate between malignant and benign tumors on physical examination, benign tumors tend to be smooth, regular, and mobile, whereas malignant masses typically are irregular and fixed to adjacent tissue. There can be associated skin or nipple retraction if an underlying malignant mass is present. One should elicit a more detailed history about fluctuations in either the size of the lesion or the nature of the discomfort, history of injury to the breast, prior similar episodes, and a family history of breast disease.

CASE CONTINUED

She does not recall trauma to the breast, and she has not noticed any change in pain or size of the lump over the last few weeks. Notable in her family history is fibrocystic disease in her mother and sister. Her other sister, maternal grandmother, and two maternal aunts have had no breast disease. Her paternal grandmother had breast cancer in her 70s and is alive and well after therapy.

 QUESTIONS

60-1. What is the most likely diagnosis for her breast lump?
A. Fibroadenoma
B. Fibrocystic disease
C. Cyst
D. Cystosarcoma phyllodes
E. Fat necrosis

60-2. You recommend:
A. Excisional biopsies of both masses
B. Mammography
C. Ductogram
D. Aspiration of the cyst
E. MRI study

60-3. The cyst on the left breast was aspirated, with resolution of pain and no residual mass. Fluid cytology report was benign, but within 6 weeks the patient returns to your office with pain and a larger mass at the same site. What has occurred, and what do you recommend now?
A. She has a cellulitis, and you start dicloxacillin therapy.
B. She has a breast abscess and needs an incision and drainage procedure.
C. She has a breast abscess, and you start oral antibiotic therapy.
D. She has a breast abscess, and you recommend follow-up with an ultrasound.
E. She has reaccumulation of fluid in the same cyst, and you recommend cyst excision.

60-4. Rank the following risk factors for breast cancer in descending order:

A. First-degree relative with bilateral premenopausal breast cancer > first-degree relative with bilateral post-menopausal breast cancer > nulliparity > menarche before age 12

B. Nulliparity > menarche before age 12 > first-degree relative with bilateral premenopausal breast cancer > first-degree relative with bilateral postmenopausal breast cancer

C. Menarche before age 12 > nulliparity > first-degree relative with bilateral premenopausal breast cancer > first-degree relative with bilateral postmenopausal breast cancer

D. First-degree relative with bilateral premenopausal breast cancer > nulliparity > first-degree relative with bilateral postmenopausal breast cancer > menarche before age 12

E. First-degree relative with bilateral premenopausal breast cancer > menarche before age 12 > first-degree relative with bilateral postmenopausal breast cancer > nulliparity

ANSWERS

60-1. C. The most likely diagnosis in this 29-year-old woman is a simple cyst. Cysts can present in any location on the breast and can grow rapidly, causing acute onset of pain and discomfort. On palpation, cysts tend to be smooth, round, and mobile. A fibroadenoma usually presents as a painless, discrete, firm, mobile mass. It is the most common benign breast tumor, occurring most frequently in young women. Fibrocystic disease, also called fibrocystic changes, describes normal physiologic changes of the breast during the menstrual cycle. Some women with fibrocystic disease complain of pain or even of a "lump" in the breast. Clinical examination findings vary from findings of a discrete, tender mass to large prominent glandular changes in the breast(s). The involved areas fluctuate in size and tenderness through the menstrual cycle. Cystosarcoma phyllodes is an uncommon tumor that presents as a well-defined, firm, rapidly growing lobulated mass. Fat necrosis describes changes in the breast, usually following a traumatic event, which can be confused with malignant lesion. Frequently a discrete, hard mass is fixed to the underlying breast tissue without associated tenderness. If a clear history of trauma to the breast is elicited, it is reasonable to observe the lesion for resolution. Otherwise, a fine-needle aspiration should be performed. Unfortunately, only 50% of women recall a history of trauma to the breast. Fat necrosis has also been seen after radiation therapy or segmental resection of the breast.

60-2. D. Aspiration of the palpable cyst is a reasonable course of action. She should have immediate relief of discomfort following decompression of the cyst. The fluid is characteristically clear with a yellow or brown tint and can be sent for cytologic study. It is reasonable to observe the patient for a short period prior to an aspiration procedure. An excision is not warranted at this stage. One would proceed to diagnostic imaging with ultrasonography if the patient declined a diagnostic aspiration or fluid was not obtained on aspiration. Ultrasound not only is a useful tool for evaluating women with breast cysts but also is ideal for guiding fine-needle aspirations of deeper, nonpalpable lesions. Mammographic imaging is limited in young women with radiographically dense breasts, although cysts usually present as smooth, round densities scattered through the breast. Ductography is useful in a patient with abnormal nipple discharge and, in particular, for evaluating for the presence of intraluminal lesions within the duct. At present, MRI does not have a role in clinical screening for breast cancer, given its cost and accessibility.

60-3. E. The event most likely to have transpired is early (<6 weeks after complete aspiration) recurrence of the cyst. Indications for excisional biopsy of the cyst are early recurrence, recurrence of the same cyst after two aspirations, or the presence of an underlying mass on examination of the breast following cyst aspiration. In the absence of a history of fevers, chills, and erythema or induration on the breast, the patient likely does not have has an abscess or cellulitis.

60-4. A. Breast cancer risk factors have been investigated extensively and relative risks calculated. Risk factors include menarche before age 12 years; older than 35 years at first pregnancy; nulliparity; older than 55 years at menopause; family history of breast cancer in mother, sister, or daughter (with greater risk if the cancer was diagnosed premenopausally, was bilateral, or was present in two or more first-degree relatives); prior history of cancer in one breast; personal or family history of ovarian or endometrial cancer; being Caucasian (in the United States); living in an industrialized nation (except Japan); and history of fibrocystic changes of the breast with papillomatosis, proliferative changes, or atypical epithelial hyperplasia (Table 60-1).

TABLE 60-1 Risk Factors for Breast Cancer

Breast Cancer Risk Factor	Relative Risk
Nulliparous vs. parous	3:1
Menarche before age 12	1.3:1
First birth after age 34	4:1
Menopause after age 50	1.5:1
First-degree relative with	
Unilateral premenopausal	1.8:1
Bilateral premenopausal	8.8:1
Unilateral postmenopausal	1.2:1
Bilateral postmenopausal	4:1
Proliferative fibrocystic change	2–5:1
White vs. Asian	3:1

SUGGESTED ADDITIONAL READING

Hindle WH, ed. *Breast care: a clinical guidebook for women's primary health care providers.* New York: Springer-Verlag; 1999.

Hindle WH, Payne PA, Pan EY. The use of fine-needle aspiration in the evaluation of persistent palpable dominant breast masses. *Am J Obstet Gynecol.* 1993;168:1814–1818.

Giuliano AE. Benign breast disease. In: Hillard PA, Berek JS, Novak E, eds. *Novak's gynecology.* 13th ed. Baltimore, Md: Lippincott Williams & Wilkins; 2002.

McCormick BM, Hudis C, Gemignani M, et al. Breast cancer. In: Hoskins WJ, Perez CA, Young RC, eds. *Principles and practice of gynecologic oncology.* 4th ed. Philadelphia, Pa: Lippincott Williams & Wilkins; 2005:1077–1170.

IX

Review
Q&A

Questions

1. A 32-year-old G_0 woman presents to your office for preconception counseling. She has been a type 1 diabetic since age 6. She has mild diabetic proliferative retinopathy and a baseline creatinine of 0.9 but no known cardiac disease. She uses an insulin pump for glycemic control. Her current hemoglobin A_{1c} (HbA_{1c}) is 12. What is the risk for fetal anomaly associated with this level of glucose control if she were to conceive now?

    A. Less than 1%
    B. 1%–4%
    C. 5%–9%
    D. 10%–15%
    E. Greater than 15%

2. A 28-year-old G_1P_0 woman with type 2 diabetes mellitus presents for her first prenatal visit. Her diabetes is controlled with metformin. You review her blood glucose values and notice her fasting values over the past 2 weeks ranged from 110 to 160. Her 1-hour postprandial values ranged from 150 to 250. She is 5 weeks pregnant by her last menstrual period (LMP). By ultrasound, you date her as 5 weeks 3 days pregnant. What is the most appropriate next step?

    A. Increase her metformin dose
    B. Change her medication to glyburide
    C. Start long-acting and short-acting insulin
    D. Start her on an insulin pump
    E. Stop all diabetic medications in the first trimester of pregnancy

3. A 39-year-old G_2P_1 woman presents at 12 weeks for fetal nuchal translucency screening. Her medical history is significant for a previous uncomplicated term delivery of a healthy boy. Her family history is unremarkable. After genetic counseling today, the patient states she desires screening given her risk for chromosomal disorders associated with advanced maternal age. The patient proceeds with the ultrasound screen, which reveals a thickened nuchal translucency. What is the most appropriate next step?

A. Repeat the test in 1 week
B. Repeat the test in 2 weeks
C. Offer chorionic villus sampling (CVS) now
D. Offer amniocentesis now
E. Offer termination of the pregnancy

4. A 37-year-old G_2P_1 woman presents at 12 weeks for karyotypic diagnosis. Her medical history is significant for a cleft lip that was repaired early in childhood. After genetic counseling, the patient states she wishes to proceed with CVS. She undergoes CVS, which reveals normal chromosomes. What further testing do you offer?

A. Maternal serum α-fetoprotein (MSAFP)
B. Amniocentesis
C. Repeat CVS
D. Fetal echocardiography
E. Cordocentesis

5. A 26-year-old G_3P_2 woman presents at 16 weeks gestation. She states she presented late because she had irregular menses and did not realize she was pregnant until recently. Her history is significant for past heroin use for which she takes methadone 80 mg PO QD. She has been on this regimen for approximately 3 years without further use of heroin or other illegal substances. She has been tested for HIV, hepatitis C, and hepatitis B within the past 6 months, with negative results. What is the most appropriate next step?

A. Stop the methadone immediately
B. Continue the methadone at the current dose
C. Taper off the methadone over 4 weeks
D. Taper off the methadone over 2 weeks
E. Stop the methadone and switch to a benzodiazepine

6. A 32-year-old G_2P_1 woman presents at 23 weeks with a monochorionic-diamniotic twin gestation. Her obstetric history is significant for a previous uncomplicated term vaginal delivery of a healthy girl. The current pregnancy is dated by her LMP consistent with an ultrasound performed at 17 weeks gestation. She states that the twins were identified at the 17-week ultrasound and reports that the ultrasound was otherwise "normal." She undergoes an ultrasound today, which reveals decreased amniotic fluid (deepest vertical pocket of 1.0) and no bladder in one twin and increased fluid (deepest vertical pocket of 10.0) in the second twin. She denies having any leakage of fluid, vaginal bleeding, or contractions. What is the next step?

    A.　Large volume amniocentesis
    B.　Amnioinfusion of the first twin
    C.　Disruption of the membrane between the twins
    D.　Amnioinfusion of the second twin
    E.　Laser ablation

7. A 22-year-old G_3P_2 woman at 38 weeks gestation with diamniotic-dichorionic twins presents in early labor. Her obstetric history is notable for two prior term vaginal deliveries of singleton gestations. This pregnancy has been uncomplicated, and the twins have been normally grown and concordant in size. Currently, the patient's cervix is 3 cm dilated and she is contracting every 3 minutes. On ultrasound the presenting twin is breech and the second twin is vertex. By ultrasound biometry the twins appear concordant in size, weighing approximately 2,500 g each. You advise which one of the following?
    A.　Vaginal delivery of both twins
    B.　External cephalic version (ECV) of the first twin followed by a vaginal delivery of both
    C.　Wait until she is completely dilated, then offer a cesarean section (C/S) if the presenting twin is still breech
    D.　Vaginal delivery of the first twin followed by extraction of the second
    E.　C/S now

8. A 28-year-old G_2P_1 woman at 37 weeks gestation presents to your office for routine prenatal care. She denies having any leakage of fluid, vaginal bleeding, or contractions. She confirms good fetal movement. On exam and confirmed on ultrasound you determine that the fetus is in the complete breech presentation with an anterior placenta. The amniotic fluid index is normal. Her history is significant for one previous NSVD. The present pregnancy has been uncomplicated. What is your first recommendation?
    A.　ECV now
    B.　Reassess the presentation in early labor and offer ECV then
    C.　C/S now; ECV is contraindicated with an anterior placenta
    D.　ECV at 39 weeks
    E.　C/S at 39 weeks

9. A 24-year-old G_1P_0 woman presents at 10 weeks gestation for her first prenatal visit. A Pap smear is performed and reveals low-grade squamous intraepithelial lesion (LGSIL). Her history is significant for occasional tobacco use, which she stopped when she found out she was pregnant. She has had three sexual partners and has no other known sexually transmitted infections. Her prenatal chlamydia, gonorrhea, RPR, and HIV tests are negative. She otherwise is healthy but has not had a Pap smear before. What do you recommend?

 A. Repeat the Pap smear in 1 month
 B. Repeat the Pap smear postpartum
 C. Colposcopy now
 D. Colposcopy postpartum as it is contraindicated during pregnancy
 E. LEEP postpartum

10. A 30-year-old G_2P_1 woman at 24 weeks gestation presents for her first prenatal visit. Her history is significant for one pack per day tobacco use. In addition, she has mild asthma requiring occasional use of an albuterol inhaler. Her obstetric history is notable for a previous uncomplicated term vaginal delivery. The patient tells you she would like to quit smoking but has not been able to quit or decrease her smoking. She feels a nicotine patch might help her stop. Which one of the following is the most appropriate recommendation?

 A. Prescribe the nicotine patch
 B. Prescribe a benzodiazepine to help her quit because the patch is contraindicated in pregnancy
 C. Recommend that she decrease the amount of cigarettes used but do not offer the nicotine patch because it is contraindicated
 D. Recommend she stop all tobacco use but do not offer the nicotine patch because it is contraindicated
 E. Recommend smoking cessation counseling only but do not offer the nicotine patch because it is contraindicated

11. A 19-year-old G_3P_1 patient with a history of a miscarriage in her last pregnancy presents to the emergency department (ED) with some vaginal spotting. She reports that her LMP was 7 weeks earlier. She has had no vaginal discharge other than the spotting, no cramping, and no abdominal pain. Her physical examination reveals a slightly enlarged uterus, no tenderness, and a closed cervical os. A β subunit of human chorionic gonadotropin (β-hCG) is sent off and returns 1,146. A pelvic ultrasound shows no intrauterine pregnancy, a 2-cm left ovarian simple cyst, and no free fluid. The patient's diagnosis is:

A. Threatened abortion/rule out ectopic pregnancy
B. Ectopic pregnancy
C. Inevitable abortion
D. Missed abortion
E. Normal pregnancy

12. In the patient in Question 11, when should a repeat β-hCG be drawn?

A. 24 hours
B. 48 hours
C. 72 hours
D. 1 week
E. It does not need to be drawn again

13. A 27-year-old G_1P_0 woman at 40 weeks gestation presents to labor and delivery with contractions every 6 to 8 minutes. She has had no vaginal bleeding and no leakage of fluid, but she has not felt fetal movement for the prior 12 hours. The fetal heart rate monitor shows fetal heart tones in the 140s with a nonreactive nonstress test but no decelerations. On sterile vaginal examination, her cervix is dilated 2 cm, 25% effaced, −2 station and posterior. Assessment and plan is:

A. Patient is in labor, admit to labor ward for delivery
B. Patient is not in labor, discharge to home
C. Patient may be in labor, but she and the fetus need further monitoring
D. Patient may be in labor, repeat cervical exam in 1 to 2 hours
E. Patient may be in labor, admit to labor ward for augmentation

14. A 19-year-old G_3P_1 woman at 31 weeks gestation presents with contractions every 3 to 4 minutes. On examination, her cervix is found to be dilated 2 cm and 50% effaced. The patient's history is remarkable for a delivery at 33 weeks gestation of a 5 lb 3 oz infant in her last pregnancy 3 years ago and a miscarriage 2 years ago. She has a history of smoking a half pack of cigarettes per day for 6 years. The most predictive risk factor for recurrent preterm labor is which of the following?

A. History of SAB
B. Prior preterm delivery
C. Large fetus
D. Cigarette smoking
E. Teenage pregnancy

15. A 19-year-old G_1P_0 woman at 38 weeks gestation presents to labor and delivery. On arrival, she is having contractions every 2 to 3 minutes, and she claims that her "water broke" 2 days earlier but that she did not come in because she had not reached her due date. She has a temperature of 101.2°F, heart rate of 110, and blood pressure of 116/72. The fetal heart rate is in the 180s with small accelerations and no decelerations. Which of the following would be normal in labor rather than a sign of chorioamnionitis?

A. Elevated maternal white blood count >20,000
B. Elevated fetal heart rate >170s
C. Severe lower back pain
D. Maternal fever
E. Uterine tenderness

16. A 37-year-old G_2P_0 woman at 42 weeks gestation with diet-controlled, class A1, gestational diabetes presents in labor. The fetal heart rate tracing is reassuring, and the patient is contracting well every 2 to 3 minutes. She progresses slowly over the course of the day until she is fully dilated. She begins the second stage of labor and pushes for 1.5 hours. Finally the head delivers, but once it does there is a shoulder dystocia. Which of the following would be most likely to worsen the situation?

A. Suprapubic pressure
B. Fundal pressure
C. Increased flexion of the hips
D. Delivery of the posterior arm
E. Episiotomy

17. A 28-year-old G_7P_5 woman at 38 weeks gestation has a history of intravenous drug abuse, hepatitis B, hepatitis C, human immunodeficiency virus (HIV), and herpes simplex virus (HSV) without any recent outbreaks and has no antibodies to rubella presents for her second prenatal visit. She currently is not undergoing treatment for any of her problems. You offer her an elective C/S at term, despite her five prior vaginal deliveries. Which of the components of her history would lead you to do this?

A. History of HIV positivity
B. History of hepatitis B
C. History of hepatitis C
D. History of HSV
E. History of lack of immunity to rubella

18. A 27-year-old G_1P_0 woman at 40 weeks gestation presents to labor and delivery with contractions every 6 to 8 minutes. Which of the following findings on the fetal heart tracing is the most worrisome?

A. Repetitive early decelerations, minimal variability
B. No heart rate decelerations, minimal variability
C. Repetitive late decelerations, absent variability
D. No heart rate decelerations, moderate variability
E. Repetitive variable decelerations, moderate variability

19. A 19-year-old primigravid patient presents for an initial prenatal visit at 7 weeks gestation. She is concerned because she used both cocaine and heroin in the month before she discovered she was pregnant. During a long discussion with her about the risks of substance abuse during pregnancy, you tell her that use of which of the following has the highest correlation with congenital abnormalities?
A. Alcohol
B. Caffeine
C. Cocaine
D. Opiates
E. Smoking tobacco

20. A patient with a dizygotic twin pregnancy presents for a routine prenatal visit at 13 weeks gestation. She is nervous about being a "high-risk" obstetric patient and wonders about the possibility of complications. When you counsel her regarding complications of pregnancy, you note she is at lowest risk for which of the following?
A. Preterm labor
B. Preterm delivery
C. Preeclampsia
D. Twin-to-twin transfusion syndrome
E. C/S for malpresentation

21. A 19-year-old G_2P_1 woman at 29 weeks gestation presents to labor and delivery with intense uterine contractions every 3 to 4 minutes. On exam, her cervix is 2 cm dilated. A variety of agents are used for tocolysis, but which of the following is the only FDA-approved tocolytic agent?
A. Hydralazine
B. Magnesium sulfate
C. Ritodrine
D. Terbutaline
E. Nifedipine

22. A 34-year-old G_1P_0 woman at 33 weeks gestation presents to labor and delivery with frequent contractions and a cervix dilated to 3 cm. By Leopold maneuvers and then on ultrasound, the fetus is noted to be a breech presentation. The following list of items are all associated with breech presentation. Which of the following would be the best setting to attempt an ECV?
   A. Preterm labor
   B. Maternal uterine abnormalities
   C. Polyhydramnios
   D. Fetal hydrocephalus
   E. Placenta previa

23. A 34-year-old G_2P_1 woman at 32 weeks gestation presents to labor and delivery with frequent contractions and a cervix initially dilated to only 1 cm. She has a history of a prior cesarean delivery at 26 weeks gestation with classic hysterotomy. She is given her first IM injection of betamethasone and a single injection of terbutaline, which slows her contractions initially. However, 2 hours later, her contractions have increased to every 2 minutes and her cervix is now 3 cm dilated. Which of the following is the best management plan for the patient?
   A. Immediate C/S
   B. Attempt tocolysis; if it fails, perform C/S
   C. Allow vaginal delivery, which is safer for the preterm infant
   D. Attempt tocolysis; if it fails, then allow vaginal delivery
   E. Augment labor

24. A 23-year-old G_1P_0 woman at 35 weeks gestation presents with a gush of fluid per vagina. On sterile speculum examination, she has a pool of clear fluid in the vagina, which is Nitrazine and fern positive. She is contracting every 3 to 4 minutes, and her cervix on visualization appears to be dilated 2 to 3 cm. Which of the following is the best course of action?
   A. Tocolysis with magnesium or terbutaline
   B. Betamethasone and tocolysis
   C. Betamethasone and no tocolysis
   D. Expectant management
   E. Amnio/dye test

25. A 26-year-old G_2P_0 patient presents for her initial prenatal visit at 8 weeks gestation by LMP. Her PE is consistent with 8 weeks gestation by bimanual exam. Which of the following is needed to complete accurate dating of the pregnancy at this point?
   A. Check fetal heart tones with Doppler
   B. Pelvic ultrasound
   C. Check fetal heart tones with fetoscope
   D. Pelvic ultrasound at 13 weeks gestation
   E. Nothing further needs to be done

26. A 36-year-old G_5P_4 woman presents at 11 weeks gestation for her first prenatal visit. She has had four prior vaginal births and a history of hepatitis C infection. Which of the following lab tests would be drawn only if she had additional symptoms?

A. RPR
B. Hematocrit
C. Blood type and antibody screen
D. Rubella titer
E. Herpes titer

27. A 27-year-old G_1P_0 woman at 40 weeks gestation presents to labor and delivery with contractions every 3 to 4 minutes. A sterile speculum examination shows positive pool, Nitrazine, and ferning. She has had no vaginal bleeding and good fetal movement. The fetal heart rate monitor shows fetal heart tones in the 140s with a reactive nonstress test. On sterile vaginal examination, her cervix is dilated 4 cm, 75% effaced, 0 station. Assessment and plan is:

A. Patient is in labor, admit to labor ward for labor and delivery
B. Patient is not in labor, discharge to home
C. Patient is not in labor, but fetus needs further monitoring
D. Patient may be in labor, repeat cervical exam in 1 to 2 hours
E. Patient may be in labor, admit to labor ward for augmentation

28. A 23-year-old G_2P_1 patient presents at 30 weeks gestation with occasional contractions and a small amount of vaginal spotting. She has had no vaginal discharge or fluid loss and can feel the fetus moving quite often. Which of the following additional complaints or history is the most reassuring in this setting?

A. Placenta previa on 20-week ultrasound
B. Prior birth of normal baby at 34 weeks gestation
C. Recent vaginal intercourse
D. Dysuria
E. Headache and right upper quadrant pain

29. A 25-year-old G_1P_0 woman at 9 weeks gestation presents for her initial prenatal visit. She has no medical or surgical history, and she has a certain LMP that is consistent with her examination. She has given blood in the past and knows that she is Rh negative. In which of the following situations could you treat with mini RhoGAM—a smaller dose of RhoGAM—with the least likelihood of Rh sensitization?

A. First-trimester bleeding
B. Second-trimester bleeding
C. Routinely at the beginning of the third trimester
D. Contractions at 34 weeks gestation
E. At the time of an amniocentesis

30. A 29-year-old G_1P_0 patient presents for her initial obstetric appointment. Since she discovered she was pregnant, she has been eating two to three times as much as she normally does and consuming high-calorie shakes because she is concerned about the fetus getting enough nourishment. How does the recommended daily caloric intake of a pregnant woman compare with that of a non-pregnant woman?

    A. Approximately the same
    B. Increase by 300 to 400 kcal
    C. Increase by 600 to 800 kcal
    D. Increase by 1,000 to 1,200 kcal
    E. Approximately double

31. A 67-year-old white woman comes to the clinic for an annual physical examination. She denies any changes in her health, but an adnexal mass is palpated upon pelvic examination. Her past gynecologic history is notable for uterine myomas. What is the next appropriate step in the management of this patient?

    A. Exploratory laparotomy
    B. Pelvic ultrasound
    C. Diagnostic laparoscopy
    D. CT-guided biopsy
    E. Bilateral salpingo-oophorectomy

32. A 23-year-old woman presents with recurrent biopsy-confirmed cervical intraepithelial neoplasia 2 (CIN2). She has had a history of treated *Chlamydia* infections and admits to smoking since age 15. What is the next appropriate step in her management?

    A. Reassurance and continued observation
    B. Chemotherapy
    C. Colposcopic examination and rebiopsy
    D. Loop electrosurgical excision procedure of the cervix
    E. Extrafascial hysterectomy

33. A 28-year-old woman who is 14 weeks pregnant presents with a Pap smear showing high-grade intraepithelial neoplasia (HSIL). She denies prior history of abnormal Pap smears. She has no abnormal vaginal discharge or postcoital bleeding. Which of the following is appropriate?

    A. Follow up in the postpartum period
    B. Endocervical curettage
    C. Colposcopic examination and biopsy of lesions suspicious for cancer
    D. Excisional procedure of the cervix and cerclage placement
    E. Hysterectomy

34. A 35-year-old white woman with a strong family history of breast and ovarian cancer comes to clinic and wishes to discuss her management options. Her 38-year-old sister recently was diagnosed with early-stage breast cancer and is considering a prophylactic oophorectomy. What would you recommend first?

- A. Screening mammogram
- B. Pelvic ultrasound
- C. Cancer antigen 125 (CA-125) measurement
- D. Genetic counseling
- E. Prophylactic surgery

35. A 56-year-old woman presents with a painless mass in the vulva. On examination it appears to be in the posterior vestibule at 4 o'clock. She recollects a similar event that occurred when she was in her 30s was treated with a minor procedure. What do you recommend?

- A. Excision and biopsy
- B. Observation as she is asymptomatic
- C. Placement of Word catheter
- D. Marsupialization
- E. Incision and drainage with antimicrobial therapy

36. A 68-year-old postmenopausal female presents with complaints of vulvar pruritus. On examination she has a well-defined erythematous lesion on the vulva, which the patient states has been present for several years. Previously she had used topical steroids with no improvement in her symptoms. A vulvar biopsy is performed with findings of Paget cells. What is the treatment of choice?

- A. Topical 5-fluorouracil
- B. Continued topical corticosteroids
- C. Radiotherapy
- D. Wide surgical excision
- E. Laser ablation

37. A 73-year-old woman presents with abnormal vaginal bleeding. She also reports profuse malodorous discharge. She denies hematuria or leg/back pain. Pelvic examination reveals an immobile, ulcerated cervix with extension to the parametria. You perform a biopsy, which shows invasive squamous cell carcinoma. What is the most appropriate next step?

- A. Preoperative evaluation for radical hysterectomy and pelvic lymphadenectomy
- B. Intravenous pyelogram
- C. Embolization
- D. Initiation of chemotherapy
- E. Cystoscopy and proctoscopy

38. A 62-year-old woman is undergoing chemotherapy for advanced ovarian cancer. She complains about increasing numbness and tingling in her hands and feet. She is concerned about losing her ability to play the piano. Which medication is most responsible for her symptoms?

- A. Carboplatinum
- B. Cisplatinum
- C. Paclitaxel
- D. Liposomal doxorubicin
- E. Growth factors

39. A 60-year-old postmenopausal woman with a history of estrogen receptor–positive breast cancer has been taking tamoxifen for 3 years. She now has new-onset abnormal vaginal bleeding. She denies heavy bleeding or clots but reports staining of her undergarments. What do you recommend with regard to her bleeding?

- A. She should discontinue tamoxifen
- B. Pelvic ultrasound
- C. CA-125 measurement
- D. Hysterectomy and bilateral salpingo-oophorectomy
- E. Endometrial biopsy

40. A 47-year-old patient with ovarian cancer is suffering from chemotherapy-induced anemia and fatigue. She denies dizziness or lightheadedness. Her blood pressure and heart rate are within normal limits. How best can you address her problem?

- A. Recombinant human erythropoietin
- B. Packed red blood cell transfusion
- C. Filgrastim injections
- D. Delaying the next cycle of treatment
- E. Group support

41. A 53-year-old woman presents with complaints of a rapidly inflamed, swollen right breast. On examination the skin has a pitted appearance, and the breast is warm and thickened. She seems to recall onset of the symptoms over the last couple of weeks. Which diagnostic test will be most informative?

- A. Needle biopsy
- B. Mammogram
- C. Ultrasound
- D. MRI
- E. PET

42. A 48-year-old Hispanic woman is diagnosed with a stage IA2 squamous cell carcinoma of the cervix. She is aware of her treatment alternatives but is afraid of radiation therapy and wishes to have the tumor excised. Which procedure do you discuss in detail?
A. Radical trachelectomy
B. Cold knife conization of the cervix
C. Radical hysterectomy
D. Radical hysterectomy, bilateral salpingo-oophorectomy, pelvic lymphadenectomy
E. Simple hysterectomy, bilateral salpingo-oophorectomy

43. Multiple factors contribute to women's risk of developing invasive breast cancer. Which of the following risk factors confers the highest risk of developing breast cancer?
A. First-degree relative with unilateral premenopausal breast cancer
B. Ashkenazi-Jewish descent
C. BRCA1/BRCA2 mutation carrier
D. Ataxia telangiectasia heterozygote
E. Nulliparity

44. A 63-year-old woman presented with vulvar pruritis. She has tried topical antifungals and Aveeno bath salt soaks to no avail. Following a biopsy, she is diagnosed with lichen sclerosus (LS) of the vulva. What is the most appropriate next step?
A. Topical corticosteroids
B. Simple vulvectomy
C. Photodynamic therapy
D. Topical testosterone
E. Focal ultrasonography

45. A 25-year-old white woman has the hereditary nonpolyposis colon cancer (HNPCC) gene. A family history of numerous male and female family members having colon cancer in their early 40s prompted genetic counseling and testing. Which gynecologic cancer is she at the greatest risk of developing?
A. Epithelial ovarian cancer
B. Adenocarcinoma of the cervix
C. Uterine sarcoma
D. Vaginal squamous cell carcinoma
E. Endometrial adenocarcinoma

46. A 7-year-old girl presents with gradually increasing pelvic discomfort and urinary frequency. Her parents have noted a gradual increase in her abdominal girth. She appears well and is afebrile. On exam, you feel a large mass in the LLQ. She has minimal abdominal tenderness and no rebound or guarding. An abdominal US reveals an 8-cm pelvic mass with both solid and cystic components. The most likely diagnosis is:

A. Pedunculated uterine fibroid
B. Follicular ovarian cyst
C. Urethral obstruction causing bladder distention
D. Germ cell tumor of the ovary
E. Tubo-ovarian abscess (TOA)

47. A 41-year-old $G_2P_0T_2$ woman presents to your office for a fertility consultation. She and her partner have been trying to conceive for the last 6 months. Her cycles are regular and every 27 to 29 days. She recently saw her primary care physician, who obtained the following labs during the follicular phase of her cycle: FSH 5.1 (normal follicular range 3.0–12 pg/ml), estradiol 99 (normal follicular phase 25–75 pg/ml). TSH and prolactin levels are normal. Which of the following statements about this patient is true?

A. Because her menstrual cycles are regular, she is likely ovulating regularly.
B. FSH level of 5.1 indicates that she has good ovarian reserve.
C. Her per cycle fecundity rate is 20% to 30%.
D. If a semen analysis and hysterosalpingogram are normal, she and her partner should continue trying to conceive for 6 more months before a diagnosis of unexplained infertility can be made.
E. A likely cause of her infertility is Asherman syndrome resulting from her two prior pregnancy terminations.

48. A 30-year-old G_0 woman presents to your office concerned that she is not ovulating. Her menstrual cycles occur every 28 to 30 days, and they usually are light and last no more than 3 days. She and her partner have been attempting to conceive for the last 3 months, and this month she used an ovulation predictor kit she purchased at the pharmacy to measure the timing of her urine LH surge. However, despite using the kit every day from days 9 through 19 of her cycle, the test never registered positive. The most reasonable next step is to:

A. Assume that she had a false-negative result and counsel her that her peak fertile period likely is between days 12 and 17 of her cycle.
B. Check serum FSH and estradiol levels to confirm your suspicion that she is undergoing premature ovarian failure.

C. Prescribe clomiphene citrate (Clomid) to help the patient ovulate more frequently.

D. Check a serum progesterone level on day 21 of her cycle to rule out a luteal phase defect.

E. Refer her for in vitro fertilization.

49. A 27-year-old woman with a long history of severe dysmenorrhea presents with progressively worsening pelvic pain. She states that her symptoms have worsened in the last 3 months. She is afebrile. Her exam is notable for mild diffuse abdominal tenderness and moderate tenderness in the left adnexa by bimanual exam. An ultrasound reveals a 4-cm heterogeneous mass of the left ovary with a trace amount of free fluid in the cul-de-sac. A CA-125 level is 47 (normal <35). The most likely diagnosis is:

A. Ovarian cancer

B. Ovarian torsion

C. Ruptured ovarian cyst

D. Endometriosis

E. Endometrial cancer

50. A 27-year-old G_0 woman presents with a several-year history of irregular menses. Her LMP was 5 months ago. In the past 5 to 7 years she has had erratic cycles that vary from 2 to 8 months in interval, but recently the intervals have become longer. Her cycles are not particularly heavy or lengthy. She denies recent weight changes. She used Depo-Provera as a teenager but now uses condoms for birth control. She uses no medications, and her medical history and review of systems are otherwise negative. On physical exam her height is 5 feet 4 inches and weight 174 lb. Her exam is normal. In addition to follicle-stimulating hormone (FSH) level and thyroid-stimulating hormone (TSH) levels, the most appropriate additional laboratory testing to obtain for this patient at this juncture is:

A. Serum progesterone level on day 21 of her cycle

B. Fasting insulin and glucose levels

C. A prolactin level

D. FSH/LH ratio

E. Testosterone level

51. A 31-year-old G_0 woman presents with a several-year history of irregular menses. Her LMP was 3 months ago. In the past 4 years she has had irregular cycles, but recently the intervals have become longer. She denies recent weight changes. She is sexually active and uses condoms for birth control. She uses occasional albuterol for mild asthma. Her medical history and review of systems are otherwise negative.

On physical exam her height is 5 feet 4 inches and weight 174 lb. Her exam is normal. You obtain an initial set of labs on this patient:

TSH: 2.35
FSH: 5.1
PRL: 84
LH: 8.3

You repeat an early AM PRL level and again it is elevated. On further evaluation of the patient you confirm that she uses no medications or recreational drugs. Her exam, including a neurologic exam, is normal. The best next step is to:

A. Prescribe combination OCPs
B. Prescribe bromocriptine
C. Obtain a head MRI
D. Obtain a chest CT
E. Prescribe levothyroxine

52. A 26-year-old G_0 woman presents with infertility. She and her partner have been trying to conceive for 14 months but have difficulty timing intercourse because of her irregular cycles. Her menses occur every 23 to 50 days and are at times very heavy. On physical exam, her height is 5 feet 5 inches and weight is 165 lb. She exhibits central obesity. Her pelvic exam is normal. Her lab results are as follows:

TSH: 1.35
FSH: 6.3
PRL: 21
Fasting glucose: 83
Fasting insulin: 26

Of the following interventions, which will most likely help her conceive?

A. Three-month cycle of a GnRH agonist
B. Intrauterine insemination on day 14 of her cycle
C. Metformin taken every day
D. Spironolactone taken every day
E. Monthly 10-day course of progesterone treatment

53. A 54-year-old woman reports a continuous watery discharge from her vagina. She denies any pelvic or vaginal discomfort. Her history is notable only for a diagnosis of endometrial cancer 1 year ago for which she underwent total abdominal hysterectomy, bilateral salpingo-oophorectomy, surgical staging, and postsurgical pelvic radiation therapy. Your exam reveals a pale yellow, watery vaginal discharge with a pH of 7 and normal epithelial cells and rare leukocytes on wet mount. The most likely cause of her vaginal discharge is:

A. Atrophic vaginitis
B. Vesicovaginal fistula
C. Detrusor hyperreflexia
D. Urethral diverticulum
E. Vaginal dysplasia

54. A 2-week-old girl is brought to your office by her mother because she noticed some blood on her daughter's diaper earlier in the day. The infant was delivered by uncomplicated vaginal delivery and has done well since. The mother has been breastfeeding exclusively and has not noticed that her baby has been spitting up a lot. On exam the infant is afebrile and appears well. Inspection of the vulvar and perianal area reveals normal skin without evidence of rash and a trace amount of bloody fluid near the vaginal introitus. The most likely cause of the bloody fluid is:

A. Estrogen withdrawal
B. Endometrial polyps
C. Anovulation
D. Vaginal foreign body
E. Precocious puberty

55. A 62-year-old woman presents to your office with complaints of pain with intercourse and a bloody, watery discharge after intercourse. She occasionally is sexually active with her husband and states that her dyspareunia consists of a burning sensation upon penetration. She has been menopausal for 11 years and took hormone replacement for several years, but she stopped a few years ago on the advice of her physician that time. On exam, you note a mildly inflamed and unrugated vaginal mucosa and a normal appearing cervix. Testing of the vaginal sample reveals the following:

Whiff test: negative
pH >5.0
KOH prep: negative
Wet smear: Marked WBCs, rare clue cells

The best next step is to:

A. Prescribe oral fluconazole
B. Prescribe an estradiol vaginal cream
C. Prescribe one time doses of azithromycin and cefixime
D. Prescribe metronidazole vaginal gel
E. Prescribe clindamycin vaginal ovules

56. A 25-year-old woman presents to the office complaining of breakthrough bleeding while taking oral contraceptive pills (OCPs). She has been on the same low-dose combined OCP for the last 4 years. Review of her history is unremarkable except that she recently increased her tobacco use to half pack per day. She has used other methods of contraception including Depo-Provera but did not tolerate them. Other than counseling her on the health benefits of tobacco cessation, your best intervention is to:

A. Advise her to use a backup method of birth control such as condoms.
B. Change her to an OCP with a higher progesterone dose.
C. Change her to an OCP with a higher estrogen dose.
D. Do nothing because it will get better.
E. Discontinue OCPs because of her smoking history.

57. A 43-year-old G_3P_3 woman with progressively heavy and painful menses presents to your office. Her menses occur regularly every 28 to 30 days and last approximately 7 days, with two of the days having very heavy flow. Over the last 2 years she started having cramping pain 4 to 5 days before her menses. She denies fevers or chills. Her last pregnancy was 16 years ago. Her LMP was 7 days ago. On physical exam, her uterus is approximately 8 weeks size, non-tender, and anteverted and feels soft. There is no cervical motion tenderness or adnexal tenderness. You do an office ultrasound, which reveals a mildly enlarged uterus with regular contours. The endometrial lining is 7 mm thick and homogenous. Both ovaries have several small simple-appearing cysts. The most likely diagnosis is:

A. Uterine fibroids
B. Adenomyosis
C. Endometrial polyp
D. Ovarian endometrioma
E. Polycystic ovary syndrome (PCOS)

58. A 67-year-old woman presents with vulvar irritation that has progressively worsened over the last 6 months. She has tried various over-the-counter creams but has had no relief. She has been postmenopausal for 15 years and has never taken hormone therapy. Pelvic exam reveals thin, white vulvar skin with areas of excoriation. There is fusion of the labia near the clitoris. A biopsy of the areas reports a thinned epidermis with acanthosis and areas of hyperkeratosis. Appropriate initial treatment for this patient is:

A. Oral estrogen and progesterone therapy
B. Estradiol cream
C. Clobetasol ointment
D. Testosterone cream
E. Metronidazole gel

59. A 24-year-old G_0 woman presents to your office stating that she has noted some lesions on the vulva. She first noticed them approximately 4 months ago, and they have been growing slowly since. She denies any pain or abnormal bleeding. On exam you see several small verrucous lesions on the posterior fourchette of the vaginal introitus. The most appropriate treatments for this lesion is:

A. Acyclovir topical cream
B. Imiquimod cream
C. Miconazole cream
D. Estrogen cream
E. Clindamycin cream

60. A 23-year-old G_0 woman presents with complaints of postcoital bleeding. In addition she has noted a watery, greenish vaginal discharge. She is sexually active with a new partner. They both were screened for sexually transmitted diseases 2 months ago, and all results were negative. She started OCPs at that time, and they do not use condoms. On speculum exam you find a cervix that appears strawberry red and bleeds easily on contact. You perform at wet smear and KOH prep. The most likely finding(s) on this slide is(are):

A. Pseudohyphae
B. Motile trichomonads and WBCs
C. Clue cells and WBCs
D. Normal because this patient's diagnosis likely is cervical dysplasia
E. Cells with increased mitotic activity

61. A 51-year-old woman presents to your office complaining of hot flashes and trouble sleeping at night. Her LMP was 6 months ago, and her periods had been irregular for the year prior to that. Which of the following tests confirms your diagnosis?

A. HCG
B. TSH
C. FSH
D. PRL
E. LH

62. A 71-year-old woman presents with complaints about vulvar pruritus. She has had these symptoms for approximately 3 months and has not responded to treatment with an over-the-counter anti-fungal medication. On physical exam, she has an atrophic vulva with fusion of the labia majora and minora. A biopsy is performed and the result returns lichen sclerosus. Which of the following is the treatment?

A. Topical estrogen
B. Topical testosterone
C. Topical ketoconazole
D. Oral estrogen supplementation
E. Oral ketoconazole

63. A 23-year-old woman presents with a single papule on her right labia. It is nontender and approximately 1 cm in diameter. The rest of her physical exam is negative except for palpable inguinal adenopathy. She last had intercourse 2.5 weeks ago, and she wants to be tested for STIs. Which of the following organisms is the most likely causal agent?

A. *Neisseria gonorrhoeae*
B. *Chlamydia trachomatis*
C. *Treponema pallidum*
D. HIV
E. HSV

64. A 23-year-old woman presents with a single lesion on her right labia. It is tender and approximately 0.5 cm in diameter. It initially presented as a papule and now is a nonindurated ulcer. The rest of her physical exam is negative except for palpable inguinal adenopathy. A Gram stain of the lesion reveals an organism with a "school of fish" appearance. She is treated with an IM injection of ceftriaxone. The most likely causative organism is:

A. *T. pallidum*
B. *Phthirus pubis*
C. *C. trachomatis*
D. HSV-1
E. *Haemophilus ducreyi*

65. A 27-year-old woman presents to the ED with complaints of vaginal discharge. On speculum exam, she has a mucous yellow discharge, and her cervix appears erythematous. On bimanual exam, she has cervical motion tenderness, no uterine tenderness, and no adnexal tenderness. Her temperature is 98.6°F and WBC 8.4. The rest of her vital signs and laboratory results are within normal limits. Her most likely diagnosis is:

A. Vaginitis
B. Cervicitis
C. Endomyometritis
D. PID
E. TOA

66. A 27-year-old woman presents to the ED with complaints of vaginal discharge and abdominal pain. On PE she has a temperature of 100.5°F, and on abdominal exam she has tenderness in the RUQ and bilateral lower quadrants (BLQs) with minimal peritoneal signs. On speculum exam, she has a mucous yellow discharge. On bimanual exam, she has cervical motion tenderness and bilateral

adnexal tenderness. WBC is 14.3, and a pelvic ultrasound shows a normal uterus and normal ovaries bilaterally. Her most likely diagnosis is:
   A. Cervicitis
   B. Endomyometritis
   C. PID
   D. TOA
   E. Appendicitis

67. A 27-year-old woman presents to the ED with complaints of abdominal pain. On history she has some nausea and anorexia. On PE she has a temperature of 100.5°F, and on abdominal exam she has tenderness in the RLQ with minimal peritoneal signs. On bimanual exam, she has cervical motion tenderness and right adnexal tenderness. WBC is 14.3, and a pelvic ultrasound shows a normal uterus and normal left ovary with some signs of inflammation around the right ovary. Her most likely diagnosis is:
   A. Cervicitis
   B. Endomyometritis
   C. PID
   D. TOA
   E. Appendicitis

68. A 52-year-old woman presents after 7 months of amenorrhea, hot flashes, mood swings, and poor sleep. Her medical history is otherwise without complications. Her physical examination is within normal limits. Because of her menopausal state, you counsel her that combination estrogen and progesterone replacement therapy can:
   A. Decrease her risk of cardiovascular disease
   B. Increase her risk of osteoporosis
   C. Decrease her risk of breast cancer
   D. Decrease her menopausal symptoms
   E. Increase her risk of colon cancer

69. A 37-year-old G_1P_1 woman presents complaining of amenorrhea and mild hot flashes. These symptoms remind her of her mother's symptoms in menopause 10 years prior, but she is too early for menopause. Which of the following is least likely to be associated with premature ovarian failure?
   A. Turner syndrome
   B. Radiation
   C. Chemotherapy
   D. Fragile X syndrome premutation carrier
   E. Use of OCPs

70. A 17-year-old ballet dancer presents in routine state of health except for absence of menses. She states that she developed breasts later than her friends and never began menstruation. For her ballet, she watches her diet and weight, but she is not as concerned about it as are most of her friends in her company. On physical examination, she is 5 feet 7 inches tall with a BMI of 20. You note no changes in dentition and no lanugo hair. She has Tanner stage 5 development of her breasts and pubic hair. On speculum exam, her cervix appears normal and she has a normal bimanual exam. The most likely etiology of her primary amenorrhea is:

- A. Anorexia nervosa
- B. Gonadal agenesis
- C. Transverse vaginal septum
- D. Testicular feminization
- E. Hypogonadotropic hypogonadism

71. A 32-year-old G_1P_1 woman presents with complaints of severe cramps with her menses. The pain is so bad that it keeps her out of work 3 to 4 days each month. In addition, she has regular periods and the amount of flow during menses has decreased since her delivery 1 year ago. She notes no intermenstrual bleeding and no symptoms except during menses. Her delivery was uncomplicated. However, her postpartum Pap smear showed signs of cervical dysplasia, and she underwent a cone biopsy with an electrocautery loop 8 months ago. On physical exam she has no palpable masses other than her uterus, which is normal in size, nontender, and slightly anteroflexed. Her most likely diagnosis is:

- A. Asherman syndrome
- B. Endometriosis
- C. Adenomyosis
- D. Cervical stenosis
- E. Uterine fibroids

72. A 68-year-old woman presents with light vaginal bleeding. She has no other complaints. The bleeding started 30 days ago, and she has bled three or four times since then. She has no other medical history. On physical exam she is a thin woman with no obvious findings. Her uterus is small and postmenopausal, and her ovaries are not palpable. Her vagina and introitus are slightly atrophic with no lesions, and she has no obvious hemorrhoids. She had a normal Pap smear result 8 months ago. On pelvic ultrasound, there is a 1-cm × 1.2-cm lesion in her intrauterine cavity. What is the most likely cause of her bleeding?

A. Atrophy
B. Cervical cancer
C. Endometrial polyp
D. Endometrial cancer
E. Excess hormones

73. A 19-year-old woman presents with complaints of no periods for the past 7 months. During this time she started college. She feels her stress has increased and she has changed her eating habits, which has led to her decreasing her weight from 120 to 105 lb. You administer a progesterone challenge test. After 14 days of 10 mg Provera, she has no withdrawal bleed. In addition to these complaints, she is interested in contraception. Which of the following regimens would be the best treatment?
   A. IUD
   B. Depo-Provera
   C. Combination OCP
   D. Premarin 0.625 mg and Provera 10 mg
   E. Cyclic Provera 10 mg for 10 days

74. A 19-year-old woman presents with a complaint of amenorrhea for 7 months. She notes that she has not had a period since 2 to 3 months after starting college. She notes no weight loss during that time; in fact, her weight has increased from 123 to 131 lb over the past few months, but she believes the weight gain is secondary to change in diet during college. She notes no other symptoms. Which of the following tests is most likely to indicate her diagnosis?
   A. TSH
   B. FSH
   C. PRL
   D. LH
   E. β-hCG

75. A 19-year-old woman presents with a complaint of amenorrhea for 7 months. She notes that she has not had a period since 2 to 3 months after starting college. She notes weight loss during that time from 131 to 114 lb over the past few months, but she believes the weight loss is secondary to change in diet during college. She also has insomnia, heat intolerance, and occasional hot flashes. Which of the following tests is most likely to indicate her diagnosis?
   A. TSH
   B. LH
   C. PRL
   D. β-hCG
   E. ACTH stim test

76. A 19-year-old woman presents with a complaint of amenor-rhea for 7 months. She notes that she has not had a period since 2 to 3 months after starting college. She notes no change in weight and no change in appetite, and she is not taking any medications. She actually does not mind the loss of menses; however, she notes that over the past month she has had increasing bilateral breast discharge that occasionally stains her shirts. She is concerned about breast cancer. On physical exam she has no abdominal masses. Which of the following tests is most likely to indicate a diagnosis?

A. TSH
B. FSH
C. PRL
D. β-hCG
E. LH

77. A 67-year-old woman presents vulvar pruritus for the prior year that has been increasing over the past few months. She went through menopause at age 49 and has been on estrogen and progesterone since then. On physical examination velvety-red lesions are noted bilaterally on the vulva. There are also some white plaques. The first step in the management of this patient is to:

A. Treat with antifungals
B. Treat with topical steroids
C. Wide local excision of the lesions
D. Punch biopsy
E. Cryotherapy

78. The patient in Question 77 undergoes a biopsy of the lesions. The carcinoembryonic antigen returns positive but the S-100 antigen returns negative. The final diagnosis is:

A. Adenocarcinoma of the vulva
B. Squamous cell carcinoma of the vulva
C. Vulvar intraepithelial neoplasia
D. Melanoma of the vulva
E. Paget disease of the vulva

79. A 33-year-old woman presents with vulvar pruritus for the last 3 months. She has been treated once with oral fluconazole (Diflucan), which decreased the symptoms for 1 week, but they returned. She is quite concerned about her risk for cancer because her mother underwent mastectomy for breast cancer at age 38. You tell her that vulvar cancer is most closely associated with which of the following cancers?

A. Ovarian cancer
B. Cervical cancer

C. Endometrial cancer
D. Breast cancer
E. Colon cancer

80. A 19-year-old woman presents for a routine examination. Her physical examination is entirely normal; however, her Pap smear returns with CIN1. On subsequent colposcopy, there are a few lesions on the anterior aspect of the cervix entirely visualized that turn white after treatment with acetic acid and have atypical vascularity. A biopsy returns CIN2 or HGSIL. She does not return for treatment and, despite efforts to contact her, does not return for follow-up. Two years later, she presents to a physician complaining of spotting after intercourse and throughout her menstrual cycle. On physical examination she has a 1-cm lesion that is eroding into her anterior cervix. A biopsy returns squamous cell carcinoma. Which of the following is used to stage her disease?
A. Physical exam
B. Margins at time of hysterectomy
C. Lymph node dissection
D. MRI
E. All of the above

81. A 24-year-old woman found a firm rubbery 1.5-cm mass on self breast exam. On examination in your office there is no skin change, nipple discharge, enlarged lymph nodes, or tenderness. She has no know family history of breast cancer. Ultrasound reveals a solid 2-cm mass. Recommended management at this point should be:
A. Diagnosis is fibroadenoma; no further follow-up necessary
B. Mammography
C. Wide local excision
D. Observation or fine-needle aspiration (FNA)
E. Genetic screening for BRCA1

82. A 57-year-old Caucasian woman is found to have a cluster of microcalcifications with a speculated mass in the outer, upper quadrant (OUQ) on screening mammography. The mass is not palpable on physical examination, and there are no skin changes or nipple discharge. The next step in management should be:
A. Follow with clinical exams for mass or skin changes
B. Stereotactic FNA
C. Ultrasound to localize tumor
D. Mastectomy for probable malignancy
E. BRCA1 screening

83. A 56-year-old G_2P_0 Caucasian female weighing 250 lb is concerned about her risks for breast cancer. Her history includes prior OCP use and hormone replacement therapy (HRT) for 3 years since she reached menopause. Her mother was diagnosed with unilateral breast cancer at age 37. Which is the correct decreasing order of relative risk factors?

A. Nulliparous > OCP use > family history > late menopause
B. OCP use > obesity > nulliparous > late menopause > family history
C. Nulliparous > obesity > family history > late menopause > OCP use
D. Family history > nulliparous > late menopause > OCP use > obesity
E. Family history > OCP use > obesity > nulliparous > late menopause

84. A 36-year-old woman was diagnosed with metastatic breast cancer. She underwent mastectomy and axillary node dissection. Estrogen and progesterone receptor status were both negative. The next step in her treatment should be:

A. Tamoxifen alone
B. Chemotherapy followed by tamoxifen
C. No further therapy
D. Chemotherapy alone
E. Hysterectomy and bilateral salpingo-oophorectomy

85. A 27-year-old G_2P_1 woman presents to labor and delivery at 37 2/7 weeks GA complaining of leaking of fluid per vagina for 14 hours. On physical exam, temperature is 98.4°F, BP 123/77, HR 90, RR 18. Speculum exam reveals Nitrazine and fern positive status. Fetal heart rate tracing is in the 130s and reactive without decelerations. On tocometer, she has no contractions. Which of the following is your recommended management plan?

A. Intravenous oxytocin
B. Expectant management
C. Intramuscular betamethasone
D. Subcutaneous terbutaline
E. Intravenous cefotetan

86. A 28-year-old G_1P_0 woman presents at 10 weeks gestation for her initial prenatal visit. In addition to the routine prenatal screening tests, she wishes to obtain screening for aneuploidy. The prenatal diagnostic screening modality for Down syndrome that will give the highest sensitivity is:

   A. CVS

   B. Combined screening (nuchal translucency + PAPP-A and free β-hCG) at 12 weeks

   C. Maternal serum triple screen (MSAFP + estriol + β-hCG) at 17 weeks

   D. Second trimester ultrasound

   E. Amniocentesis at 16 weeks

87. A 29-year-old G_3P_1 woman with a history of a prior cesarean delivery for breech presents at 34 weeks gestation to discuss mode of delivery. A trial of labor carries the lowest risk for uterine rupture or other major complications in a patient with a history of a prior cesarean in which of the following scenarios?

   A. Prior classic hysterotomy

   B. Placenta previa

   C. Twin pregnancy, vertex-vertex positions, laboring at 37 weeks gestation

   D. Two or more prior cesareans

   E. Preeclampsia at 38 weeks requiring induction of labor with prostaglandin

88. A 33-year-old G_2P_1 woman with a history of a prior cesarean delivery presents for a trial of labor. She is contracting every 2 to 3 minutes; cervical exam reveals she is 3 cm dilated. During management of labor and delivery, you will need to pay attention to possible signs and symptoms of uterine rupture. The most common finding associated with uterine rupture in a patient undergoing a trial of labor after cesarean is:

   A. Nonreassuring fetal heart tracing

   B. Vaginal bleeding

   C. Hypovolemic shock

   D. Loss of presentation

   E. Sharp suprapubic pain

89. A 37-year-old G_1P_0 woman presents in early labor at 2 cm dilated. She wishes to review her options for pain control. With regard to epidural analgesia during labor, please select the best answer:

   A. Maternal request is sufficient medical indication for epidural analgesia pain relief in labor.

   B. Use of epidural in labor has shown to have no impact on the length of second stage.

   C. Use of epidural analgesia is generally contraindicated before 4- to 5-cm dilation.

   D. C/S rates are higher in women who use epidural analgesia.

   E. Neonatal asphyxia is more common in women who received epidural analgesia in labor.

90. A 32-year-old G_1P_0 patient at 28 weeks gestation should be advised to discontinue moderate aerobic exercise in which of the following settings?

  A. Twin pregnancy
  B. Soccer or other contact sports
  C. Premature labor
  D. Preeclampsia
  E. All of the above

91. A pregnant woman at 10 weeks gestation is concerned about x-ray exposure to her fetus after she had a CT scan of her abdomen after a motor vehicle accident (MVA) She should be advised that:

  A. Exposures of < 5 rads are not associated with teratogenic effects
  B. Termination of the pregnancy is indicated because of the risk of cancer to the fetus
  C. CT scans of the abdomen usually require >5 rads of exposure
  D. Risk of childhood leukemia after in utero exposure is increased 10-fold to 20-fold over the baseline
  E. X-ray diagnostic procedures should not be done in pregnant women

92. A 23-year-old G_3P_1 woman at 16 weeks gestation wants more information about vaccinations during pregnancy. You should advise her that:

  A. MMR vaccine during the first trimester is teratogenic
  B. Influenza vaccine should be offered only if there is underlying cardiopulmonary disease
  C. Varicella vaccine is contraindicated in pregnancy
  D. Hepatitis B vaccine is contraindicated in pregnancy
  E. Pneumococcus vaccine should be offered in the second and third trimesters during flu season

93. A 28-year-old G_2P_1 woman at 38 weeks gestation with a prior history of a low transverse C/S at term has been diagnosed with preeclampsia. On exam, her cervix is long and fingertip dilated. Labor induction in this patient should be:

  A. Contraindicated
  B. Considered only if she has a favorable cervix
  C. Started with misoprostol
  D. Begun with Foley bulb
  E. Induced with artificial rupture of the membranes only

94. During a routine prenatal visit of an 18-year-old G_1P_0 woman at 36 weeks gestation, you suspect that the fetus is in breech presentation. After ultrasound confirmation of the fetal lie, you recommend:

A. Await spontaneous onset of labor; allow vaginal breech delivery

B. Attempt ECV; allow vaginal breech delivery if version is unsuccessful

C. Attempt ECV; elective C/S at 39 weeks if version unsuccessful

D. Attempt ECV in labor

E. Elective C/S at 39 weeks

95. A 37-year-old G_6P_3 woman at 36 weeks gestation with a complete anterior placenta previa is scheduled to undergo an elective cesarean. She has a history of three prior low transverse cesareans. The serious complication that is increased the most for this patient compared to women undergoing a first cesarean is:

A. Risk of RDS

B. Risk of blood loss secondary to placenta previa

C. Risk of surgical injury to intra-abdominal organs

D. Risk of placenta accreta/percreta

E. Risk of postoperative wound infection and dehiscence

96. A 26-year-old G_3P_2 woman at 32 weeks gestation is brought by ambulance after a head-on MVA collision where she was the restrained driver. Upon arrival, the first step in management should include:

A. Continuous fetal heart rate monitoring

B. Administration of 300 µg D immune globulin if she is Rh negative

C. Ultrasound to establish gestational age (GA), placental location, amniotic fluid volume, and fetal condition

D. Maternal stabilization

E. All of the above

97. A 22-year-old G_2P_0 woman at 38 weeks gestation is a diet-controlled gestational diabetic with an estimated fetal weight (EFW) of 4,600 g by Leopold maneuvers and obstetric ultrasound. The best course of action is:

A. Immediate induction for impending macrosomia

B. Await the onset of labor and then perform a cesarean

C. Offer an elective cesarean at 39 weeks gestation

D. Be prepared to assist with forceps in the second stage of labor

E. Review shoulder dystocia maneuvers

98. A 19-year-old G_2P_0 woman presents at 9 weeks gestation unable to keep anything down orally. In considering her management, which of the following interventions is most likely based on false-positive findings?

    A. Vitamin B_6 for extreme nausea

    B. Hyperthyroidism treatment in cases of suppressed TSH levels

    C. Nasogastric feeds for intolerance of oral intake

    D. IV fluids for dehydration on urinalysis

    E. Metoclopramide for vomiting

99. A 33-year-old G_3P_0 woman is recovering from a pregnancy loss at 11 weeks gestation. She had two prior losses at 10 and 9 weeks. Which test do you recommend?

    A. Parental karyotype

    B. Lupus anticoagulant

    C. Hysterosalpingography (HSG)

    D. Anticardiolipin antibodies

    E. All of the above

100. You are caring for a 28-year-old G_4P_2 woman who is HIV positive. Which of the following policies and guidelines effectively reduce the vertical transmission of HIV?

    A. Use of rapid HIV testing in women in labor with a undocumented HIV status

    B. Wait for confirmatory test before initiation of antiretroviral prophylaxis

    C. Breastfeeding is allowed unless confirmatory tests are also positive for HIV

    D. Neonatal prophylaxis is not necessary if maternal prophylaxis was initiated 4 hours before delivery

    E. If maternal prophylaxis for HIV transmission was not given in labor, neonatal prophylaxis is of no benefit

Answers and Explanations

1. E	26. E	51. C	76. C
2. C	27. A	52. C	77. D
3. C	28. C	53. B	78. E
4. A	29. A	54. A	79. B
5. B	30. B	55. B	80. A
6. A	31. B	56. C	81. D
7. E	32. D	57. B	82. B
8. A	33. C	58. C	83. C
9. C	34. D	59. B	84. D
10. A	35. A	60. B	85. A
11. A	36. D	61. C	86. B
12. B	37. E	62. B	87. C
13. C	38. C	63. C	88. A
14. B	39. E	64. E	89. A
15. C	40. A	65. B	90. E
16. B	41. A	66. C	91. A
17. A	42. D	67. E	92. C
18. C	43. C	68. D	93. D
19. A	44. A	69. E	94. C
20. D	45. E	70. E	95. D
21. C	46. D	71. D	96. D
22. C	47. A	72. C	97. C
23. B	48. A	73. C	98. B
24. D	49. D	74. E	99. E
25. E	50. C	75. A	100. A

1. E. Poor glucose control is associated with fetal anomalies, especially CNS and cardiac anomalies. HbA_{1c} of 12 represents poor chronic glucose control. At the time of conception, this degree of control is associated with a high rate of fetal anomalies with estimates as high as 20% to 25%.

2. C. Conversion to short-acting and long-acting insulin often provides better glucose control compared to oral hypoglycemic agents in pregnant diabetic patients. Optimal glucose control is of prime importance to this patient because she is still early in pregnancy and thus in the period of fetal organogenesis. Good glucose control during this period can significantly decrease the risk for fetal anomalies. In addition, subcutaneous insulin has been proven to be safe in pregnancy; some oral hypoglycemic agents have been used safely in pregnancy, but their long-term effects are still unproven. Switching this patient to an insulin pump immediately could be challenging. It is generally safer to first put a patient on an insulin regimen, educate the patient on how to control blood sugar levels, then switch the patient to a pump when she is more experienced and knowledgeable about her individual needs.

3. C. Fetal nuchal translucency screening in the first trimester offers an evaluation of risk of trisomy 21, 13, and 18 early in pregnancy between 11 and 14 weeks. One of the benefits of this early test is the allowance for invasive diagnostic testing. CVS and amniocentesis can both provide diagnostic testing for chromosomal disorders, but CVS can be done much earlier in pregnancy. Offering CVS testing to this patient is the most appropriate next step. Repeating the ultrasound is not an appropriate option if the nuchal region of the fetus was adequately seen. In addition, CVS cannot be performed beyond 13 weeks, so waiting 1 to 2 weeks to repeat the test would limit the patient's options. She does have the option to wait until 15 to 16 weeks GA and obtain an amniocentesis, which is associated with a slightly lower rate of pregnancy loss than CVS. However, an amniocentesis usually is not done at the current GA and prior to 15 weeks is associated with a higher pregnancy loss rate. Termination of a desired pregnancy without definitive diagnostic testing would not be the most appropriate next step.

4. A. The patient's normal karyotype as obtained via CVS is entirely reassuring regarding aneuploidy. However, she still needs a screening test for neural tube defects, so she should undergo the MSAFP screen between 15 and 20 weeks gestation. She does not need to bear the risk of an amniocentesis unless the MSAFP level is elevated. Fetal echocardiography is used to rule out fetal cardiac anomalies in women who are at increased risk for such anomalies (e.g., pregestational diabetes). CVS does not need to be repeated. A cordocentesis or percutaneous umbilical blood sampling (PUBS) is used to obtain fetal cells when obtaining a karyotype immediately is important or if one needs to know the fetal hematocrit, as in Rh alloimmunization.

Abnormal first-trimester nuchal translucency measurements are associated with chromosomal disorders, specifically trisomy 21, 13, and 18. However, in the face of invasive testing that reveals normal chromosomes, these fetuses appear to have a slightly increased rate of cardiac anomalies. Therefore, the current recommendation for patients with abnormal first-trimester nuchal translucency measurements is evaluation with fetal echocardiography in the second trimester. Of note, however, the nuchal translucency measurement cutoff for this recommendation is controversial but generally between 3.5 and 4.0 mm. Repeating the CVS is not recommended because this diagnostic test is not associated with false-negative results. Amniocentesis and cordocentesis would provide the same information about the chromosomes as CVS and are not appropriate.

5. B. Immediate cessation of methadone and even rapid dose tapering with or without the addition of a benzodiazepine are associated with poor fetal prognosis including intrauterine fetal demise. Therefore, most centers continue patients on their current methadone dose. Highly motivated patients may be able to taper their methadone dosing, but the taper must be slow and the patient followed closely with antenatal fetal surveillance.

6. A. The most likely diagnosis in this scenario in a patient who has not had rupture of membranes (ROM) is twin-to-twin transfusion syndrome (TTTS). TTTS is a condition seen almost exclusively in monochorionic twin gestations. The condition is poorly understood but is believed to stem from unbalanced arteriovenous vascular anastomoses within the placenta that connects the twin gestations and disrupts the pressure balance between the twins. The first recommended management step in a patient with this diagnosis is large-volume amniocentesis. Disruption of the membrane between the twins, amniotic septostomy, and laser ablation of the communicating vessels have been used but currently are not the first recommended step in management. Amnioinfusion to either fetus is not recommended.

7. E. C/S now is the most appropriate recommendation. ECV is contraindicated (and not feasible) in a twin gestation. In addition, vaginal delivery typically is not recommended for breech presentation in the presenting twin; however, if the first twin is vertex and the second is breech, vaginal delivery of the first followed by breech extraction of the second is recommended in well-counseled patients. The presentation of the first twin is unlikely to change once the patient is term and in labor; therefore, waiting until she is completely dilated to assess presentation is not appropriate.

8. A. ECV now is appropriate for breech presentation of a nonanomalous fetus in this scenario. ECV is generally performed at 36 to 37 weeks gestation, although there is some controversy surrounding the most optimal GA for ECV. Most agree that waiting until 39 weeks can risk spontaneous ROM or labor, both of which are relative contraindications to the procedure. An anterior placenta is not a contraindication. Offering ECV in a well-counseled patient is more appropriate than proceeding directly with a C/S. However, ECV does have some associated risk (ROM, abruption, fetal bradycardia, onset of labor, failure of the provider to rotate the fetus, and/or return of the fetus to a malpresentation after being rotated to vertex), and some patients may choose not to undergo the procedure. Overall, however, ECV is an effective means for decreasing, but not eliminating, the rate of cesarean delivery for breech presentation.

9. C. The most appropriate step is evaluation with colposcopy to rule out invasive disease, which would require more aggressive management during pregnancy. Waiting and repeating the Pap smear (especially until postpartum) are less appropriate. The patient has not had a Pap smear before and is a previous smoker, making the scenario more concerning. Colposcopy is not contraindicated in pregnancy. LEEP is not an appropriate step without definitive testing.

10. A. The nicotine patch is not contraindicated in pregnancy; however, its use is most appropriate during pregnancy when the patient is smoking 10 or more cigarettes per day. At this level of tobacco use, the nicotine exposure from the patch is approximately equivalent. Given her history of asthma and her use of more than 10 cigarettes per day, a nicotine patch is an appropriate option for her. In addition, smoking cessation counseling and buproprion are useful adjuncts appear to have an additive effect.

11. A. This patient has the diagnosis of a threatened abortion. A patient with an early pregnancy who presents with abdominal or pelvic pain and vaginal bleeding is at risk for ectopic pregnancy. The diagnostic workup includes a history, physical examination, β-hCG, CBC, type and screen (T&S), and pelvic ultrasound. If the physical exam shows a closed cervical os in the setting of vaginal bleeding and either a viable intrauterine pregnancy (IUP) or a pelvic ultrasound and β-hCG are too early to show a viable IUP, the diagnosis is *threatened abortion.* If the IUP cannot be seen but there is not enough evidence to confirm an ectopic pregnancy, the patient is also considered to have a rule-out ectopic pregnancy. If the cervical os is open but the products of conception (POC) have not passed, this is called an *inevitable abortion.* If some, but not all, of the POCs have passed, this is an *incomplete abortion.* If all of the POCs have passed, this is called a *complete abortion.* Finally, if the POCs have not passed but the pregnancy is not viable, this is called a *missed abortion.*

12. B. In patients who have the diagnosis of rule-out ectopic because their β-hCG is still too low for an IUP to be seen on pelvic ultrasound, the β-hCG should be checked every 48 hours. The β-hCG of a normally developing IUP should double every 48 hours or at least increase by a minimum of 60%. Once the β-hCG level reaches 1,600 to 2,000, known as the *discriminatory zone,* an IUP should be able to be seen via transvaginal ultrasound. The discriminatory zone is much higher, often >6,000 for transabdominal ultrasound, which is much more dependent upon patient habitus.

13. C. This patient may be in labor, which can be confirmed with repeat cervical examination in 1 to 2 hours. However, the fetus has had nonreassuring fetal testing in this presentation and needs further testing. The fact that the patient has felt decreased or absent fetal movement needs to be taken seriously, and any patient with this complaint in the third trimester needs to have fetal testing. In this setting with a nonreactive NST, a biophysical profile (BPP) or CST may be performed. In this patient whose contractions are 6 to 8 minutes apart, a CST could be achieved by augmenting the contractions with intravenous oxytocin (Pitocin) until she is having at least three in 10 minutes. A fetal heart rate that has good variability and shows no decelerations can be considered reassuring. BPP, an ultrasound evaluation of the fetus looking for fetal breathing, fetal movement, fetal tone, and amniotic fluid level, is a reasonable alternative to the CST.

14. B. Preterm labor is described as contractions leading to cervical change before 37 weeks gestation. Risk factors include prior preterm delivery, prior preterm labor, PPROM, uterine abnormalities, polyhydramnios, bacterial vaginosis, placental abruption, preeclampsia, chorioamnionitis, and pregestational weight <50 kg. Prior dilation of the cervix in a therapeutic or spontaneous abortion, particularly in the second trimester, has been associated with cervical incompetence. This would be unlikely in this patient, who has reached 31 weeks gestation. A large fetus can be associated with polyhydramnios, which is correlated with preterm labor, but this association is far weaker than prior preterm delivery. Teenage pregnancy is correlated with lower socioeconomic status, which is correlated with many complications of pregnancy, including preterm delivery, but again this is weaker than prior preterm delivery. Smoking has a stronger association with low birth weight rather than preterm delivery itself.

15. C. Chorioamnionitis is an infection of the fetal membranes and amniotic fluid that usually involves the uterus and the fetus as well. The five diagnostic signs are elevated maternal white blood count and temperature, fetal tachycardia, uterine tenderness, and vaginal discharge. If diagnosis is uncertain, amniocentesis can be performed and tested for Gram stain, glucose, white blood count, and culture. Neither the sensitivity nor the specificity of the first three tests is >80%, and although culture is the gold standard, it can take several days to obtain results. Recently, it has been suggested that interleukin (IL)-6 in the amniotic fluid is a more sensitive marker for intrauterine infection. Unfortunately, it has not been adopted at most institutions and remains experimental. Intense lower back pain is not uncommon in labor and usually is attributed to the malposition of occiput posterior (OP).

16. B. The management of shoulder dystocia, as with any emergency situation, should be discussed and considered frequently so that clinicians can react quickly and efficiently to its occurrence. A common algorithm is to begin with suprapubic pressure to dislodge the anterior shoulder and the McRobert maneuver to increase the pelvic diameter. An episiotomy is commonly performed if these maneuvers fail. This usually is followed with the Wood screw maneuver, delivery of the posterior arm, or the Rubin maneuver. If none of these maneuvers is successful after several attempts, more aggressive interventions include fracturing the fetal clavicle. A final maneuver that has been described, the Zavanelli maneuver, is to place the fetal head back into the maternal pelvis and perform a cesarean delivery. Fundal pressure, which would likely further impact the anterior fetal shoulder behind the maternal pubic symphysis, is not recommended.

17. A. C/S is offered as the mode of delivery in patients with active herpes lesions at term and to HIV patients. It has not been shown to change the transmission of hepatitis B or C virus and would not be an issue in a rubella nonimmune patient. This patient has no active lesions, so the indication to offer her a cesarean delivery is her HIV positivity. The evidence of decreased vertical transmission of HIV has been demonstrated primarily in women who have been on no treatment or AZT alone. In patients on triple therapy with undetectable viral loads, it is unclear whether C/S offers any benefit because these patients are likely to have quite a low transmission rate anyway. The patient in this question is not on antiretroviral therapy, so her fetus is likely to benefit from the protective effect of a C/S.

18. C. Fetal heart rates are evaluated, paying attention to baseline rate, variability, accelerations, and decelerations. The baseline rate should be between 110 and 160 bpm. Minimal and absent variability are worrisome for hypoxia and acidemia of the fetus, with absent variability being worse than minimal. Three types of decelerations have been described—early, variable, and late. *Early decelerations* begin and end with contractions and are thought to be a result of fetal head compression. *Variable decelerations* are sharp drops in the fetal heart rate with quick return to baseline and can be either isolated or correlated with contractions; they are thought to result from compression of the umbilical cord. *Late decelerations* begin after the contraction has begun and end after it has ended. They usually are shallow and can be quite subtle and difficult to detect. They are indicative of decreased placental perfusion, which can be secondary to inadequate blood flow to the uterus or increased vascular resistance of the placenta.

19. A. Although none of the substances are recommended in pregnancy, only alcohol, which is associated with fetal alcohol syndrome and with cardiac defects in particular, is associated with congenital anomalies. Cocaine use during pregnancy has been correlated with central nervous system effects and developmental delay in the exposed child. Tobacco use has been correlated with small for GA fetuses and increased respiratory disease in childhood. Caffeine and opiates do not have particularly noted fetal effects, although fetuses exposed to opiates throughout pregnancy will need to be weaned off the drug postpartum.

20. D. Twin gestations are more likely to have a variety of complications in pregnancy, including preterm labor, preterm delivery, preeclampsia, malpresentation, and postpartum hemorrhage. TTTS is an unfortunate complication of the vascular connections in a shared placenta that leads to a plethoric recipient twin that can become hydropic and a donor twin that can have such severe oligohydramnios that it may appear "stuck" against the uterine wall. This syndrome is seen in approximately 10% to 15% of monochorionic-diamnionic twins. However, it has never been described in dichorionic/diamnionic (di/di) twins who have different placentas.

21. C. Tocolytics are used to decrease or halt contractions with the intent of prolonging pregnancy. A variety of agents are currently used for tocolysis, including calcium channel blockers (nifedipine), β-agonists (terbutaline, ritodrine), prostaglandin inhibitors (indomethacin), and magnesium sulfate. In addition, intravenous hydration is used to decrease contractions secondary to dehydration. A new class of agents, oxytocin receptor antagonists, are currently being studied, although early results do not indicate any improvement over existing medications. Ritodrine is the only tocolytic that is FDA approved. Unfortunately, both ritodrine and the other tocolytics have generally not been demonstrated to prolong pregnancy more than 48 hours. Hydralazine is an α-blocker used for blood pressure control. It is particularly effective in the intravenous form in the acute setting.

22. C. Alone and of itself, preterm labor is not a risk factor for breech presentation; however, because preterm infants are breech more often than term infants, it is seen more often than at term. Uterine anomalies, placenta previa, fetal anomalies, including hydrocephalus, and polyhydramnios are all risk factors for breech presentation. Breech vaginal delivery has been associated with fetal head entrapment and neonatal morbidity and is being used as an option for delivery in fewer cases. Thus, ECV, in order to convert the fetal presentation from breech to cephalic, is commonly used so that women may undergo labor. Several relative contraindications include fetal anomalies, ROM, preterm gestation, placenta previa, and need for urgent delivery. Polyhydramnios, because of the increased fluid in which to maneuver the fetus, is the best setting to attempt ECV.

23. B. The two salient issues here are the management of preterm labor and the mode of delivery and management of a prior classic cesarean. Because the patient is in preterm labor with a cervix dilated to 3 cm but is not definitely beyond the point of unstoppable preterm labor, she should undergo tocolytic therapy. If this fails to stop the cervical change and she rapidly progresses to beyond 5 cm, most obstetricians would consider it a failed intervention. At this point, plans for delivery should be made. In the setting of a prior cesarean birth with either a low transverse or low vertical hysterotomy, a trial of labor would be reasonable. However, in this woman with a prior classic hysterotomy, generally trial of labor is not used because of the increased risk for uterine rupture. Thus, a repeat cesarean would be the mode of delivery of choice.

24. D. The management of PPROM is widely debated. Before 32 to 34 weeks gestation, most institutions use betamethasone to help induce fetal lung maturity; however, it is rarely used beyond 34 weeks gestation. The use of tocolysis varies greatly, ranging from no use to tocolysis at less than 26 to 28 weeks gestation to tocolysis until 34 weeks, as in preterm labor. Many patients with PPROM go into labor within 48 to 72 hours; for those who do not, the risks of prolonged ROM include chorioamnionitis, abruption, and cord prolapse. With these risks weighed against the risks of prematurity, induction of labor has been considered between 32 and 36 weeks gestation. Some institutions send the amniotic fluid for fetal lung maturity testing and induce labor if it is mature. Tocolysis at 35 weeks gestation would not be used in this patient; thus, the most appropriate plan presented would be expectant management. If the patient stopped contracting, many practitioners would induce or augment at that point.

25. E. Dating of a pregnancy is important to establish as soon as possible. For example, the Nägele rule of dating a pregnancy is based on the fact that the estimated date of confinement (EDC) is 280 days from the LMP. On average, that is 9 months 1 week from the LMP. Thus, the Nägele rule is to subtract 3 months and add 7 days (and 1 year). Usually, 280 days from the LMP is used as the EDC, which is confirmed by physical examination and eventually a second-trimester ultrasound. However, physical examination is not a particularly accurate way to date a pregnancy, and ultrasound becomes less accurate as a pregnancy continues. Ultrasound is considered to have a 7% to 10% range of accuracy, and a rule of thumb is that it can be off by up to 1 week in the first trimester, 2 weeks during the second trimester, and 3 weeks during the third trimester. Thus, in a patient who had no clear LMP to date the pregnancy, an ultrasound performed as early as possible would be the best way to date the pregnancy. Dating by LMP consistent with physical examination is the most accurate way to date a pregnancy and generally all that is done in this setting. Ultrasound actually is quite poor at 12 to 14 weeks gestation because the crown–rump length becomes a poorer indicator at that point. Biometry, which uses the biparietal diameter, abdominal circumference, and femur length, is not as accurate as it is later in pregnancy.

26. E. A variety of prenatal specimens are drawn at the initial prenatal visit. An RPR is drawn to screen for syphilis. Because syphilis still can be easily treated with IM benzathine penicillin, congenital syphilis syndrome can be prevented. The rubella screen tests for immunization for rubella; if the titer is low or negative, the vaccine can be given postpartum, rather than during pregnancy, because it is a live virus. Knowing the blood type is important because of the possibility of Rh isoimmunization. The risk of iron deficiency anemia increases during pregnancy because of the increased production demands; thus, a first-trimester hematocrit is important to establish a baseline. All of these tests are drawn in everyone despite their history or symptoms. Although it is important to know of a history of genital herpes, because the antibody titer will be positive with oral or genital herpes, the antibody titer is generally sent only for a woman with new onset symptoms of genital herpes to determine whether it is first outbreak of HSV. Of note, some authors have started recommending routine HSV titer screens to identify women who have been infected but have never had an outbreak. However, it is unclear what benefit this would confer and whether it is cost effective, and the practice has not been adopted by the American College of Obstetricians and Gynecologists (ACOG).

27. A. This patient's contraction pattern is regular and more frequent than every 5 minutes. In addition, she has ruptured membranes and her cervix has advanced to 4 cm and 80% effacement, which are all consistent with ongoing labor. Patients usually are admitted at this time, particularly in the setting of ruptured membranes. There is a small chance that her contractions will decrease; however, at that point, augmentation with oxytocin could be used. In a patient with ruptured membranes without contractions, admission is still indicated. In one study of this question, patients managed expectantly had higher rates of chorioamnionitis than those augmented immediately, whereas the rates of cesarean delivery were the same.

28. C. Vaginal bleeding in the third trimester can be a sign of abruption, placenta previa, PPROM, or preterm labor, as well as indicative of cervical or vaginal injury and needs to be investigated. Thus, a history of a placenta previa on ultrasound would not be reassuring. A prior preterm birth, even though the child is normal, puts her at increased risk for subsequent preterm birth. Dysuria is a sign of a urinary tract infection, which commonly can be the cause of preterm contractions. Although not as worrisome as preterm labor, a urinary tract infection certainly is not reassuring. Headache and right upper quadrant pain are hallmarks of severe preeclampsia and would require complete workup to rule out preeclampsia and HELLP syndrome. Recent vaginal intercourse could cause both the vaginal spotting and the contractions; thus, giving an etiology for these symptoms which, alone, are not associated with poor outcomes.

29. A. Management of the Rh-negative patient with RhoGAM has led to a marked reduction in women who have been sensitized to the

Rh antigen. The recommendations for treatment with RhoGAM include use anytime in the first two trimesters with vaginal bleeding or amniocentesis, at the beginning of the third trimester at approximately 28 weeks gestation, during the third trimester if there are signs of a fetal–maternal hemorrhage that is greater than can be negated by the 28-week dose of RhoGAM, and postpartum if the infant is Rh positive. RhoGAM is not routinely given during preterm labor unless the patient has not yet received a dose in the pregnancy. Because the dose of RhoGAM is dependent upon the measured or theoretical volume of exposure to fetal red blood cells, treatment in the first trimester, when the fetal blood volume is extremely low, only requires administering a smaller dose of RhoGAM. Of note, some have used the micro dose in the second trimester as well. However, this would be less reassuring than in the first trimester because the fetal blood volume increases between these two times.

30. B. During pregnancy, the average woman needs to increase her caloric intake by approximately 300 to 400 kcal per day. Postpartum, women who are breastfeeding need to increase their caloric intake by 500 to 600 kcal per day. If a women is grossly underweight, she may need to further increase her caloric intake to make up for the existing deficiency. However, women who are overweight should not particularly attempt to lose the weight during pregnancy. In 1990 the Institute of Medicine made recommendations for weight gain in pregnancy of 25 to 30 lb in women of normal weight. It has been found that women who gain significantly more than this have higher rates of cesarean delivery and macrosomic (large, >4,500 g) babies.

31. B. The most common postmenopausal adnexal mass is a benign serous cystadenoma. However, the overall risk of malignancy in an ovarian cystic mass is 45% in a postmenopausal woman compared to 13% in a premenopausal woman. Ultrasonography has complemented clinical identification of pelvic masses by using various parameters to distinguish benign from malignant masses, including size, presence of excrescences, number of loculations, overall density, and pulsatility. Although its specificity for prediction of malignancy is low, ultrasonography is useful in the counseling of a patient with regard to operative intervention approaches. Biopsy or aspiration of ovarian masses is not recommended because of the issue of possible tumor spill. Radiographic information can help determine the operative approach: laparoscopy versus laparotomy, as well as possible extent of surgery, and simple oophorectomy versus ovarian cancer staging.

32. D. Both excision and ablation are acceptable for women with CIN2 and satisfactory colposcopy. However, recurrent moderate dysplasia (CIN2) warrants excision of cervical lesions. The general consensus is that ablation or excision of CIN2/CIN3 lesions reduces the incidence and mortality of invasive cervical cancer.

CIN2/CIN3 lesions tend to persist or progress. Therefore, continued observation is not an appropriate management decision. Cryotherapy is acceptable in the setting of satisfactory colposcopy. Hysterectomy or chemotherapy is unacceptable as primary therapies for CIN2/CIN3.

33. C. Colposcopic evaluation of pregnant women with HSIL should be conducted by clinicians experienced in the evaluation of colposcopic changes induced by pregnancy. Cervical biopsy during pregnancy is associated with an increased risk for minor bleeding but not with increased risk for major bleeding or pregnancy loss. In fact, failure to perform biopsies has been associated with missed cancers. Because unsatisfactory colposcopy may become satisfactory as the pregnancy progresses, women with unsatisfactory colposcopic findings should undergo repeat colposcopy in 6 to 12 weeks. Endocervical curettage is prescribed in pregnant women because of risk for injury to the fetus. Use of diagnostic excisional procedures during pregnancy is limited to cases where invasive cancer cannot be ruled out.

34. D. Among women with an inherited susceptibility to breast and ovarian cancer, there is a role for prophylactic surgery. However, prophylactic mastectomy and oophorectomy do not guarantee the absence of future cancer. Prior to performance of such procedures, a detailed family history must be documented, the patient counseled in detail about her risk for inherited cancers, and thoughtful consideration given to the consequences of such drastic risk reduction techniques.

Current care for women at increased risk for cancer includes periodic screening with mammogram, pelvic ultrasound, CA-125, chemoprophylaxis, and prophylactic surgery.

35. A. The Bartholin glands are located at the base of the labia minora and drain into the vestibule at the 4 and 8 o'clock positions. They usually are not palpable except in the presence of infection or disease. Excision of an enlarged Bartholin gland in a postmenopausal woman is performed because of concern about possible neoplastic growth. If infected, incision and drainage are discouraged because of the tendency for the cyst or abscess to recur. The preferred method involves placement of a Word catheter or marsupialization.

36. D. Extramammary Paget disease occurs most commonly in women in the sixth and seventh decades. Treatment of noninvasive extramammary Paget disease involves wide surgical excision, particularly because the disease usually extends well beyond the gross lesion. Recurrence rates are lowest for patients undergoing vulvectomy, followed by Mohs micrographic surgery and wide local excision.

A history of unchanged symptoms or lesion appearance despite extended topical steroid therapy is not uncommon in patients with vulvar Paget disease. Laser ablation is best used in the case of recurrent disease. Radiotherapy, topical chemotherapy, and photodynamic therapy are under investigation.

37. E. Cervical cancer is a clinically staged disease. This patient has advanced cervical cancer, which must be properly staged with an examination under anesthesia, cystoscopy, and proctoscopy. Treatment options for stage IB and early stage IIA cervical cancer include either a primary surgical approach with radical hysterectomy and pelvic lymphadenectomy or primary radiation therapy with concurrent chemotherapy. The 5-year survival rates approximate 87% to 92% with either approach. Radical surgery is not appropriate treatment for bulky or locally advanced cervical cancer.

38. C. Symptoms of numbness, tingling, or burning in the hands or feet occur often with paclitaxel. They usually improve or resolve within several months of completing therapy. Alopecia almost always occurs with paclitaxel. Cisplatinum may cause irreversible peripheral neuropathies that are manifested as paresthesias in a stocking-glove distribution, loss of proprioception and vibratory sensation, and areflexia. Unlike cisplatinum, carboplatinum confers more hematologic than neurologic toxicity.

39. E. Use of the antiestrogen tamoxifen for treatment of breast cancer is associated with a twofold to threefold increased risk for endometrial cancer development. Endometrial aspiration is the accepted first step in evaluating a patient with abnormal uterine bleeding. Its diagnostic accuracy is 90% to 98% compared with subsequent findings on dilation and curettage or hysterectomy. Despite the identification of multiple risk factors for endometrial cancer, routine screening currently is not recommended because of the lack of an appropriate and cost-effective test that reduces mortality. It has been shown that women taking tamoxifen receive no benefit from routine screening with pelvic ultrasonography or endometrial biopsy. CA-125 level may be elevated in advanced endometrial cancer and therefore is useful as a marker of disease progression or recurrence.

40. A. Anemia frequently results from cancer treatment, leading to fatigue, poor exercise tolerance, disturbed sleep, and lack of appetite. Following a basic workup to rule out treatable causes of anemia, initiation of erythropoietic agents improves hemoglobin levels, decreases the risk of transfusions, and improves quality of life.

Blood transfusions are indicated for acute symptomatology. Filgrastim stimulates myelopoiesis.

41. A. This patient's presentation is concerning for inflammatory breast cancer, one of the most aggressive manifestations of primary breast carcinoma. The erythema and pitted skin appearance are consistent with peau d'orange changes typically associated with inflammatory breast cancer. The median age at diagnosis is younger than seen with other breast cancers. Needle biopsy is the most definitive test to determine the histologic diagnosis. Imaging studies are very useful, but the presence of cancer cells can only be determined histologically.

42. D. The definitive surgical therapy for stage IA2 cervical cancer (depth of invasion >3 mm and <5 mm, width <7 mm) involves a radical hysterectomy, pelvic lymphadenectomy, and bilateral salpingo-oophorectomy.

Selected patients with stage IA1 cervical cancer can be treated with cold knife conization or extrafascial hysterectomy. Recent reports have described the use of radical trachelectomy with lymphadenectomy for patients of reproductive age with stage IA2 cancers.

43. C. Carriers of BRCA1/BRCA2 mutations have an up to seven-fold increase in the risk for breast cancer development and 10-fold increased risk for ovarian cancer development compared to women who do not carry these mutations. BRCA1/BRCA2 mutations also increase the risk for early-onset breast cancer. History of a first-degree relative with premenopausal breast cancer increases the relative risk to 1.8, whereas Ashkenazi-Jewish descent increases the relative risk twofold. The risk of breast cancer development is increased fourfold in women who are heterozygotes for ataxia telangiectasia. Nulliparity increases the relative risk threefold.

44. A. Patients with LS typically present with thin, parchmentlike skin that is a poor barrier to moisture loss. In addition to use of bland emollients, a potent topical corticosteroid is recommended for definitive therapy generally over 2 to 3 weeks. Maintenance therapy with small amounts is generally satisfactory, as well.

Vulvectomy is not indicated for treatment of this disease unless there is associated dysplasia or invasive cancer. Photodynamic therapy and focal ultrasonography are being studied for efficacy. Testosterone or estrogen creams have no role in treating LS.

45. E. Endometrial cancer is the most common gynecologic cancer in women with HNPCC. Women with HNPCC syndrome have a similar lifetime risk for colon and endometrial cancer of 40% to 60%. In addition to the high risk for colon and endometrial cancers, they are at increased risk for developing ovarian cancer. The other extra-colonic sites include breast and stomach.

46. D. In prepubertal girls, the most common ovarian tumor is a germ cell tumor. Given that these tumors can grow to a large size relatively quickly, the typical presentation is of increasing discomfort and girth and possible urinary frequency due to compression of the bladder.

Fibroids grow in an estrogen environment and have not been described in prepubertal girls. A follicular cyst occurs from normal ovulatory function of the ovary. This would require this patient to show signs of precocious puberty. Urethral obstruction typically does not cause urinary frequency. Moreover, an enlarged bladder on ultrasound would not have solid components within it. A TOA usually results from an infectious process, usually as a result of PID. Less commonly, a TOA results from a ruptured appendix. Neither of these is likely given the patient's presentation.

47. A. In the setting of normal ovarian reserve, an early follicular (day 3) FSH level should be at its highest during the cycle, whereas estrogen levels should be low (Figure A47-1). As the follicle matures and estrogen rises, FSH level falls via the feedback effect on the pituitary gland. This patient's FSH level is relatively low. However, this is a false result because the estradiol level drawn at the same time is high. Although it is true that she is ovulating regularly because her menstrual cycles are regular, given her age she likely

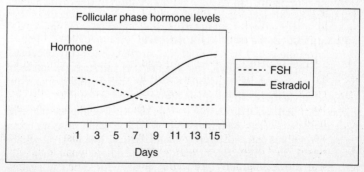

FIGURE **A47-1**

has diminished ovarian reserve. A repeat day 3 FSH level likely would indicate an elevated FSH level and would confirm the diagnosis of diminished ovarian reserve. This couple should immediately be referred for consultation for assisted reproduction if they wish to maximize their chances of pregnancy. After age 40, a woman's per cycle fecundity rate is 9%, whereas the same rate for those under age 40 is 21% (*Hum Reprod.* 1994;9:2284-2286). Asherman syndrome is the term used to describe intrauterine scarring. It is a rare complication of dilation and curettage procedures .

48. A. Ovulation predictor kits use a monoclonal antibody that measures urinary LH, which increases rapidly 24 to 36 hours before ovulation. Although this method can be easier and more accurate in predicting ovulation than other monitoring methods (e.g., changes in basal metabolic temperature), urinary LH monitoring has its limitations. False-negative results can occur if peak LH concentrations are <40 IU/L, which may occur in up to 35% of ovulatory cycles. Common factors that affect the likelihood of a false negative are:

- Checking the urine early in the morning. LH is produced by the body in the morning and usual shows up in the urine by midafternoon.
- Not holding the urine for long enough, hence obtaining a dilute sample.
- Excessive hydration at the time of testing.

This patient has regular cycles and is ovulating regularly. There is no indication of premature ovarian failure. Clomid will not help her ovulate more frequently because she ovulates normally now.

49. D. This patient's history of dysmenorrhea is most consistent with endometriosis. With endometriosis, inflammation from the peritoneal implants can cause a mild elevation in the CA-125 level. The mass in the left ovary is likely an endometrioma.

50. C. PCOS is the most common cause of anovulatory, irregular cycles in women. An LH/FSH ratio >2:1 suggests PCOS, but because it is not particularly sensitive, the diagnosis is increasingly made by excluding other causes of anovulation. Abnormal thyroid function and elevated prolactin levels can affect pituitary production of FSH; hence, serum TSH and prolactin should be checked in all young women with irregular menses. One variant of PCOS is an insulin-resistant form. Women with this form of PCOS have a relatively low glucose/insulin ratio. The elevated insulin level stimulates the ovaries to produce more androgens, which in turn inhibit normal egg maturation and ovulation. A glucose/insulin ratio <4.5 suggests insulin-resistant PCOS. Because PCOS is the result of excess androgen production, a mild elevation in testosterone is common. A day 21 progesterone level can help determine whether the patient has ovulated but is not a practical test to perform in this patient because her cycles are very irregular.

51. C. This patient is having anovulatory cycles due to hyperprolactinemia. The most common cause of hyperprolactinemia is a pituitary tumor, usually a prolactinoma. Other causes are:

- Primary hypothyroidism due to increased TRH resulting in increased TSH and prolactin
- Ingestion of certain drugs, including phenothiazines, certain high blood pressure medications (especially α-methyldopa), tranquilizers, opioids, antinausea drugs, oral contraceptives
- Breast stimulation can cause a modest increase in the amount of prolactin in the blood
- Other tumors arising in or near the pituitary may block the flow of dopamine from the brain to the prolactin-secreting cells
- Unexplained in approximately 30%

An MRI is the most sensitive test for detecting pituitary tumors and determining their size and should be the first step in the management of this patient. Ultimately this patient will require treatment, the goal of which is to return prolactin secretion to normal, reduce tumor size, correct any visual abnormalities, and restore normal pituitary function. Because dopamine is the chemical that normally inhibits prolactin secretion, bromocriptine or cabergoline (dopamine agonists) is used for medical treatment.

52. C. This patient's history and physical exam findings are consistent with PCOS. Moreover, her glucose/insulin ratio is <4.5, indicating an insulin-resistant form of PCOS. This patient may have a return to normal ovulation if she is treated with an oral hypoglycemic such as metformin. Spironolactone is used to treat the hirsutism caused by PCOS. Although a 10-day course of progesterone would provoke a withdrawal bleed, it would not promote ovulation. GnRH treatment will suppress ovulation by inhibiting FSH secretion. IUI on day 14 of her cycle would be ineffective because she does not ovulate on her own on day 14.

53. B. In the United States, the most likely cause of vesicovaginal fistula is surgery or pelvic irradiation. Women with vesicovaginal fistula present with painless, continuous loss of urine. You can confirm the diagnosis but instilling methylene blue dye into the bladder and seeing if the dye leaks onto a sanitary pad.

54. A. Within the few weeks of birth, some newborn girls will have a small amount of bleeding from the vagina. In utero, the fetus was exposed to maternal estrogen, which in turn stimulated the fetus's endometrium. After birth, the level of the mother's hormones in the baby's system gradually decreases, which can result in a small withdrawal bleed. This type of vaginal bleeding usually lasts less than 1 day and is not painful. No special evaluation or treatment is needed.

Table A54-1 lists the common causes of abnormal genital bleeding by age group.

55. B. This patient's physical exam findings are consistent with vaginal atrophy. The vaginal epithelium thins and becomes unrugated when estrogen levels fall. This epithelial thinning can cause a watery discharge and inflammation of the vaginal tissues. Common complaints are vaginal dryness and dyspareunia. Postcoital spotting can

TABLE A54-1 Common Causes of Abnormal Genital Bleeding by Age Group

Neonates	Reproductive Years
Estrogen withdrawal	Anovulation
	Pregnancy
Premenarchal	Cancer (cervical, uterine, vaginal, vulvar)
Foreign body	Polyps (endometrial or cervical), fibroids, adenomyosis
Trauma	Infection
Infection	Endocrine (PCOS, thyroid, pituitary adenoma)
Urethral prolapse	Bleeding diathesis
Sarcoma botryoides	Medication related (e.g., irregular use of OCPs)
Ovarian tumor	
Precocious puberty	**Perimenopausal**
	Anovulation
Early postmenarche	Polyps, fibroids, adenomyosis
Anovulation (hypothalamic immaturity)	Cancer
Bleeding diathesis	
Stress (psychogenic, exercise induced)	**Menopausal**
Pregnancy	Atrophy
Infection	Cancer
	Hormone therapy

occur as a result of trauma to the thinned epithelium. All components of vaginal testing are normal except for the presence of WBCs on the wet smear. The components are as follows:

> *Wet mount:* Sample of the vaginal discharge is placed on a slide and mixed with saline. The slide is examined under a microscope for bacteria, yeast cells, trichomonads, white blood cells, or clue cells (bacterial vaginosis).
> *KOH slide:* Sample of the vaginal discharge is placed on a slide and mixed with a solution of potassium hydroxide (KOH). KOH destroys bacteria and cells from the vagina, leaving yeast hyphae and spores (if present) that indicate a yeast infection.
> *Vaginal pH:* Normal vaginal pH is 3.8 to 4.5. Bacterial vaginosis, trichomoniasis, and atrophic vaginitis often cause a vaginal pH >4.5.
> *Whiff test:* Several drops of KOH solution are added to a sample of the vaginal discharge. A strong fishy odor from the mixture suggests bacterial vaginosis.

The appropriate treatment for atrophic vaginitis is vaginal administration of estrogen. This can be prescribed as a cream, tablet, or vaginal ring.

56. C. Intermenstrual bleeding is the most common side effect of OCPs and is related to a relatively high progesterone/estrogen ratio. This patient has been doing well on her current OCP for several years. Because the only change in her history is an increase in tobacco use, this is the likely culprit. Studies show that breakthrough bleeding is increased in women who smoke, likely due to an increased estrogen metabolism. Although this patient almost has a relative contraindication for OCP use due to her tobacco use (relative contraindication in this case is for women under 35 who smoke more than one pack per day), she can still use OCPs safely. Increasing her to a 35-μg estrogen pill may decrease her likelihood of breakthrough bleeding.

57. B. Adenomyosis is the term used to describe the presence of endometrial glands and stroma within the uterine musculature. The tissue causes hypertrophy within the surrounding endometrium, producing a diffusely enlarged uterus. Adenomyosis typically causes menorrhagia and dysmenorrhea, although approximately one third of women are asymptomatic. The characteristic findings are a soft, diffusely enlarged uterus. Uterine fibroids typically would be seen on ultrasound as a mass within or arising from the myometrium. An endometrial polyp, which may not be seen on ultrasound because of its small size, is most commonly associated with intermenstrual spotting and rarely causes pain. Endometriosis would not cause menorrhagia. The most common symptom of PCOS is irregular menses, and this patient's cycles are regular.

58. C. This patient's history, physical exam findings, and biopsy are consistent with a diagnosis of lichen sclerosus (LS). LS is a chronic skin condition that occurs most commonly in the anogenital area but it can occur elsewhere, such as on the gums. Vulvar LS usually occurs in postmenopausal women and is marked by inflammation and epithelial thinning, which in turn causes itching and pain. Thin, white skin is localized to the labia majora and minora. Chronic inflammation can cause the labia to fuse. High-potency topical steroid ointments, such as clobetasol, are the treatment of choice. Multiple studies have shown that there is no role for use of estrogen, progesterone, or testosterone in the treatment of LS.

59. B. The lesions described here are most consistent with condyloma (genital wart). Condyloma is caused by infection by low-risk type human papilloma viruses (most commonly types 6 and 11). The lesions are benign but can get quite large. They are contagious. Treatments can involve:

> Tissue destruction
> - Repeated application of trichloroacetic acid
> - Cryotherapy to freeze the affected areas
> - Laser removal
> Surgical excision
> Immune modulators
> - Imiquimod cream: Applied at home three times per week up to 16 weeks
> - Podophyllin
> - Interferon-α: Injection given intralesionally or intramuscularly

Acyclovir is used to treat HSV lesions, which are painful papular lesions that become ulcerated.

60. B. A strawberry-red cervix that bleeds on contact is pathognomonic for *Trichomonas* vaginitis. Findings on wet prep are trichomonads (although not always motile) and a high number of WBCs. Treatment is with metronidazole. Clue cells are seen in the setting of bacterial vaginosis. Postcoital bleeding can be associated with cervical cancer, not usually cervical dysplasia, but this is an unlikely diagnosis in this woman.

61. C. An elevated FSH level is used to confirm menopause in a patient with whom the diagnosis is uncertain. In a patient such as the one described, a diagnosis usually would be made on a clinical basis. Determination of hCG would be used for a younger woman to rule out pregnancy with secondary amenorrhea of 6 months. TSH and PRL levels also would be determined to rule out sources of secondary amenorrhea in a patient with an unknown etiology.

62. B. Postmenopausal women presenting with vulvar pruritus or vulvodynia usually should have a biopsy to rule out vulvar dysplasia or cancer. If vulvar candidiasis seems to be the etiology of the symptoms, topical antifungals such as ketoconazole may be used first. If the diagnosis is LS, a topical 2% testosterone cream is used. If the etiology is hypertrophic, a topical hydrocortisone should be used. If it is secondary to atrophy, topical estrogen is the treatment of choice. In a patient with vulvar atrophy who is not on HRT, oral supplementation should be offered as well.

63. C. This patient's history is most consistent with syphilis *(T. pallidum)* and is least consistent with genital herpes. Because of concern for other STIs with the transmission of syphilis, the battery of tests sent would include those for Gonorrhea (GC), *Chlamydia*, HIV, hepatitis B, and hepatitis C. The syphilis would be screened for with an RPR or Venereal Disease Research Laboratory (VDRL) test and confirmed with fluorescent treponemal antibody absorption test (FTA-ABS) or microhemagglutination assay for *Treponema pallidum* (MHA-TP). Once the patient is diagnosed with *T. pallidum*, it is imperative to determine whether this is primary, secondary, or tertiary syphilis because this determines the management. Because of the single chancre, the most likely diagnosis is primary syphilis. However, when primary or secondary status cannot be confirmed by physical exam, a lumbar puncture is a necessary part of the diagnosis to rule out neurosyphilis.

64. E. The patient's history is most consistent with chancroid, which is confirmed with the Gram stain of *Haemophilus ducreyi*. The Gram stain often may not reveal a diagnosis, and culture of this organism can be difficult; thus, the diagnosis usually is made by history and physical examination and by excluding other possible diagnoses.

65. B. Cervical motion tenderness with no other findings on exam is most consistent with cervicitis. The two most common organisms that cause cervicitis are *N. gonorrhoeae* and *C. trachomatis*. Cultures or DNA tests for these organisms should be sent to the lab. However, because the results usually will not return for 48 to 96 hours, the patient should be treated for both to prevent infection progression. The treatment of cervicitis should cover both gonococcus and chlamydia. The most common method of treatment is a single IM dose of ceftriaxone and 1 week of PO doxycycline. Because of concern for patient compliance, a single dose of azithromycin is often used to treat chlamydia rather than the week-long course of doxycycline.

66. C. This patient's constellation of findings is most consistent with PID, likely complicated by Fitz-Hugh and Curtis syndrome with a perihepatitis leading to RUQ tenderness. TOA should be on the differential diagnosis but is unlikely with a normal pelvic ultrasound. Appendicitis should be considered; if the appendix is not visualized on ultrasound, a CT would more definitively rule out appendicitis. Because the patient will be managed in the hospital, she can be followed with serial exams as well. Treatment of PID usually involves a second-generation cephalosporin and doxycycline. The oral absorption of doxycycline is excellent, so IV administration is necessary only if the patient is strictly NPO or cannot tolerate PO medications. Triple antibiotics with amp/gent/clinda will be effective in this patient but is usually reserved for PID not responsive to first-line therapy or TOAs. Other regimens include clindamycin and ofloxacin, which is particularly effective in non-parenteral or home Rx, because both medications are equally efficacious given PO compared to IV.

67. E. Appendicitis usually is diagnosed by general surgeons, but because most women with abdominal pain are seen by gynecologists, it is important to keep appendicitis on the differential. This patient with localizing RLQ pain and a h/o nausea and anorexia is at high risk for appendicitis. Her cervical motion tenderness is consistent with this diagnosis, particularly in the setting of an appendix that has burst or is sitting in the posterior cul-de-sac behind the cervix.

68. D. Estrogen replacement in a postmenopausal patient has been shown to decrease the risk of osteoporosis and urogenital atrophy, as well as decrease menopausal symptoms. However, the recent Women's Health Initiative (WHI) trial demonstrated an increase in cardiovascular events as well as breast and uterine cancer, which contradicted longstanding beliefs regarding HRT. Because isolated estrogen can increase the risk for endometrial cancer, it is given in conjunction with either continuous or cyclic progesterone to protect the uterus. There is no long-term evidence that combination HRT changes the risk for colon cancer. Given these findings, many clinicians have stopped recommending HRT altogether. A more sensible approach might be to utilize the hormones only in the setting of women with moderate to severe symptoms for shorter courses rather than the years of treatment previously recommended.

69. E. Patients with Turner syndrome undergo rapid ovarian atresia, usually prior to puberty, and along with radiation therapy and chemotherapy can lead to premature failure of the ovaries. Ovarian surgery can lead to devascularization of the ovary and early failure as well. A recent finding is that women who have the fragile X syndrome premutation are at increased risk for premature ovarian failure. OCP use will not lead to failure of the ovary; the hormones simply suppress ovulation while they are being used as a contraceptive.

70. E. This patient likely has primary amenorrhea due to a lack of GnRH pulsatility, which likely is secondary to the exercise and stress from her ballet. Primary amenorrhea is the absence of menses prior to age 16. Anatomical etiologies include vaginal agenesis, transverse vaginal septum, Mayer-Rokitansky-Kuster-Hauser syndrome, and other müllerian anomalies that lead to no development of either the vagina or uterus. Hormonal etiologies are related to the lack of either release or response to GnRH, FSH, or LH. Noninherited etiologies of hypogonadotropic hypogonadism include anorexia, stress, and athletics. Asherman syndrome, which is intrauterine scarring, usually is secondary to infection or instrumentation and rarely causes primary amenorrhea.

In this young woman, the absence of GnRH pulsatility leads to hypogonadotropic hypogonadism. Anorexia nervosa should be considered in all women with primary and secondary amenorrhea, but there is no other evidence supporting this diagnosis in this patient. The diagnosis of an eating disorder usually will not be made based on history because many of these women will be evasive; however, there usually are some physical findings, such as lanugo hair, poor dentition secondary to vomiting in bulimics, and extremely low BMI <17. The anatomical causes were each ruled out on physical exam. A transverse vaginal septum was ruled out by visualization of the cervix. In testicular feminization, the patient will have breast development but no uterus. Thus, a normal bimanual exam of the pelvic organs and a visualized cervix rules out this diagnosis. Patients with gonadal agenesis with either 46,XY or 46,XX karyotypes will not have breast development, although those with 46,XX will have a uterus.

71. D. Cervical stenosis can be congenital but more likely is secondary to scarring from a surgical procedure of the cervix. It leads to decreased menses and severe menstrual cramps. It can be treated by dilation of the cervix but often needs multiple treatments.

Endometriosis commonly presents prior to pregnancy. Fibroids and adenomyosis more commonly present later in life. Uterine fibroids are more commonly associated with increase in menstrual flow but occasionally compress the cervix, leading to cervical stenosis. Adenomyosis also could present as in this patient; however, on exam the uterus is commonly tender and slightly enlarged and feels boggy.

72. C. In patients with postmenopausal bleeding, it is imperative to make a diagnosis because they are considered to have cancer until proven otherwise. The lesion in this woman's uterus is most likely to be an endometrial polyp; rarely endometrial cancer presents this way. However, this patient has none of the risk factors for endometrial cancer, such as obesity, hypertension, or diabetes. Cervical cancer would be unlikely to present this way and would not be likely to occur so soon after a normal Pap smear. Excess endogenous or exogenous hormones could cause irregular postmenopausal bleeding; however, this patient is unlikely to be taking hormones given that she has mild atrophy. Finally, the atrophy itself can cause postmenopausal bleeding; however, the eroded site of the bleeding usually would be visualized and would be rare with mild atrophy.

73. C. This patient needs both contraception and estrogen supplementation. Only the combination OCP would give her both. The IUD is made with and without progesterone but not estrogen. Depo-Provera and cyclic Provera are progesterone only. Premarin 0.625 mg is used for postmenopausal women but may not be adequate estrogen supplementation in a young woman and does not offer contraception. Adequate estrogenization is important for maintaining bone density and for its cardioprotective effect.

74. E. The most common cause of secondary amenorrhea is pregnancy, which is the most likely diagnosis that can be made from the tests being ordered. She does not have symptoms of hypothyroidism, hyperthyroidism, or elevated prolactin level, but these tests usually are ordered as well. LH and FSH levels would not be ordered and offer no helpful information for making a diagnosis. Many women who become pregnant may not realize they are until quite late into the pregnancy.

75. A. This patient has signs and symptoms of hyperthyroidism: weight loss, insomnia, and heat intolerance. These could also be put together as a constellation of stress or even anorexia; however, there is no specific test to diagnose either of these conditions.

76. C. This patient most likely has a prolactinoma that is causing both her amenorrhea and the breast discharge. The fact that her breast discharge is bilateral is suggestive of elevated prolactin level rather than a focal breast disease. It is best to send a prolactin level without having done a breast exam, so it is important to ask her whether she has done one prior to the appointment. If so, a fasting prolactin level the next morning would be the best test to send. TSH and β-hCG levels still should be sent, particularly because breast discharge is seen in pregnancy. Pregnancy is less likely here because of the 7 months of amenorrhea with no palpable uterus abdominally.

77. D. When a postmenopausal patient presents with vulvodynia or vulvar pruritus, cancer must be ruled out by biopsy of any visualized lesions. If there are no obvious lesions, colposcopy can be performed with acetic acid and any aceto-white lesions can be biopsied. Even in this patient in whom Paget disease should be suspected, a diagnosis should be made before more aggressive surgical therapy is attempted.

78. E. As mentioned above, even prior to the biopsy, Paget disease is the leading diagnosis with the description of velvety-red lesions. Vulvodynia and vulvar pruritus can be symptoms of candidal infection, vulvar atrophy and dystrophies, vulvar cancer, and vulvar Paget disease. The positive test for carcinoembryonic antigen makes the diagnosis. Once diagnosis is made, a wide local excision is performed and often is curative.

79. B. Vulvar cancer is most closely related to cervical cancer, and HPV DNA is commonly found in both of these cancers. However, this patient is unlikely to have vulvar cancer from an epidemiologic viewpoint. The fact that she obtains some relief from the single dose of Diflucan particularly increases the likelihood of this being a candidal infection. However, biopsy of any visual lesions will help to reassure this patient and help to make any other diagnosis.

80. A. Cervical cancer is staged clinically. Commonly this is an exam performed under anesthesia and deals with the extent of the disease down to the vagina and laterally to the pelvic sidewalls. Intravenous pyelogram (IVP), ultrasound, or CT can be used to ensure there is no retroperitoneal disease obstructing the ureters. MRI is not commonly used. Checking the disease-free margins and lymph node dissection occasionally is performed but is not a standard part of the clinical staging.

81. D. In a low-risk patient without worrisome family history or signs of malignancy on physical exam, breast masses can be followed clinically with frequent follow-up exams. Mammography is a poor study in young patients because of dense breast parenchyma leading to poor sensitivity. Definitive diagnosis can be made with FNA for cytology, which has >90% sensitivity for breast disease.

A lumpectomy or wide local excision is unnecessary if FNA is diagnostic. In this patient, the most likely diagnosis is fibroadenoma; however, many patients will want a biopsy to make sure they do not have cancer. Although a patient with BRCA1 or BRCA2 would be more worrisome, it is uncommon to obtain such genetic screens without a family history or actual breast cancer.

82. B. Identification of nonpalpable lesions by mammography is critical for earlier diagnosis. Although these microcalcifications can be due to a benign condition, 25% to 30% of such characteristics on mammography are associated with an invasive breast cancer. If the cluster of microcalcifications is associated with a well-demarcated mass, it is more likely to be benign. The chance of benign diagnosis is much lower when associated with an irregular speculated mass. Ultrasound is not useful because the mass is not palpable, so a stereotactic FNA would be necessary for sampling. Tissue diagnosis is recommended prior to major surgical treatments. Although a patient with BRCA1 or BRCA2 would be more worrisome, it is uncommon to obtain such genetic screens without a family history or actual breast cancer.

83. C. Nulliparous women are at 3:1 relative risk of parous women. Obesity is her next risk factor putting her at two times the risk. A first-degree relative who developed unilateral breast cancer premenopausally has 1.8 relative risk. One who reaches menopause after age 50 is at 1.5 times the risk, whereas OCP use has no evidence of increasing breast cancer risk. Of note, the recent WHI study revealed that estrogen replacement therapy in postmenopausal women is associated with an increased risk for breast cancer.

84. D. In advanced-stage breast cancer in premenopausal women, chemotherapy regardless of hormone receptor status has been shown to significantly improve survival. The current chemotherapy regimen is six cycles of some combination of doxorubicin (Adriamycin), cyclophosphamide (Cytoxan), fluorouracil, and methotrexate. Chemotherapy offers a response rate varying from 15% to 40%. Node-positive women are treated with tamoxifen for 2 to 5 years if estrogen receptor (ER) status is positive and no further therapy if ER status is negative. In premenopausal women with BRCA1, BRCA2, or ER-positive status, a bilateral salpingo-oophorectomy occasionally is used to prevent ovarian cancer or to achieve lower estrogen levels. However, this would not be indicated in this setting without knowing the BRCA status.

85. A. In a patient presenting with term PROM or ROM beyond 37 weeks, consensus management is to proceed with induction/

augmentation of labor with oxytocin or prostaglandin agents. This management plan does not lead to an increase in cesarean deliveries and decreases the rate of chorioamnionitis. Some patients decline such management in favor of expectant management. In this setting, they should receive extensive counseling regarding the risks of prolonged (>18 hours) ROM. Betamethasone is given to women <34 weeks gestation at risk for preterm delivery to enhance fetal pulmonary maturation. Terbutaline is give as a tocolytic agent to women in preterm labor or with preterm contractions. Cefotetan is a second-generation cephalosporin usually used in women who have chorioamnionitis. This woman is afebrile without fetal tachycardia.

86. B. Nuchal translucency screening with or without serum screening and second-trimester maternal serum screening are two accepted strategies for Down syndrome screening among women at low risk for chromosomal abnormalities. When using the combined first-trimester screen using nuchal translucency plus the serum screens of Pregnancy Associated Plasma Protein A (PAPP-A) and free β-hCG, 80% sensitivity is reached. The second-trimester triple screen has only approximately 50% sensitivity in women under age 35. A level II ultrasound has only approximately 50% sensitivity for Down syndrome as well, and routine obstetric ultrasounds probably are even less sensitive. CVS and amniocentesis are invasive, definitive, diagnostic tests that carry a procedure-related risk of miscarriage (CVS 1/150; amnio 1:200).

87. C. Most women who had a prior lower uterine segment cesarean delivery may undergo a trial of labor after proper counseling on the risks and benefits of this approach compared to an elective repeat cesarean. However, important contraindications to a trial of labor after a cesarean delivery include prior classic or vertical uterine incision (risk of uterine rupture 10%); complete or partial placenta previa (risk of bleeding); or two or more cesareans without prior vaginal deliveries (risk of uterine rupture five times greater compared to women with only one prior cesarean). In addition, induction of labor increases the risk of uterine rupture twofold to fivefold. Use of prostaglandin agents for cervical ripening, in particular, appears to increase this risk. Few and only small trials have evaluated the safety of vaginal birth after cesarean (VBAC) in twins; however, there is no existing evidence that twin gestations increase the risk of uterine rupture.

88. A. Uterine rupture is a serious complication that affects approximately 0.5% of patients with one prior low uterine segment C/S undergoing a trial of labor (VBAC). Uterine rupture carries significant morbidity for the mother and fetus, including permanent disability and death. Prompt recognition and intervention are key to minimize serious injury. A prerequisite to allow offering VBAC to women is the availability of staff and infrastructure capable of performing an emergency C/S. The most common sign after uterine rupture in labor is a nonreassuring fetal heart tracing. Vaginal bleeding, persistent pain between contractions, signs and symptoms of hypovolemia, and loss of fetal station are all classic signs and symptoms associated with rupture but often are not present.

89. A. Epidural analgesia is generally safe and provides effective means of pain relief for many women in labor, a process that may cause severe pain among many parturients. Some, but not all, studies have found that epidural pain relief may prolong labor, particularly if given before 5-cm dilation. For this reason, other forms of analgesia are often used during early labor. However, there is no contraindication for its use, and it should not be withheld from women experiencing significant pain no matter their stage of labor. During the second stage of labor, maternal pushing efforts are generally less efficient with epidural use, so this stage of labor typically is longer when an epidural was used. C/S rates are not different with or without epidurals. Although transient fetal heart tracing abnormalities, including bradycardia, may be seen with hypotension following epidural use, there is no evidence of an increase rate of neonatal asphyxia with epidural use in labor.

90. E. Women with uncomplicated pregnancies should be encouraged to participate in moderate aerobic exercise on a frequent, if not daily, basis for at least 30 minutes per session. There is scarce information regarding the general safety of strenuous exercise in pregnancy; women engaged in such activities warrant close medical supervision. Contact sports and scuba diving are generally contraindicated during pregnancy given the potential for harm to the mother and/or fetus. All conditions associated with an increased risk for preterm labor are believed to be contraindications to moderate or intense physical activities.

91. A. Exposures of ionizing radiation of <5 rads are generally *not* associated with harmful fetal effects. However, studies have shown that exposure of the fetus to 1 to 2 rads may result is a small but statistically significant risk of leukemia by 1.5- to 2.0-fold over baseline (risk of 1:2,000 vs. background risk of 1:3,000). Concerns about possible fetal effects of high-dose radiation exposure should not prevent medically indicated diagnostic imaging procedures, such as the one depicted in the example above.

92. C. Because rubella vaccine is made with live attenuated virus, concern about teratogenic effects to the fetus existed. However, no reported case of teratogenicity has ever been documented; nonetheless, as a precaution, rubella-nonimmune women should be vaccinated with MMR in the postpartum. Influenza vaccine is recommended for *all* pregnant women if their second or third trimester of pregnancy occurs during flu season. Varicella vaccine also is made from live attenuated virus; susceptible women should be vaccinated postpartum, as a precaution. Hepatitis B vaccine can and should be considered in pregnant women at risk. *Pneumococcus* vaccinate indications are the same as in nonpregnant individuals.

93. D. Induction of labor in a patient with a prior uterine scar is not contraindicated, but the risks of uterine rupture may be slightly higher (7.7:1,000) compared to the risk of rupture in cases with spontaneous onset of labor (5.2:1,000). A favorable (ripe) cervix is a good predictor of successful induction and length of induction but is not an absolute requisite for labor induction, with or without a prior uterine scar. Misoprostol, a PGE_1 analogue, has been shown to be an excellent induction of labor agent, but its use is contraindicated in cases of prior uterine scar because of a high risk of uterine rupture (15-fold higher compared to elective C/S). Oxytocin, artificial ROM, and Foley bulb balloon catheter can be used alone or in combination for labor induction in a patient with a prior low transverse C/S scar. In this patient with an unfavorable cervix, the Foley bulb would be an excellent way to begin induction of labor.

94. C. A recent large multicenter RCT showed that vaginal breech deliveries at term are associated with a significantly higher risk of serious perinatal morbidity and mortality, without any differences in terms of maternal morbidity. As a result of this trial, vaginal breech deliveries are no longer recommended in most hospitals in the United States. Patients identified in breech presentation near term (36–38 weeks) should be offered the possibility of an ECV, which has a success rate of approximately 50%, in order to avoid a cesarean. If the version is unsuccessful or the patient declines, an elective cesarean is recommended at 39 weeks.

95. D. Patients with two or more C/Ss with an anterior or central placenta previa have a 33% to 50% chance of having a placenta accreta. Placenta accreta occurs when there is a defect in the decidua basalis resulting in an abnormally invasive implantation of the placenta. When the placenta invades though all three layers of the uterus, it is called *percreta*. Placenta accreta carries an increased maternal mortality rate due to massive blood loss, intraabdominal organ injury, fistula formation, and other postoperative complications. Ultrasound and MRI might be helpful in the diagnosis, but neither tool has sufficient sensitivity or specificity to completely exclude or confirm the diagnosis. When the diagnosis is suspected antenatally, care should be taken to allow for proper location and timing of delivery in a setting with adequate surgical staff and resources, including blood products available. Patients should be informed and provide consent for the possible need for hysterectomy. All other complications listed can be encountered in this example but are generally of less serious consequences.

96. D. Physical trauma complicates one in 12 pregnancies and is a leading cause of maternal morbidity and mortality. Management of the seriously injured woman after physical trauma requires a multidisciplinary approach, where the first priority is treatment and stabilization of the woman. Only then should attention be directed to the fetus. Continuous fetal heart rate monitoring and ultrasound assessment are important components in the evaluation of the pregnancy and fetus after significant abdominal trauma. Administration of RhoGAM is important in any Rh-negative pregnant woman after abdominal trauma.

97. C. Macrosomia and diabetes are independent variables associated with shoulder dystocia. Clinical estimation of fetal weight is equivalent to ultrasound EFW prediction, both with an estimated ±10% to 15% error. Even with this poor estimate of fetal weight, these estimates are associated with increased risk of shoulder dystocia. Thus, ACOG recommends that woman with EFW ≥5,000 g (or 4,500 g if diabetic) be offered an elective cesarean to avoid a potential serious shoulder dystocia and its sequelae. Immediate induction of labor is also used in this setting but has not been studied carefully, so it is unclear whether it improves outcomes. Certainly in this setting with a macrosomic fetus, operative vaginal delivery is not advised because this increases the risk of shoulder dystocia. If cesarean delivery is chosen, it is better to do so in the elective setting rather than await labor once the fetus is at 39 weeks gestation.

98. B. Nausea and vomiting of pregnancy affects approximately 70% of pregnant women; when severe, it may compromise the health of both mother and fetus. Mild cases of nausea and vomiting may be managed with lifestyle and dietary changes. In more severe cases, prompt recognition and treatment are efficacious and may prevent more serious complications, including the need for hospitalization. It is important to exclude other conditions that present with nausea and vomiting before attributing symptoms to nausea and vomiting of pregnancy. Vitamin B_6 (pyridoxine), antihistamine H_1 receptor blockers, phenothiazines, and benzamides have been shown to be both safe and effective in the treatment of nausea and vomiting in pregnancy. In addition, several small studies have shown ginger, acupuncture, and acupressure to be potentially efficacious in decreasing vomiting and the symptoms of nausea. TSH is suppressed in many pregnant patients up to 20 or more weeks of pregnancy, a common false-positive test in pregnancy because the pregnancy hormone hCG is structurally similar to TSH. In the absence of goiter and with confirmation of hyperthyroidism by FT_4 and FT_3, nausea and vomiting of pregnancy cannot be attributed to a suppressed TSH level. The rest of these findings, the patient's symptoms, and the urinary concentration indicative of dehydration are unlikely to be false-positive findings.

99. E. Recurrent pregnancy loss is defined as two or three consecutive spontaneous abortions, most of which occur prior to 12 weeks gestation. Recurrent pregnancy loss affects approximately 1% of women of reproductive age. The underlying etiology is not identified in more than half of the cases. Common accepted causes of recurrent pregnancy loss include antiphospholipid antibody syndrome (lupus anticoagulant, anticardiolipin antibodies), uterine cavity abnormalities (HSG), parental structural chromosome abnormalities (balanced translocations; parental chromosome studies), overt diabetes and other metabolic disorders, as well as other causes. Many other etiologies have been implicated in recurrent pregnancy loss, but the data supporting the association are weak and/or no known effective intervention is available. Hence, testing for this subgroup of conditions is not recommended, including testing for cultures for viruses and bacteria of the reproductive tract, antithyroid antibodies, glucose tolerance testing, antinuclear antibodies, and maternal antipaternal antibodies.

100. A. Rapid HIV testing can be used effectively in labor and delivery to test women with undocumented HIV status and provide an opportunity to start antiretroviral prophylaxis of a previously undiagnosed infection. Rapid HIV test is a screening test with results available in 1 hour or less. If a rapid HIV test is positive, the patient should be encouraged to start antiretroviral prophylaxis without delay because the confirmatory test will not be available for several days. In some cases, cesarean delivery can provide additional benefit in decreasing the risk of transmission and should be considered, particularly if labor has not begun and the membranes are intact. Other programmatic efforts that have shown to be effective in preventing HIV transmission in pregnant women to their newborns include opt-out prenatal HIV testing where legally feasible, and repeat HIV testing in the third trimester to women at high risk for HIV or in areas of high HIV prevalence. Neonatal prophylaxis is beneficial and should contribute to the efforts in decreasing vertical transmission of HIV. Breastfeeding should be postponed until a confirmatory test is available and has ruled out HIV infection.

Index

Page numbers followed by italic *f* or *t* refer to illustrations or tables, respectively.